Encyclopedia of Colorectal Cancer: Epidemiology, Psychology and Nutrition

Volume III

Encyclopedia of Colorectal Cancer: Epidemiology, Psychology and Nutrition Volume III

Edited by **Teresa Young**

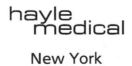

New York

Published by Hayle Medical,
30 West, 37th Street, Suite 612,
New York, NY 10018, USA
www.haylemedical.com

Encyclopedia of Colorectal Cancer: Epidemiology, Psychology and Nutrition
Volume III
Edited by Teresa Young

© 2015 Hayle Medical

International Standard Book Number: 978-1-63241-136-5 (Hardback)

Printed in the United States of America.

Contents

Preface

Every book is initially just a concept; it takes months of research and hard work to give it the final shape in which the readers receive it. In its early stages, this book also went through rigorous reviewing. The notable contributions made by experts from across the globe were first molded into patterned chapters and then arranged in a sensibly sequential manner to bring out the best results.

Colorectal cancer is one of the most common cancers found in many parts of the world. The challenges and mortality that this disease accompany, call for better and improved methods for patient care and treatment. This book presents the essential work that scientists and experts have done in this field covering patient care methods, the disease epidemiology, psychology and nutrition. This book provides a valuable and rich account of information to the students, clinicians and medical professionals.

It has been my immense pleasure to be a part of this project and to contribute my years of learning in such a meaningful form. I would like to take this opportunity to thank all the people who have been associated with the completion of this book at any step.

Editor

Part 1

Introduction

Tumor Engineering: Finding the Brakes

Rajunor Ettarh
Department of Structural and Cellular Biology,
Tulane University School of Medicine, New Orleans,
USA

1. Introduction

There is sufficiently detailed understanding about how an automobile works such that starting or running the engine can be selectively disabled. Applying this analogy to colorectal cancer, the question researchers and clinicians ask is: can colorectal cancer be prevented from starting? Once started, can the disease be prevented from running? These two aims fall broadly into the categories of prevention and treatment respectively. Many of the aspects of colorectal cancer that provide focal points for clinical management of patients of the disease are included in Figure 1 (below). This volume provides insights into aspects of disease incidence and presentation, some of the advances and developments in diagnosis and patient management, and examines prevention and therapeutic targets and regimes. This chapter provides a general overview of some of the aspects of colorectal cancer that affect clinical management of the disease and explores incidence of the disease, diagnosis and treatment as well as preventive screening programs.

2. Epidemiology

As a disease, the statistical data for colorectal cancer are disturbing. Every year, there are over 1 million new cases worldwide, half of them in men; over 200,000 new cases in Europe; and 1.5 million new cases in the United States (Jemal et al, 2010). Over 700,000 patients die each year.

Expanded surveys and studies show that the incidence of colorectal cancer is increasing worldwide, along with cancer detection rates. Other studies suggest that these rates may also be dependent on anatomic site along the intestine at which the cancer occurs. However, although absolute numbers of patients affected by the disease is increasing in the US, the trend for colorectal cancer is downward: age adjusted incidence has declined steadily since 1976 (Ji et al, 1998; Chen et al, 2011; Eser et al, 2010; Merrill & Anderson, 2011). Genomic instability is present in 15% of colorectal cancer, and forms the basis for those who advocate the need for screening programs for colorectal cancer patients (Geiersbach et al, 2011).

Incidence of colorectal cancer around the world per 100,000 of population varies between 3-43 and is influenced by age, gender, socioeconomic status, and ethnicity (Center et al, 2009; Hao et al, 2009). Younger patients have greater susceptibility if there is an associated family history and tend to present at a more advanced stage of the disease. Long and short-term incidence of colorectal cancer is also affected by aspirin intake and this effect may be dependent on dosing regime and patient history (Dube et al, 2007; Flossmann et al, 2007; Rothwell et al, 2010).

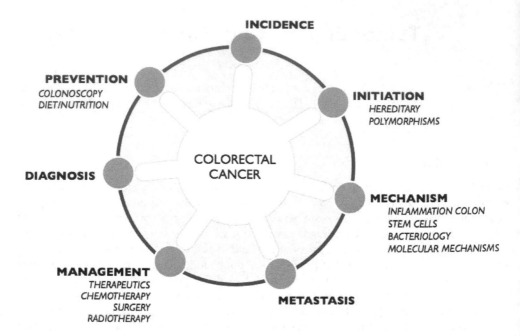

Fig. 1. Basic science studies and clinical management continue to improve our understanding of colorectal cancer. This volume considers incidence, diagnosis and clinical management of the disease as well as metastatic disease. Aspects of initiation and mechanisms are dealt with in the first volume of the book.

3. Diagnosis and treatment

There has been steady improvement in survival rates in colorectal cancers that are diagnosed early. Prognosis for patients who present with late stages of the disease remains poor. Treatment options include surgery for localized tumors, chemotherapy and immunotherapy. When resectable, surgical removal of the tumor remains the treatment of choice for localized colorectal disease. Surgery may be curative or palliative and is sometimes combined with chemotherapeutic regimes to achieve pre-operative tumor shrinkage (Zhao et al, 2010). Minimally invasive approaches such as laparoscopic surgery for colonic tumors are reported to offer improved short-term clinical outcomes (Hiranyakas & Ho, 2011). Chemotherapeutic regimes include infusional combination therapies such as FOLFIRI that combine irinotecan, 5-fluorouracil and leucovorin, and FOLFOX that combines oxaliplatin, 5-fluorouracil and leucovorin (Lee & Chu, 2007; Garcia-Foncillas & Diaz-Rubio, 2010). Studies suggest that overall survival time and progression-free survival are significantly improved with the addition of cetuximab to FOLFIRI.

Better understanding of some of the molecular mechanisms in colorectal cancer has led to the development of targeted therapy that modulate specific pathways and pathway components. Biological treatment with bevacizumab, a recombinant antibody to vascular endothelial growth factor (VEGF) receptor, cetuximab and panitumumab has improved clinical outcomes for patients, prolonged survival times and is recommended in metastatic disease (Koukourakis et al, 2011). Despite these improvements in treatment, the number of patients who develop metastatic disease is significant and the prognosis for such patients is poor. Metastatic disease is thought to be related to epigenetic mechanisms and the development of cancer stem cell-mediated chemoresistance (Anderson et al, 2011). Treatment for metastatic disease is complex and requires careful patient evaluation and selection from single and combination treatment options that include surgery for resectable metastases, chemotherapy and biological therapy. Fluoropyrimidine 5-fluorouracil (5-FU) has been joined by cetuximab, an IgG antibody whose efficacy has been documented in several clinical trials (Lee & Chu, 2007). Improving regimes have led to better 2-year survival rates in patients.

New therapeutic approaches and targets are emerging from research studies. One promising approach currently being explored is the prospect of therapeutic vaccines to combat colorectal cancer (Kabaker et al, 2011; Kameshima et al, 2011).

4. Screening for prevention

A reduction in the morbidity and mortality from colorectal cancer can only be achieved through effective screening for the disease. Screening allows for early detection of cancer and early treatment of detected cancers. It is estimated that up to 60% of deaths from colorectal cancer could be prevented by routine screening after the age 50 years (Byers, 2011; He & Efron, 2011). Approaches to screening for colorectal cancer include stool-based tests (fecal immunochemical testing FIT, fecal occult blood testing FOBT), endoscopy (sigmoidoscopy and colonoscopy) and radiologic examinations (barium radiography, and colonography) (de Wijkerslooth et al, 2011). Studies suggest that stool-based testing is more cost effective than colonoscopy (Hassan et al, 2011; Wilschut et al, 2011).

Colonoscopy remains the gold standard for screening and while it offers advantages for treatment such as removal of premalignant lesions, this approach may not be as protective for right-sided disease as it is for left sided disease (Baxter et al, 2009; Brenner et al, 2010; Singh et al, 2010). Other advanced colonic imaging techniques include capsule colonoscopy, computed tomographic colonography, virtual colonoscopy and magnetic resonance colonography (Liu et al, 2011). All screening programs are complicated by social and community factors (such as culture, level of knowledge about the disease) that affect participation rates (O'Donnell et al, 2010; Ramos et al, 2011; Reeder, 2011).

5. Conclusion

Colorectal cancer remains a major health challenge. Trends for geographically distributed fluctuations in incidence point towards the need for developing strategies to tackle increasing colorectal disease in the population under age 50 years, the relationship of the disease with socioeconomic status, and the increasing incidence of the disease in Asia.

Treatment options are still dictated by the stage of the disease in the patient at presentation but evidence from basic science research studies are providing a better understanding of the disease process, drivers for improvements in therapeutic options for patients, and new therapeutic targets for impeding the progression of the disease.

Despite the remarkable improvement in our understanding of certain aspects of colorectal cancer, the best approach to combating the disease remains a preventive one. Prevention and screening programs need to be more efficient and more effective. Cost benefit analyses preclude early adoption of newer screening methods but advances in colonoscopic and colonographic approaches are helping to reduce morbidity and mortality for colorectal cancer.

6. References

Anderson EC, Hessman C, Levin TG, Monroe MM, Wong MH. (2011). The Role of Colorectal Cancer Stem Cells in Metastatic Disease and Therapeutic Response. *Cancers (Basel)*, Vol.3, No.1, pp. 319-339.

Baxter NN, Goldwasser MA, Paszat LF, Saskin R, Urbach DR, Rabeneck L. (2009). Association of colonoscopy and death from colorectal cancer. *Ann Intern Med*, Vol.150, pp. 1-8

Brenner H, Hoffmeister M, Arndt V, Stegmaier C, Altenhofen L, Haug U. (2010). Protection from right- and left-sided colorectal neoplasms after colonoscopy: population-based study. *J Natl Cancer Inst*, Vol.102, pp. 89-95.

Burke CA, Choure AG, Sanaka MR, Lopez R. (2010). A comparison of high-definition versus conventional colonoscopes for polyp detection. *Dig Dis Sci*, Vol.55, pp. 1716-1720.

Byers T. (2011). Examining stools for colon cancer prevention: what are we really looking for? *Cancer Prev Res (Phila)*, Vol.4, No.10, pp. 1531-1533

Center MM, Jemal A, Ward E. (2009). International trends in colorectal cancer incidence rates. *Cancer Epidemiol Biomarkers Prev*, Vol.18, pp. 1688-1694.

Chen HM, Weng YR, Jiang B, Sheng JQ, Zheng P, Yu CG, Fang JY. (2011). Epidemiological study of colorectal adenoma and cancer in symptomatic patients in China between 1990 and 2009. *J Dig Dis*, Vol.12, No.5, pp. 371-378.

de Wijkerslooth TR, Bossuyt PM, Dekker E. (2011). Strategies in screening for colon carcinoma. *Neth J Med*, Vol.69, No.3, pp. 112-119.

Dubé C, Rostom A, Lewin G, Tsertsvadze A, Barrowman N, Code C, Sampson M, Moher D; U.S. Preventive Services Task Force. (2007). The use of aspirin for primary prevention of colorectal cancer: a systematic review prepared for the U.S. Preventive Services Task Force. *Ann Intern Med*, Vol.146, No.5, pp. 365-375.

Eser S, Yakut C, Özdemir R, Karakilinç H, Özalan S, Marshall SF, Karaoğlanoğlu O, Anbarcioğlu Z, Üçüncü N, Akin Ü, Özen E, Özgül N, Anton-Culver H, Tuncer M. (2010). Cancer incidence rates in Turkey in 2006: a detailed registry based estimation. *Asian Pac J Cancer Prev*, Vol.11, No.6, pp. 1731-1739.

Flossmann E, Rothwell PM; British Doctors Aspirin Trial and the UK-TIA Aspirin Trial. (2007). Effect of aspirin on long-term risk of colorectal cancer: consistent evidence from randomised and observational studies. *Lancet*, Vol.369, No.9573, pp. 1603-1613.

García-Foncillas J, Díaz-Rubio E. (2010). Progress in metastatic colorectal cancer: growing role of cetuximab to optimize clinical outcome. *Clin Transl Oncol*, Vol.12, No.8, pp. 533-542.

Geiersbach KB, Samowitz WS. (2011). Microsatellite instability and colorectal cancer. *Arch Pathol Lab Med*, Vol.135, No.10, pp. 1269-1277.

Hao Y, Jemal A, Zhang X, Ward EM. (2009). Trends in colorectal cancer incidence rates by age, race/ethnicity, and indices of access to medical care, 1995–2004 (United States). *Cancer Causes Control*, Vol.20, No.10, pp. 1855-1863

Hassan C, Benamouzig R, Spada C, Ponchon T, Zullo A, Saurin JC, Costamagna G. (2011). Cost effectiveness and projected national impact of colorectal cancer screening in France. *Endoscopy*, Vol.43, No.9, pp. 780-793.

He J, Efron JE. (2011). Screening for colorectal cancer. *Adv Surg*, Vol.45, pp. 31-44.

Hiranyakas A, Ho YH. (2011). Surgical treatment for colorectal cancer. *Int Surg*, Vol.96, No.2, pp. 120-126.

Jemal A, Siegel R, Xu J, Ward E. (2010). Cancer statistics, 2010. *CA Cancer J Clin*, Vol.60, No.5, pp. 277-300.

Ji BT, Devesa SS, Chow WH, Jin F, Gao YT. (1998). Colorectal cancer incidence trends by subsite in urban Shanghai, 1972-1994. Cancer Epidemiol Biomarkers Prev, Vol.7, No.8, pp. 661-666.

Kabaker K, Shell K, Kaufman HL. (2011). Vaccines for colorectal cancer and renal cell carcinoma. *Cancer J*, Vol.17, No.5, pp. 283-293.

Kameshima H, Tsuruma T, Torigoe T, Takahashi A, Hirohashi Y, Tamura Y, Tsukahara T, Ichimiya S, Kanaseki T, Iwayama Y, Sato N, Hirata K. (2011). Immunogenic enhancement and clinical effect by type-I interferon of anti-apoptotic protein, survivin-derived peptide vaccine, in advanced colorectal cancer patients. *Cancer Sci*, Vol.102, No.6, pp. 1181-1187.

Koukourakis GV, Sotiropoulou-Lontou A. (2011). Targeted therapy with bevacizumab (Avastin) for metastatic colorectal cancer. *Clin Transl Oncol*, Vol.13, No.10, pp. 710-714.

Lee JJ, Chu E. (2007). An update on treatment advances for the first-line therapy of metastatic colorectal cancer. *Cancer J*, Vol.13, No.5, pp. 276-281.

Liu J, Kabadi S, Van Uitert R, Petrick N, Deriche R, Summers RM. (2011). Improved computer-aided detection of small polyps in CT colonography using interpolation for curvature estimation. *Med Phys*, Vol.38, No.7, pp. 4276-4284

Merrill RM, Anderson AE. (2011). Risk-adjusted colon and rectal cancer incidence rates in the United States. *Dis Colon Rectum*, Vol.54, No.10, pp. 1301-1306.

O'Donnell S, Goldstein B, Dimatteo MR, Fox SA, John CR, Obrzut JE. (2010). Adherence to mammography and colorectal cancer screening in women 50-80 years of age the role of psychological distress. *Womens Health Issues*, Vol.20, No.5, pp. 343-349.

Ramos M, Llagostera M, Esteva M, Cabeza E, Cantero X, Segarra M, Martín-Rabadán M, Artigues G, Torrent M, Taltavull JM, Vanrell JM, Marzo M, Llobera J. (2011). Knowledge and attitudes of primary healthcare patients regarding population-based screening for colorectal cancer. *BMC Cancer*, Vol.11, No.1, pp. 408.

Reeder AI. (2011). "It's a small price to pay for life": faecal occult blood test (FOBT) screening for colorectal cancer, perceived barriers and facilitators. *N Z Med J*, Vol.124, No.1331, pp. 11-17.

Rothwell PM, Wilson M, Elwin CE, Norrving B, Algra A, Warlow CP, Meade TW. (2010). Long-term effect of aspirin on colorectal cancer incidence and mortality: 20-year follow-up of five randomised trials. *Lancet*, Vol.376, No.9754, pp. 1741-1750.

Siegel RL, Jemal A, Ward EM. (2009). Increase in incidence of colorectal cancer among young men and women in the United States. *Cancer Epidemiol Biomarkers Prev*, Vol.18, No.6, pp. 1695-1698.

Singh H, Nugent Z, Demers AA, Kliewer EV, Mahmud SM, Bernstein CN. (2010). The reduction in colorectal cancer mortality after colonoscopy varies by site of the cancer. *Gastroenterology*, 139, pp. 1128–1137.

Tribonias G, Theodoropoulou A, Konstantinidis K, Vardas E, Karmiris K, Chroniaris N, Chlouverakis G, Paspatis GA. (2010). Comparison of standard vs high-definition, wide-angle colonoscopy for polyp detection: a randomized controlled trial. *Colorectal Dis*, 12, e260–e266.

van den Broek FJ, Reitsma JB, Curvers WL, Fockens P, Dekker E. (2009). Systematic review of narrow-band imaging for the detection and differentiation of neoplastic and non-neoplastic lesions in the colon (with videos). *Gastrointest Endosc*, Vol.69, pp. 124–135

Wilschut JA, Hol L, Dekker E, Jansen JB, van Leerdam ME, Lansdorp-Vogelaar I, Kuipers EJ, Habbema JD, van Ballegooijen M. (2011). Cost-effectiveness Analysis of a Quantitative Immunochemical Test for Colorectal Cancer Screening. *Gastroenterology*, Vol.141, No.5, pp. 1648-1655.

Zhao R, Zhu J, Ji X, Cai J, Wan F, Li Q, Zhong B, Tucker S, Wang D. (2010). A phase II study of irinotecan and capecitabine for patients with unresectable liver-only metastases from colorectal cancer. *Jpn J Clin Oncol*, Vol.40, No.1, pp. 10-16.

Part 2

Epidemiology and Psychology

2

Early Detection of Colorectal Cancer and Population Screening Tests

Christos Lionis and Elena Petelos
Clinic of Social and Family Medicine,
Faculty of Medicine, University of Crete,
Greece

1. Introduction

Issues of early detection of colorectal cancer with reference to the value of screening programmes and the role of the primary care practitioner

Colorectal cancer (CRC) is the most common newly-diagnosed cancer, one of the leading causes of illness and death in the Western world, and the second most common cause of cancer morbidity in Europe. Yet, CRC is a preventable disease and, if detected early, highly treatable. Early detection and prevention are health care strategies of critical importance for the reduction of CRC morbidity and mortality. In a number of countries, screening programmes have been implemented on nationwide scale since the 1960s for other forms of cancer. The early detection of cancer increases the likelihood of successful outcomes, but in order to have early detection, education and training promoting early diagnosis and resulting in increased screening, participation is needed. Additionally, the effectiveness of screening can be measured by the reduction on mortality, but it greatly depends upon tangible and sometimes intangible factors, contingent on setting and target population; it is essential, for example, to identify and screen the appropriate target population and to overcome implementation and uptake barriers. All of these issues, with emphasis on obstacles encountered at the level of general and family practice are highlighted in a recent editorial in Family Practice (Lionis and Petelos, 2011).

Although the screening is performed in the context of public health, and for the benefit of the community, the rights and welfare of the individual should also be respected. The role of the General Practitioner/Family Practitioner (GP/FP) and generally of the Primary Care Provider (PCP) is challenging yet instrumental in achieving this balance, as it is at that level screening is initiated (Viguier et al, 2011). The involvement and the role of GPs and PCPs in convincing patients to participate and initiate CRC screening should be further explored and elucidated, as it is of key importance in cultural and organisational context and health policy issues (Sarfaty, 2006). CRC screening of asymptomatic population groups is currently recommended in the USA and many European countries, and a number of pilot and nationwide programmes have been developed for this purpose. More specifically, mass screening programmes are currently established in 13 of 39 European countries (Pox et al, 2007; Manfredi et al, 2011) with feasibility studies undertaken as pilot actions in many more.

Although many of these screening programmes, both opportunistic and population-based are already implemented, and screening and early detection of adenomatous polyps has been shown to be effective in the reduction of CRC morbidity and mortality, the rate of screening participation remains low in many population groups at risk for the disease. Good news have recently arrived from across the Atlantic, where decision analysis tools were employed to inform recommendation updates and "microsimulation modelling demonstrated that declines in CRC death rates are consistent with a relatively large contribution from screening" (Edwards et al, 2010), nevertheless, similar efforts are lacking in some European countries, an issue that is given its due importance in this chapter. The success in the US can be attributed to the efforts of international organisations and national task forces, as they have resulted in a level of high awareness of CRC screening among US primary care providers (PCPs) in the US (Klabunde et al, 2003; Levin et al, 2008), but also in certain European countries. However, there is a variation in the evidence that explains the low rate of CRC screening, especially in younger patients (Walsh et al, 2009), while, few physicians recommend screening for the majority of their patients (McGregor et al, 2004). Compounding this effect is evidence that close to a quarter of physicians report not following national screening guidelines, and only half reported the adoption of recommendations that was consistent with the guidelines (Meissner at al, 2006), another key issue that requires special attention.

Additionally, very few PCPs use chart reminders or outreach programmes to contact patient populations most likely to benefit from screening (Klabunde et al, 2009). There is limited research focusing on obstacles and barriers, and the role of the physician-patient relationship plays in determining participation in screening programmes, especially when it comes to ethnic and culturally diverse groups (Lionis and Petelos, 2011). The importance of culturally relevant strategies for designing and implementing screening programmes has been already highlighted (Tu et al, 2006). Additionally, the role of socioeconomic disparities in CRC screening has been highlighted and documented (Meissner et al, 2011) if not explored in detail (Aubin-Auger et al, 2011), thus indicating a need for a close collaboration between medical and social care scientists in order to improve the requisite understanding for increased compliance to CRC screening recommendations. To compound the increasing complexity of national guidelines and the sensitivity of implementing them to culturally and linguistically varied patients, support through interventions focusing on organizational changes and further education and training for PCPs on early diagnosis, prevention and health promotion is needed. These are all issues that this chapter attempts to address. All of these factors are relevant for and have an impact on the ongoing debate about the role of GPs/FPs and PCPs, as well as the contribution these have on the effective implementation of screening programmes, opportunistic and population-based.

From all of the above one can surmise that the early detection of CRC is an issue of complexity requiring clear messages to increase the awareness and performance of the health care actors. This is another objective of the present chapter. Thus, the particular aims of this chapter are: (a) to provide information about the recommendations issued by certain large national and international organizations, including those issued by the U.S. Preventive Services Task Force (US PSTF) on the use of the available screening tests for the early detection of CRC and adenomas for average-risk subjects, (b) to critically review the role of clinical physicians and mainly PCPs in the early detection of CRC, (c) to explore issues with an impact on CRC screening, and, finally, (d) to highlight some quality issues relevant to CRC screening and relevant guidelines for quality assurance mechanisms in the relevant processes. The chapter starts with concepts and definitions, proceeds with the recommended screening tests and concludes by outlining main points of interest and corresponding recommended tasks and actions for PCPs, for the purpose of increasing uptake and facilitating implementation of CRC screening programmes.

2. Concepts and definitions

Population screening is the systematic application of a suitable test with the aim of identifying individuals at a risk of a specific condition or disorder, but who have not sought medical attention on account of symptoms for that particular condition or disorder, and who can benefit from further investigation or direct preventive action (Wald, 1994). The notion differs from opportunistic screening, and it is a systematic process that includes certain steps from call or recall to screening, feedback of the results and follow-up in well-defined intervals. For population screening, the organised framework in which it takes place provides opportunities for more effective management, quality assurance and evaluation.

In our empirical view, understanding of the notion of screening, population or opportunistic, greatly varies between health care practitioners with the result of adversely impacting the effective implementation of the early detection programmes for CRC. It is for this reason we have decided to provide an extensive review on the existing literature and consensus criteria to define screening, focusing on CRC screening.

As stated by Wilson and Jungner in their seminal paper (Wilson and Jungner, 1968) *"the central idea of early disease detection and treatment is essentially simple. However, the path to its successful achievement (on the one hand bringing to treatment those with previously undetected disease, and, on the other, avoiding harm to those persons not in need of treatment) is far from simple though sometimes it may appear deceptively easy"*. On the basis of whether early detection is possible at an early stage of the disease and taking into consideration whether an appropriate treatment is available, they attempted to formulate criteria that could help guide the selection of conditions and population groups suitable for screening. They also noted case-finding differences, depending on whether it is performed by a public health agency or by a general practitioner, and, almost four decades ago, emphasised the aspect of cost by underlining the importance of assessing effectiveness not only from an individual, but also from a public health perspective.

The fast pace of genetic research and the advent of new therapies has resulted in the generation of many other lists of screening criteria; most of them based to a greater or lesser degree on the Wilson-Jungner criteria. Additionally, even when consensus at the national or regional level is reached on which set of criteria to apply, there are other social, ethical and even logistical considerations to be examined. More recent trends on patient-centric and evidence-based health care, as well as cost-effectiveness and quality assurance, have resulted through a series of consultations to the modified Wilson and Jungner criteria (Andermann et al, 2008). In these amended criteria, opportunistic screening, essentially case-finding performed outside a framework of an organised programme as the one required to ensure such criteria are met, is, therefore, not a valid alternative; additionally to being less efficient it is also more costly, and, most importantly, quality assurance mechanisms cannot be embedded in a standardised fashion in such a process.

The definition of an "organised" screening programme according to the International Agency for Research on Cancer (IARC) includes: 1) an explicit policy with specified age categories, method and interval for screening; 2) a defined target population; 3) a management team responsible for implementation; 4) a health-care team for decisions and care; 5) a quality assurance structure; and 6) a method for identifying cancer occurrence and death in the population (IARC 2005). Such organised population-based screening programmes have a predefined specific population, according to epidemiological data and on the basis of target age and geographical area, and during all the stages, from the invitation of the eligible individuals to the assessment procedures following testing, a specific protocol is followed. As mentioned, quality aspects of the process can be better addressed, as for example during follow-up (Miles et al, 2004). Furthermore, such screening programmes usually do not incur any costs for the participants.

It is important to have also a concrete idea regarding more abstract terms determining the usefulness and, even, the effectiveness of screening tests, and to keep such definitions in mind. Although these terms have been widely used, there is also great variation of their understanding and usage in clinical decision-making. For example, the ability of a measure or test to predict a subsequent event is a form of validity. On the basis of such a criterion we determine the predictive value of a test. The positive predictive value (PPV) in terms of detection through FOBT screening is defined as "*the percentage of people with detection of at least one lesion/adenoma/advanced adenoma/cancer at follow-up colorectal screening among those with positive tests who have attended follow-up colorectal screening*" [Adapted from the European guidelines for quality assurance in colorectal cancer screening and diagnosis. 2011. European Commission, Directorate General for Health and Consumers, EAHC — Executive Agency for Health and Consumers, World Health Organisation], whereas a positive test is, effectively, an abnormal result leading to further investigation (i.e. colonoscopy) or the removal of a lesion, for example, according to the protocol of the organized screening programme. By alluding to a false-positive result, we effectively mean that although the test indicated disease is present this is not the case. In a true-positive test, the result is correct and the disease is really present. Similarly a false-negative test indicates a disease-free subject has been tested, but the disease is present and might remain undetected if there is no further testing, symptoms, etc., whereas a true-negative test indicates a disease-free subject has been tested. Prevalence of the disease affects not only the positive predictive value of a screening test but also its negative predictive value, i.e. the probability that the person subjected to the screening test is truly free from the disease when a negative (normal) test result is obtained.

Two concepts often discussed in relation to true- and false- positive and negative results are sensitivity and specificity and both terms have an important impact on the PCP decisions on which of the available tests for the early detection of CRC should be recommended. The sensitivity refers to the number of cases the test can identify or in more simple words the probability of one diagnostic test telling the truth when the disease exists. It gives us a certainty that true positives will not be missed. Specificity refers to the accuracy of the finding or in simple words the probability in telling the truth when the disease is absent. Ideally, a test should be both highly sensitive and specific. To that direction, the US Preventive Services Task Force and the Institute of Medicine (IoM) recommend the fecal occult blood test (FOBT) test, and more specifically the guaiac test (gFOBT) for screening programmes. Nevertheless, when used on its own, it has relatively low sensitivity, whereas the a combination with a more sensitive test, such as the fecal immunochemical test (FIT) could help to render screening programmes more effective (Allison, et al, 2007). Another interesting consideration, especially given the public health context of mass screening, is cost-effectiveness and how it correlates to specificity and sensitivity. Although uncertainty remains, the assessment of a screening program based on FIT for a one-year period in France seemed to be the most cost-effective approach (Hassan, et al, 2011). More research is necessary, as for example indicating what the best cut-off levels for colonoscopy referral are, without compromising sensitivity, to determine optimal public health approaches.

3. Screening tests, guidelines for CRC and the importance of early detection

As previously mentioned, CRC can be curable when diagnosed at an early stage. Also, CRC mostly develops from colorectal non-malignant precursor lesions, thus, rendering it a preventable disease through the removal of premalignant lesions. Systematic early detection and removal at the "adenoma-phase" can prevent the occurrence of CRC and markedly decrease overall population incidence (Winawer et al, 1993), as human colon carcinogenesis progresses to the carcinoma pathway via the dysplasia-adenoma phase.

The readers of this chapter are aware from previous chapters of this book that there are various tumour staging systems, the ones mainly used in Europe being Duke's classification and TNM (Tumour, Node, Metastasis) classification of malignant tumours, introduced by the Union Internationale Contra le Cancer (UICC) and the American Joint Committee on Cancer (AJCC). Despite the fact TNM yields greater information, there are several major issues due to the reclassification of the system. Most importantly, there seems to be great disparity between the therapeutic decision-making and the TNM staging, with multiple TNM staging versions being used in different countries and great variance in reporting. It has been argued that changes should only occur after extensive discussion within the scientific community (Quirke et al, 2010), and it is essential to note that the reporting on a nationwide scale for any given CRC screening programme should be performed on the basis of the same staging system. Lesion reporting within the frame of the screening programme should be standardized to allow for better evaluation and reporting, and, consequently, improved outcomes. TNM stages and version, frequency of CRC and distribution of TNM stages should be reported along with the presence of non-neoplastic lesions. According to the report of the EU on CRC quality guidelines (European Commission, Directorate General for Health and Consumers, EAHC − Executive Agency for Health and Consumers, World Health Organisation, 2011), without explicit criteria for the diagnosis and staging of early adenocarcinoma unnecessary radical resection would result in severe overtreatment, raising the morbidity and mortality in the context of the programmes.

Various screening technologies are currently available, from the more established Guaiac faecal occult blood tests (gFOBT) and immunochemical FOBT to sigmoidoscopy and colonoscopy, as well as combinations (i.e. combined FOBT with sigmoidoscopy) to the new screening technologies, as CT colonography, stool DNA and capsule endoscopy. Early reports during the previous decade suggested that biennial screening by FOBT reduces CRC mortality, as for example in the French (Faivre et al, 2004) and Danish populations (Jørgensen et al, 2002). This fact lead WHO (World Health Organization) and OMED (World Organization for Digestive Endoscopy) to suggest a choice of FOBT that should take into account dietary compliance to recommendations, but also colonoscopy resources (Young et al, 2002). Prior to any recommendation for screening tests for CRC, the PCPs should be able to recognise whether the individual visiting the practice/office is at average, increased or at high risk for CRC. In other words, to be able to identify whether the particular individual truly belongs to the target population of the screening programme or –should there not be one available– whether there is reason for referral in the context of opportunistic screening.

In Australia, the Department of Health and Aging has issued clinical practice guidelines for the prevention, early detection and management, and national population-based screening programs are in place for various cancers, from breast cervix and to bowel (CRC) (Australian DoHA, 2011). Also, the National Bowel Cancer Screening Program Register plays an important role in the programme, as it assists participants through the screening pathway, allows for reminders and follow-ups without taxing local resources and GPs. There are online tools and decision-aids available to GPs and information in twenty languages targeted at patients. Pre-invitation, invitation, follow-up letters, FOBT kit instructions and an information booklet are all provided in all of these languages and are also available online. Additionally, a qualitative evaluation of opinions, attitudes and behaviours influencing CRC were examined in the pilot phase of the national screening programme and the report was published and integrated in future planning [A Qualitative Evaluation of Opinions, Attitudes and Behaviours Influencing the Bowel Cancer Screening Pilot Program: Final Report August 2005]. Most interestingly, the invitation is sent directly to the candidate participant and it is not necessary to nominate a physician in the forms submitted, although participants are encouraged to nominate a doctor in the context of follow-up if the FOBT is positive:

a. If no doctor is nominated, the FOBT results will only be sent to the participant.
b. If a doctor is nominated, the results of the FOBT will be sent to the participant and their doctor.
c. If the FOBT result is positive it is explained that it will be necessary to discuss the result with a doctor.

The American Cancer Society (ACS) and the National Colorectal Cancer (NCC) in cooperation with the Thomas Jefferson University have edited a Primary Care Clinician's Evidence-Based Toolbox and Guide (Sarfaty, 2008). According to this guide, an individual is at an average risk when s/he has no first-degree relatives with a history of either CRC or adenomatous polyps and no illness or past health problems have been reported (Sarfaty, 2008). For individuals at average risk, GPs are recommended to initially take a medical history, including age, symptoms, family medical history, and also individual history with a focus on bowel diseases and dietary habits, and to perform a clinical examination including a digital rectal examination. Also, various CRC screening guidelines and recommendations have been issued, both by national and international organisations and institutions. In 2008, a joint effort of the ACS and the American Gastroenterology Association was released regarding certain modalities including stool tests, flexible sigmoidoscopy (FS), colonoscopy (CS), double-contrast barium enema (DCBE), computer tomography, colonography (CTC) (McFarland, et al 2008). Those joint guidelines also stressed the importance of prevention of CRC important tasks for PCPs. The US Preventive Services Task Force (US PSTF) recommends routine asymptomatic screening for three cancer sites, including that of breast, CRC and cervix, mainly because they are asymptomatic to a high degree in early staging, have a high 5-year survival rate when the cancer is localised, and as there is a strong evidence on the screening effectiveness (Cardarelli, 2010).

In terms of a recommended start and stop age for screening, the ACS has issued guidelines for the early detection of CRC and polyps with recommended screening beginning at age 50 for both men and women (ACS, 2011). The US PSTF recommends a screening for average-risk men and women 50 years of age and older, with colonoscopy every 10 years, flexible sigmoidoscopy or DCBE every five years and faecal occult blood test every year (U.S. Preventive Services Task Force, 2011). In a supporting document, this Task Force summarises its recommendations and recommends screening for CRC using an FOBT, sigmoidoscopy, or colonoscopy in adults beginning at the age of 50 years and continuing until the age of 75 (Grade: A Recommendation). However, US PSTF recommends against screening for CRC in adults over 85 (Grade: D Recommendation), while it concludes that the evidence is insufficient to assess the benefits of CT colonography and faecal DNA testing for CRC as screening modalities. Judging the benefits against harms, the American Task Force discusses among the benefits of the less invasive CRS screening the number of colonoscopies that may be reduced. However, it recommends that for any positive test there is a follow-up with colonoscopy. The Task Force Recommendation statement underlines that the benefits of CRC detection and early intervention decline at the age of 75 years, thus it leaves the decision for a routine screening at individual level. There is, as described, a lot of information, but slightly conflicting evidence and advice. Nevertheless, participation of the 50-75 years age group increased by 13.1% reaching 65.4%, whereas a significant CRC incidence decline was noted in 35 states and mortality declined in 49 states and DC (CDC, 2011). Further efforts are currently being made in the field of patient engagement and patient-reported outcomes, and in the context of comparative effectiveness research (PCORI, 2011).

In the United Kingdom, Cancer Research UK underlines the importance of screening for the reduction of CRC mortality and has elaborated upon the role of FOBT and flexible sigmoidoscopy (Cancer Research UK, 2011). This institute refers to evidence provided by four RCTs where the use of FOBT every two years reduced CRC mortality by 15% to 18% in people aged 45-74 years. Centralised systems, such as the Australian and, to a certain extent, the UK system, remove pressure from the individual GP and the organisational capacity at practice level, but could potentially result in a loss of involvement and a lowered feeling of responsibility.

An individual is at increased risk when s/he has a personal and family history of CRC or adenomatous polyps but without reporting any of the high-risk familiar syndromes. Those hereditary syndromes include: the hereditary non-polyposis CRC (HNPCC), the familiar adenomatous polyposis (FPP) and the attenuated PAP (APAP). In this group, the clinical physicians and the PCP should change their strategy from screening to regular surveillance, and the tests that primarily detect cancer should be replaced by more sensitive diagnostic approaches and particularly colonoscopy, which should start at age 40 or younger (Sarfaty, 2008). The National Institute for Health and Clinical Excellence (UK) has recently published a new guideline on colonoscopic surveillance for the prevention of people with ulcerative colitis, Crohn's disease or adenomas (NICE, 2011). At the third category where the probability of developing CRC is high, the PCPs should be more cautious when recommending screening and surveillance. A family history of an adenomatous polypus or CRC in a relative under the age of 50 is suggesting a high probability of the presence of any of the above high-risk hereditary syndromes and the clinical physician requires genetic testing; a close collaboration with hospital specialists at a centre with expertise should be established (Sarfaty, 2008).

In Europe, the high degree of heterogeneity in health care systems, policy, roles, screening programme resources and very different values in local and regional settings had previously created a rather fragmented picture. There are ongoing efforts toward harmonisation, for example, recently developed guidelines (2011) in an effort under the auspices of the European Commission, focus on quality assurance and provide clear and concise information to facilitate decision-making at the GP/FP and PCP levels. As illustrated by

Table 1, an evidenced-based brief overview of various conventional screening methods is given, although new technologies resulting in more modern forms of screening are not assessed for lack of evidence; some information regarding cost-effectiveness is provided along with the recommendations and examined in more details in the report (European Commission, Directorate General for Health and Consumers, EAHC — Executive Agency for Health and Consumers, World Health Organisation, 2011)

Finally, it is important to underline that early detection is directly dependent on acceptance of the screening test by both provider and patient, as well as the uptake of the screening programme. For example, early versions of stool DNA (sDNA) testing lacked the requisite sensitivity and markers, but improved sDNA tests are now available. It is important to understand patient preferences regarding screening options for selecting the right tool for a given population; for example, whether a non-invasive test is preferred to colonoscopy or whether accuracy is considered much more important than discomfort. In a study by Schroy et al, (2002), those preferring colonoscopy to sDNA or FOBT rated accuracy as the most important factor, whereas those rating concerns about discomfort or frequency of testing as the most important parameter preferred sDNA. Most subjects preferred a shared (54%) or patient-dominant (34%) decision-making process.

As previously highlighted, removal of all adenomas, without accurately distinguishing between those which will become malignant and those which will not, will effectively result in excessive overtreatment, and it is for this reason that newer screening tests, such as the sDNA, focusing on genomic changes affecting associated biological and metabolic processes should not be overlooked as options necessitating further research -particularly because of their potential to avoid iatrogenic care, but also because they might better reflect patient preferences for certain population groups (Sillars-Hardebol, et al, 2012).

[Adapted from the European guidelines for quality assurance in colorectal cancer screening and diagnosis. 2011. European Commission, Directorate General for Health and Consumers, EAHC — Executive Agency for Health and Consumers, World Health Organisation.]

Guaiac FOBT

There is good evidence that invitation to screening with FOBT using the guaiac test reduces mortality from colorectal cancer (CRC) by approximately 15% in average risk populations of appropriate age

RCTs have only investigated annual and biennial screening with guaiac FOBT (gFOBT) (II). To ensure effectiveness of gFOBT screening, the screening interval in a national screening programme should not exceed two years

Circumstantial evidence suggests that mortality reduction from gFOBT is similar in different age ranges between 45 and 80 years. The age range for a national screening programme should at least include 60 to 64 years in which CRC incidence and mortality are high and life expectancy is still considerable. From there the age range could be expanded to include younger and older individuals, taking into account the balance between risk and benefit and the available resources

Immunochemical FOBT

There is reasonable evidence from an RCT that iFOBT screening reduces rectal cancer mortality, and from case control studies that it reduces overall CRC mortality; Additional evidence indicates that iFOBT is superior to gFOBT with respect to detection rate and positive predictive value for adenomas and cancer

Given the lack of additional evidence, the interval for iFOBT screening can best be set at that of gFOBT, and should not exceed three years

In the absence of additional evidence, the age range for a screening programme with iFOBT can be based on the limited evidence for the optimal age range in gFOBT trials

Sigmoidoscopy

There is reasonable evidence from one large RCT that flexible sigmoidoscopy (FS) screening reduces CRC incidence and mortality if performed in an organised screening programme with careful monitoring of the quality and systematic evaluation of the outcomes, adverse effects and costs

The available evidence suggests that the optimal interval for FS screening should not be less than 10 years and may even be extended to 20 years

There is limited evidence suggesting that the best age range for FS screening should be between 55 and 64 years. After age 74, average-risk FS screening should be discontinued, given the increasing co-morbidity in this age range

Colonoscopy

Limited evidence exists on the efficacy of colonoscopy screening in reducing CRC incidence and mortality. However, recent studies suggest that colonoscopy screening might not be as effective in the right colon as in other segments of the colorectum

Limited available evidence suggests that the optimal interval for colonoscopy screening should not be less than 10 years and may even extend up to 20 years

Indirect evidence suggests that the prevalence of neoplastic lesions in the population below 50 years of age is too low to justify colonoscopic screening, while in the elderly population (75 years and above) lack of benefit could be a major issue. The optimal age for a single colonoscopy appears to be around 55 years. Average risk colonoscopy screening should not be performed before age 50 and should be discontinued after age 74

Combination of FOBT and sigmoidoscopy

The impact on CRC incidence and mortality of combining sigmoidoscopy screening with annual or biennial FOBT has not yet been evaluated in trials. There is currently no evidence for extra benefit from adding a once-only FOBT to sigmoidoscopy screening

New screening technologies under evaluation

There currently is no evidence on the effect new screening tests under evaluation on CRC incidence and mortality. New screening technologies such as CT colonography, stool DNA testing and capsule endoscopy should therefore not be used for screening the average-risk population

Cost-effectiveness

Costs per life-year gained for both FOBT and endoscopy screening strategies are well below the commonly-used threshold of US$ 50 000 per life-year gained (LYG)

There is some evidence that iFOBT is a cost-effective alternative to gFOBT

Available studies differ with respect to what screening strategies are most cost-effective. No recommendation of one screening strategy over the others can be made based on the available evidence of cost-effectiveness

Table 1. Recommendations and conclusions

Finally, the concepts of colonoscopic surveillance and screening for recurrent CRC should receive attention by PCPs. The adenomatous precursors of CRC are present in over 30% of individuals over 55 (Eide, 1991), placing them at higher risk of developing CRC, but the removal of these lesions reduces risk to that of the general population (Citarda et al, 2001). Recurrent CRC, as for example following resection, also necessitates an intensive surveillance programme, as the detection at an asymptomatic stage can result in survival benefit (Renehan, et al, 2002). This means that surveillance and follow-up programmes should also be combined or evaluated along with a screening programme.

4. Primary care and CRC: Tasks and steps for screening implementation in primary care

One of the most important factors for the effective implementation of a CRC screening programme is the involvement of a PCP, particularly of the GP or the FP, in convincing targeted individuals to participate and to initiate the screening. The PCPs have multiple and varying tasks, more specifically to (Sarfaty, 2008):

1. Assess the risk of developing CRC and increase the risk awareness, as described above.
2. Discuss options with patients/individuals and effectively engage in shared decision-making (SDM) – this would ensure patient perspectives and preferences are consistent to decisions made.
3. Convince to participate – this task requires communication and consultation skills, as well as an established continuity of care.
4. Implement the initial tests: those primarily used to detect cancer, including the annual Guaiac-based occult blood test (gFOBT), the annual faecal immunochemical test (FIT), or stool DNA test (sDNA).
5. Consider and assess the available screening resources and capacity: it is an important task for PCPs, who should be aware of the available resources in their district or health region capacity, as well as patient limitations (e.g. socioeconomic, mobility, etc.), to determine the optimal referral pathway for the test(s) that detect adenomatous polyps and CRC (FS, CS, DCBE, CRC).
6. To make the necessary arrangement to complete the CRC screening.

One of the most challenging issues that the PCPs encounter is to convince the average risk individual to use a simple and inexpensive test to initially detect if any hidden blood is present in stools, constituting a strong indication of the presence of an adenomatous polyp or CRC. To achieve it, an effective doctor-patient communication should be established, and the purpose of the GPs/PCPs might also need to be re-assessed by further education or training on early diagnosis, prevention and promotion. The role of a multidisciplinary team is also essential. FOB Testing serves this role, although it has received criticism because of the lack of specificity, particularly when the test is dehydrated, and because of the subsequent increase of the associated costs of screening programmes (WHO, Rudy and Zdon, 2000). FIT, also, fulfils this purpose; it is a simple procedure: the stool sample is collected by the individual/patient at home, and the completed test is sent to a laboratory or to the PCPs office. Usually two samples from different bowel movements are required and the instructions on sampling procedures on how the water sample should be transferred by the brush onto the test card are clear and readily understood.

Another important task for PCPs and other practitioners is to educate their patients/clients to contact the PHC services when some warning signs are experienced and among them are (Rudy and Zdon, 2000):

- Hematochezia
- Melaena
- Anaemia resulting from occult blood loss
- Change in bowel habits

Prior to the decision of the PCP to refer the subjects to either CS/FT or CT should be explored the access to that screening method and consider the existing diagnostic capacity resources (Sarfaty and Wender, 2007).

Finally, another essential consideration in the PCP decision to implement screening tests for early detection of CRC is that of quality of life. Quality of life in evidence-based medicine should always reflect the preferences of patients, as patient-centeredness is its cornerstone. Despite the fact everyone values particular aspects of life differently, all aspects of life that may be affected adversely or in a beneficial manner by aspects of health and illness should be taken into consideration. For screening programmes, it is important to understand the cultural context in which it is performed or is to be performed and to ensure the values of the patients are taken into consideration when determining and/or assessing outcomes.

5. Obstacles to implementing CRC screening in primary care

Obstacles in primary care

As mentioned above, the CRC screening rate increase does not seem to apply in many countries and regions and the associated obstacles and barriers that have already been reported in the literature (Lionis and Petelos, 2011) could be classified as follows:

- Obstacles at doctor level: Obstacles reported by the GPs were relevant to the difficulties in being convinced especially when signs and symptoms were lacking. There was, in other words, confusion in addressing difficulties stemming from conflict between personal experiences and public health implications (Aubin-Auger et al, 2011). Also, there is research indicating that even in countries with established screening programmes only 50% of the GPs considered themselves to be sufficiently trained, as for example in France (Viguier et al, 2011).

- Obstacles at patient level: Researchers examined obstacles at patient level and how these were linked to the physician-patient interaction and communication. For example, cancer screening did not fall in with the perception of some patients regarding health care, and they failed to identify benefits outside the context of familiar high-risk groups. Potentially inadvertently reflecting specificity and sensitivity issues, participants were afraid of poor technical skills, and taking ownership of the risk for performing the test, resulting in false positive or false negative results (Aubin-Auger et al. 2011). Mirroring the high number of GPs who do not feel they are sufficiently trained, patients cited the absence of recommendation as one of the most important reasons for not undergoing screening (Viguier et al, 2011).

- Obstacles at doctor-patient level: GPs and patients agreed the lack of symptoms and lack of familial risk were two of the main reasons for doubting how useful such a test could be, the GPs thought that the patients misunderstood the process and were afraid of reactions to false negative results, whereas the patients complained about time, as well as the constipation effect from repeating the test, and did not express fears about such results (Aubin-Auger et al, 2011). Further evidence (Schroy et al, 2011) indicates that screening intentions and test ordering are adversely affected when patient and provider preferences differ. Interestingly, compounding previously reported data (Serra et al, 2008), having a screening habit (e.g. mammography) proved to be a positive factor for women, whereas increased participation was reported for those with a higher educational level, particularly for male patients. Without diminishing the importance of facilitators, a patient having a relative having already performed gFOBT was more likely to accept the test, but friends and family were not identified as obstacles.

Further barriers:

Cultural and linguistic barriers were also touched upon by these researchers, but not explored in detail; it is highlighted that even the wording a doctor uses has an effect and that further research is necessary (Lionis and Petelos, 2011). There is evidence that by employing culturally and linguistically relevant approaches for FOBT promotion, screening participation increases in target populations of low-income and/or less acculturated minority patients (Tu et al, 2006). Indeed, a challenge of equal significance to guideline adherence and compliance in screening is ensuring equity of access to screening. Part of ensuring equity of access is to ensure awareness issues have been addressed for all ethnic and culturally diverse groups. A study of all the patients aged 50-60 registered in general practices for a UK region (West Midlands), with a total number of over eleven thousand respondents, examined factors that contributed positively or negatively on behaviour toward screening (Taskila et al, 2009). People without a screening habit (men), older people, and those with Indian ethnic backgrounds were more likely to have negative attitudes, whereas Black-Caribbean ethnic background people reporting abdominal pain, bleeding or tiredness were more likely to have a positive attitude. This great variation in attitudes indicates that there are different needs to be addressed for increasing awareness and highlight the importance of culturally relevant strategies for designing and implementing screening programmes (Taskila et al, 2009). Evidence amasses from various countries, with a study focusing specifically on FOBT use, along with the subsequent investigation of a positive result (Bampton et al, 2005). Researchers established that both indications for use and follow-up of a positive result varied according to the ethnicity of the GP and independently of the medical training received (Koo et al, 2011). Additionally, it was indicated that the ethnicity of the patient and, similarly to results of other research, associated linguistic and cultural barriers affect screening uptake and was noted that this may adversely affect the health of immigrant populations.

To address all the obstacles and barriers previously mentioned, it is necessary to embrace the perspective of the users of screening programmes, and also to examine screening under the prism of public health perspective. A recently conducted review highlights the need for policy supporting both screening delivery and organisational transformation in a manner that promotes improvement of operational features for preventive services (Senore et al, 2010). The researchers examined recently proposed conceptual frameworks that were aimed at identifying key elements and, thus, potential targets for interventions aiming to improve screening (Cole et al, 2009 and Federici et al, 2005). The models developed conceptualised these potential targets at various levels: the organizational context in which health care delivery and provision are taking place, the practice itself, and the structural and operational characteristics of given settings, and also examined the provider and patient levels. The researchers concluded that although a given intervention may be implemented at one or multiple levels, the factors determining uptake and participation are, indeed, correlated with all of these levels in an interconnected and interdependent manner.

In concluding this section, the role of the PCPs is extremely complex, and although research on obstacles, barriers and limitations is starting to create a more robust evidence base, further qualitative and translational research is required to identify best practices and intervention transferability. Additionally, policy measures for the purpose of supporting screening delivery mechanisms are required, and, similarly, policy should aim to facilitate the organisational changes necessary for creating and supporting the operational features of preventive services.

6. Increasing the CRC screening rate

Although messages about the effectiveness of CRC screening have been widely available, there are still concerns in terms of both physician involvement and PC user participation in CRC screening. This is not a message that concerns CRC screening per se, but prevention and health promotion activities undertaken by GPs in Europe. There are significant gaps between GP knowledge and practice in Europe, already reported upon (Brotons et al, 2005). Evidence from the literature indicates that less than one third of the PC physicians use chart reminders and 15% use outreach mechanisms to contact patients needing screening (Klabunde et al, 2009). Investment has been made on efforts and research programs to assess the impact of quality improvement intervention programs. One of them combined diverse components, such as performance activities, delivery system design, electronic medical record tools and patient activation (Ornstein et al, 2010), and reported promising results in the Evidence-Based Toolbox and Guide we currently have (Sarfaty, 2008). Thus, the implementation of educational programmes for PCPs and patients in addition to the development of shared-decision making tools, given the differing perspectives between doctor and patient, seem imperative, as otherwise lack of consensus could adversely impact the CRC screening rate (Schroy et al, 2011).

A page invitation to the health practitioners to avoid certain errors has been made and among them the following:

- To screen for CRC with only a digital rectal exam or with a single sample from a stool blood test
- Recommend screening with colonoscopy at average risk more often than every 10 years or CT colonography, DBCE or flexible sigmoidoscopy more often than five years

A toolkit for a systematic approach in tracking and increasing screening for public health improvement of CRC intervention was prepared for the Agency for Health Care Research and Quality (AHRQ). It delivers tools, process guidelines, tips and evidence of the intervention effectiveness (Harris et al, 2010). It is strongly recommended for PCPs, health care planners and managers. However, the role of PCPs in increasing the CRC screening rate remains a key component. According to the ACS and NCS, the positive impact of its advice is well documented, and the magnitude of the doctor's impact is considerable (Sarfaty, 2008).

7. Designing a national CRC screening programme/framework

We have seen the importance and potential of CRC screening in detail. The importance of screening taking place in an organised framework for optimal results, as for example in nationwide programmes, has also been examined and noted. As many European countries are still in the process of designing such a programme and many other countries globally are far from implementing such interventions, it is important to see how to best learn from other experiences and how to use lessons already learned to help us morph a flexible and robust model that can be adapted according to regional and local needs to ensure high acceptance, uptake and, indeed, equal access and reduced disparities. Thus, we decided to include in this section some key issues that health planners, health policy makers and public health decision makers should take into account when considering the design and implementation of a CRC screening programme.

Many of the countries in which a nationwide programme is implemented have extensively reported on the outcomes and evaluation of such programmes. Australia has introduced such a programme, but reporting indicated the needs and beliefs of minority groups, as for example indigenous Australians, were not always taken into consideration, with stronger drives, as for example economic benefit at country level, determining the approach undertaken and the strategy selected (Christou and Thompson, 2010).

To start, the need of conducting a feasibility study should be evaluated. According to Bowen et al, (2009) performing a feasibility study may be indicated when *"(a) community partnerships need to be established, increased, or sustained, (b) there are few previously published studies or existing data using a specific intervention technique, (c) prior studies of a specific intervention technique in a specific population were not guided by in-depth research or knowledge of the population's socio-cultural health beliefs, by members of diverse research teams, or by researchers familiar with the target population and in partnership with the targeted communities, (d) the population or intervention target has been shown empirically to need unique consideration of the topic, method, or outcome in other research or (e) previous interventions that employed a similar method have not been successful, but improved versions may be successful; or previous interventions had positive outcomes but in different settings than the one of interest"*. By quickly reviewing these grounds it becomes apparent CRC programmes, independently of whether they are still being designed or already implemented, are prime candidates for qualitative research via feasibility studies. These pilot actions can help elicit patient preferences and elucidate obstacles adversely affecting participation. In terms of results, even small modifications to existing programmes or design can greatly affect outcomes. For example, a sound review being the starting point for deploying such a pilot action, recent systematic reviews of interventions in Australia, indicated that organisational level changes were the most effective in terms of screening behaviour enhancement. It is important to note necessary modifications for increased effectiveness were those that included non-physicians in the screening process (Christie et al, 2008, Wardle et al, 2003, Vernon 1997). Language and literacy barriers are, of course, the most difficult to overcome, as illustrated by the Alaskan and Australian Aboriginal examples, and can only be adequately researched and addressed through engagement of local actors and community leaders, strong community orientation and high level of awareness of the PHPs, including most importantly nursing and all other available healthcare personnel –especially in rural or remote areas.

Additionally, elements of the care pathway ought to be assessed in context and real settings, and, especially where pragmatic trials are impossible, difficult or unethical. Participation in and completion of the screening test is not the only necessary part to ensure successful outcomes, as there has to be a follow up with the appropriate diagnostic testing. (Christou and Thompson, 2010).

Screening utilisation is also influenced by behavioural factors and health economics parameters, as well as by the organizational and cultural settings (Senore et al, 2010). A theoretical framework to explain the adoption of health-related behaviours is needed to underpin any given implementation effort. Models conceptualizing elements of the health care provision have been proposed, providing targets for intervention at patient and provider levels (Stone et al, 2002; Bastani et al, 2004, Senore et al, 2010). However, it is important to note that although any given intervention component may act upon more than one levels, screening uptake is interdependent on all these factors (Senore et al, 2010).

Consideration of multidisciplinary teams is also essential. These teams can help direct resources along a predefined, according to the evidence-base, care pathway ensuring effective, efficient and sustainable implementation and, thus, better results. As we have previously discussed, CRC screening is complex and comprises of different stages involving the participation of different health care actors. For example, all abnormal results should be followed-up and after-care service following treatment should be available. Nevertheless, only a small portion of health plans monitor follow-up care (Klabunde et al, 2003). Multidisciplinary participation can help implement interventions that have added value at patient, provider and even public health-health care system level. For example same day follow-up for abnormal FS, offering on-site colonoscopy seems to lead to better compliance (Stern et al, 2000; Senore et al, 2010). Another benefit in the involvement of nursing and clerical staff is the integration of quality indicators and quality assurance mechanisms in delivery processes and their monitoring as part of standardised care delivery without draining on valuable resources.

8. CRC screening: An issue of quality assurance in modern health care systems

Quality issues in colorectal cancer screening have been previously discussed in editorials in the journals of Quality in Primary Care and Family Practice (Lionis, 2007, Lionis and Petelos, 2011). These editorials address issues relevant to improvement of uptake of CRC screening with the use of cognitive methods and the translation of the Health Belief Model into education and training programs for health care providers. The authors call for a closer collaboration between medical and social care scientists, and reveals another important challenge that PCPs face: addressing health inequalities in a changing and financially restrained world, where for example, minority groups showcase low adoption rates of preventive measures and screening tests.

As previously mentioned, the Directorate General for Health and Consumers, with tasks funded by the EU Health programme (CRC screening grant No 2005317), led an effort aiming to develop EU guidelines on best practice in CRC screening, which resulted in the publication of the first edition of the European guidelines for quality assurance in colorectal cancer screening and diagnosis in February of 2011 (European Commission, Directorate General for Health and Consumers, EAHC — Executive Agency for Health and Consumers, World Health Organisation). The guidelines systematically examine the evidence for efficacy and effectiveness of CRC screening and outline the guiding principles for organising CRC screening programmes. Most importantly, the authors underline the importance of the availability of comprehensive, evidence-based quality assurance guidelines that address all the steps of a screening programme, including invitation, information, surveillance and any other subsequent care, as a key factor to the success of any cancer screening programme. Finally, the authors advocate the widespread application of standardised indicators, as recommended and elaborated upon in the guidelines, to facilitate quality management and promote information exchange in the context of continuous quality improvement.

9. Epilogue

This chapter serves as an overview of the guidance available for CRC screening in the US, UK, Europe and Australia and briefly discussed the important role of GPs/FPs and PCPs, in general, in increasing the CRC screening rate. Although the literature is rich in information, guidelines and recommendation for CRC screening, there is room for improvement. It is to important invest in translating primary research into practice and combine qualitative and quantitative evidence for relevant, contextualised training and educational interventions, both at patient and provider levels.

10. References and internet resources

10.1 References

Allison JE, Sakoda LC, Levin TR, Tucker JP, Tekawa IS, Cuff T, Pauly MP, Shlager L, Palitz AM, Zhao WK, Schwartz JS, Ransohoff DF, Selby JV. (2007). Screening for colorectal neoplasms with new fecal occult blood tests: update on performance characteristics. *J Natl Cancer Inst. Vol. 3;99(19):1462-70*. Epub 2007, Sep 25.

Andermann, A., Blancquaert, I., Beauchamp, S., Déry, V.. (2008). Revisiting Wilson and Jungner in the genomic age: a review of screening criteria over the past 40 years. *Bull World Health Organ. Vol. 86(4):317-9*.

Aubin-Auger, I., Mercier, A., Lebeau. J.P., Baumann, L., Peremans, L., Van Royen, P. (2011). Obstacles to colorectal screening in general practice: a qualitative study of GPs and patients. *Family Practice*. Advance Access: cmr020 first published online May 6, 2011 doi:10.1093/fampra/cmr020.

Bampton, P.A., Sandford, J.J., Cole, S.R., Smith, A., Morcom, J., Cadd, B., Young, G.P. (2005). Interval faecal occult blood testing in a colonoscopy based screening programme detects additional pathology. *Gut. Vol. 54(6):803-6*.

Bastani, R., Yabroff, K.R., Myers, R.E. and Glenn, B. (2004). Interventions to improve follow-up of abnormal findings in cancer screening. *Cancer. Vol. 101:1188-1200*.

Bowen D.J., Kreuter M., Spring B., Cofta-Woerpel L., Linnan L., Weiner D., Bakken S., (...), Fernandez M. (2009) How We Design Feasibility Studies. *American Journal of Preventive Medicine. Vol. 36(5)*:452-457.

Brotons, C., Björkelund, C., Bulc, M., Ciurana, R., Godycki-Cwirko, M., Jurgova, E., Kloppe, P., Lionis, C., Mierzecki, A., Piñeiro, R., Pullerits, L., Sammut, M.R., Sheehan, M., Tataradze, R., Thireos, E.A., Vuchak, J.; EUROPREV network. (2005) Prevention and health promotion in clinical practice: the views of general practitioners in Europe. *Prev Med. Vol. 40(5)*:595-601.

Cardarelli, R. (2010). The Role of Primary Care Providers in Cancer Screening. Primary Care Institute. (Accessed online November 10, 2011: http://www.centerforcommunityhealth.org/Portals/14/Reports/PCPCancerBrief Final%282%29.pdf).

Christie, J., Itzkowitz, S., Lihau-Nkanza, I., Castillo, A., Redd, W., Jandorf, L. (2008). A randomized controlled trial using patient navigation to increase colonoscopy screening among low-income minorities. *Journal of the National Medical Association. Vol. 100(3)*:278-284.

Christou, A., and Thompson, S.C. (2010). "How could the National Bowel Cancer Screening Program for Aboriginal people in Western Australia be improved?" Report to the WA Bowel Cancer Screening Implementation Committee, Department of Health, Western Australia and Combined Universities Centre for Rural Health.

Citarda, F., Tomaselli, G., Capocaccia, R., Barcherini, S., Crespi, M. (2001). The Italian Multicentre Study Group: Efficacy in standard clinical practice of colonoscopic polypectomy in reducing colorectal cancer incidence. GUT. *Vol. 48*:812–815

Cole, S.R., Young G.P., Byrne, D., Guy, J.R., and Morcom, J. (2002). Participation in screening for colorectal cancer based on a faecal occult blood test is improved by endorsement by the primary care practitioner. *J Med Screen. Vol (9)*:147–152.

Edwards, B.K., Ward, E., Kohler, B.A., Eheman, C., Zauber, A.G., Anderson, R.N., Jemal, A., Schymura, M.J., Lansdorp-Vogelaar, I., Seeff, L.C., van Ballegooijen, M., Goede, S.L., Ries, L.A. (2010). Annual report to the nation on the status of cancer, 1975-2006, featuring colorectal cancer trends and impact of interventions (risk factors, screening, and treatment) to reduce future rates. *Cancer. Vol. 1;116(3)*:544-73.

Eide, T.J. (1991). Natural history of adenomas. *World J Surgery. Vol. 15*:3–6.

European Commission, Directorate General for Health and Consumers, EAHC — Executive Agency for Health and Consumers, World Health Organisation. (2011). European guidelines for quality assurance in colorectal cancer screening and diagnosis. (Accessed online September 10, 2011: http://bookshop.europa.eu/is-bin/INTERSHOP.enfinity/WFS/EU-Bookshop-Site/en_GB/-/EUR/ViewPublication-Start?PublicationKey=ND3210390).

Faivre, J., Dancourt, V., Lejeune, C., Tazi, M.A., Lamour, J., Gerard, D., Dassonville, F., Bonithon-Kopp, C. (2004). Reduction in colorectal cancer mortality by fecal occult blood screening in a French controlled study. *Gastroenterology. Vol. 126(7)*:1674-80.

Federici A, Giorgi Rossi P, Bartolozzi F, Farchi S, Borgia P & Guasticchi G. (2005). Survey on colorectal cancer screening knowledge, attitudes, and practices of general practice physicians in Lazio, Italy. *Prev Med. Vol(41):*30–35.

Harris, D.M., Borsky, A.E., Stello, B. et al. (2010). *Toolkit for the System Approach to Tracking and Increasing Screening for Public Health Improvement of Colorectal Cancer Intervention.* AHRQ Publication No 11-0016.

Hassan, C., Benamouzig, R., Spada, C., Ponchon, T., Zullo, A., Saurin, J.C., Costamagna, G. (2011). Cost effectiveness and projected national impact of colorectal cancer screening in France. *Endoscopy. Vol. 43(9):*780-93. Epub 2011 May 27.

IARC (2005). *Cervix Cancer Screening.* IARC Handbooks of Cancer Prevention. Volume 10.

Jørgensen, O.D., Kronborg, O., Fenger, C. (2002). A randomised study of screening for colorectal cancer using faecal occult blood testing: results after 13 years and seven biennial screening rounds. *Gut. Vol. 50(1):*29-32.

Klabunde, C.N., Frame, P.S., Meadow, A., Jones, E., Nadel, M., Vernon, S.W. (2003). A national survey of primary care physicians' colorectal cancer screening recommendations and practices. *Prev Med. Vol. 36(3):*352-62.

Klabunde, C.N., Lanier, D., Nadel M.R, et al. (2009). Colorectal Cancer Screening by primary care physicians: recommendations and practices; 2006-2007. *Am J Prev Med. Vol.(37):*8-16.

Koo J.H., You B., Liu K., Athureliya M.D., Tang C.W., Redmond D.M., Connor S.J., Leong R. (2011). Colorectal cancer screening practices is influenced by ethnicity of medical practitioner and patient. *J Gastroenterol Hepatol.* doi: 10.1111/j.1440-1746.2011.06872.x. [Epub ahead of print]

Levin, B., Lieberman, D.A., McFarland, et al. (2008). Screening and surveillance for the early detection of colorectal cancer and adenomatous polyps, 2008: a joint guideline from the American Cancer Society, the US Multi-Society Task Force on Colorectal Cancer, and the American College of Radiology. *CA Cancer J. Clin. Vol 58:*130-160.

Lionis C, and Petelos E. (2011). Early detection of colorectal cancer: barriers to screening in the primary care setting. *Family Practice. Vol 28(6):*589-91.

Lionis, C. (2007). Colorectal cancer screening and the challenging role of general practitioner/family physician: an issue of quality. *Quality in Primary Care. Vol. 15:*129-131.

McFarland, E.G., Levin, B., Lieberman, D.A., Pickhart, P., Johnson, C.D., Glick, S.N., Brooks, D., Smith, R.A. (2008). Revised colorectal screening guidelines: Joint effort of the American Cancer Society. *CA Cancer J Clin* Vol 2008;58:160.

McGregor, S.E., Hilsden, R.J., Murray, A., Bryant, H.E. (2004) Colorectal cancer screening: practices and opinions of primary care physicians. *Prev Med. Vol 39(2):*279-85.

Meissner, H.I., Breen, N., Klabunde, C.N., Vernon, S.W. (2006). Patterns of colorectal cancer screening uptake among men and women in the United States. *Cancer Epidemiol Biomarkers Prev. Vol 15(2):*389-94.

Miles, A., Cockburn, J., Smith, R.A., Wardle J. (2004). A perspective from countries using organized screening programs. *Cancer. Vol. 101(5):*201-1213.

Ornstein, M., Nemeth, L.S., Jenkins, P.G., Nietert, P.J. (2010). Colorectal cancer screening in Primary Care: Translating Research into Practice. *Medical Care* Vol 48: 900-906.

Pox, C., Schmiegel, W., Classen, M. (2007). Current status of screening colonoscopy in Europe and in the United States. *Endoscopy 39:*168–173.

Quirke, P., Cuvelier, C., Ensari, A., Glimelius, B., Laurberg, S., Ortiz, H., Piard, F., Punt, C.J., Glenthoj, A., Pennickx, F., Seymour, M., Valentini, V., Williams, G., Nagtegaal, J.D. (2010). Evidence-based medicine: the time has come to set standards for staging, *Journal of Pathology. Vol. 221(4):*357-360.

Renehan AG, Egger M, Saunders MP, O'Dwyer ST. (2002). Impact on survival of intensive follow up after curative resection for colorectal cancer: systematic review and meta-analysis of randomised trials. *BMJ. Vol. 6;324(7341):*813.

Rudy, D.R., Zdon, M.J. (2000). Update on Colorectal Cancer. *Am Fam Physician* Vol 61:1759-70,1773-4.

Sarfaty, M. (2006) How to Increase Colorectal Cancer Screening Rates in Practice: a Primary Care Clinician's Evidence-Based Toolbox and Guide. Atlanta, GA: The American Cancer Society, National Colorectal Cancer Roundtable and Thomas Jefferson University. (Accessed online November 10, 2011: http://www.cancer.org/acs/groups/content/documents/document/acspc-024588.pdf).

Sarfaty, M., Wender, R. (2007). How to increase colorectal cancer screening rates in practice. *CA Cancer J Clin. Vol. 57(6):*354-66.

Schroy, P.C. 3rd, Lal, S., Glick, J.T., Robinson, P.A., Zamor, P., Heeren, T.C. (2007). Patient preferences for colorectal cancer screening: how does stool DNA testing fare? *Am J Manag Care. Vol. 13(7):*393-400.

Schroy, P.C., Mylvaganam, S., Davidson, P. (2011). Provider perspectives on the utility of a colorectal cancer screening decision aid for facilitating shared decision-making. Health Expect September 8 [Epub ahead of print], doi:10.1111/j.1369-7625.2011.00730.x.

Senore, C., Malila, N., Minozzi, S., Armaroli, P. (2010). How to enhance physician and public acceptance and utilisation of colon cancer screening recommendations. *Best Pract Res Clin Gastroenterol. Vol 24(4):*509-20.

Sillars-Hardebol, A.H., Carvalho, B., van Engeland, M., Fijneman, R.J., Meijer, G.A. (2012). The adenoma hunt in colorectal cancer screening: defining the target. *Journal of Pathology. Jan;226(1):*1-6. doi: 10.1002/path.3012. Epub 2011 Nov.

Stern, M.A., Fendrick, A.M., McDonnell, W.M., Gunaratnam, N., Moseley, R., Chey, W.D. A randomized, controlled trial to assess a novel colorectal cancer screening strategy: the conversion strategy–a comparison of sequential sigmoidoscopy andcolonoscopy with immediate conversion from sigmoidoscopy to colonoscopy in patients with an abnormal screening sigmoidoscopy. *Am J Gastroenterol. Vol. 95:*2074–2079.

Stone, E.G., Morton, S.C., Hulscher, M.E., Maglione, M.A., Roth, E.A., Grimshaw, J.M., Mittman, B.S., Rubenstein, L.V., Rubenstein, L.Z., Shekelle, P.G. (2002).

Interventions that increase use of adult immunization and cancer screening services: a meta-analysis. *Ann Intern Med. Vol. 136*:641–651.

Sung, J.J., Lau, J.Y., Goh, K.L., Leung, W.K.; Asia Pacific Working Group on Colorectal Cancer. (2005) Increasing incidence of colorectal cancer in Asia: implications for screening. *Lancet Oncol.* Vol 6(11):871-6.

Taskila T., Wilson S., Damery S., Roalfe A., Redman V., Ismail T., Hobbs R. (2009). Factors affecting attitudes toward colorectal cancer screening in the primary care population. *Br J Cancer. Vol 21;101(2):*250.

Tu S.P., Taylor V., Yasui Y, Chun A., Yip M.P., Acorda E. et al. (2006). Promoting culturally appropriate colorectal cancer screening through a health educator: a randomized controlled trial. *Cancer. Vol 107*:959–966.

Vernon SW. (2003). A national survey of primary care physicians' colorectal cancer screening recommendations and practices. *Prev Med. Vol. 36(3)*:352-62.

Viguier J, Calazel-Benque A, Eisinger F, Pivot X. (2011). Organized colorectal cancer screening programmes: how to optimize efficiency among general practitioners. *Eur J Cancer Prev. Vol. 20 Suppl 1:S*26-32.

Wald N.J. (1994). Guidance on terminology. *J Med Screen.* 1: 76.

Walsh, J.M., Posner, S.F., Perez-Stable, E.J. (2002) Colon cancer screening in the ambulatory setting. *Prev Med. Vol 35(3):*209-18.

Wardle, J., Williamson, S., McCaffery, K. (2003). Increasing attendance at colorectal cancer screening: testing the efficacy of a mailed, psychoeducational intervention in a community sample of older adults. *Health Psychology. Vol. 22*:99-105.

Wilson, J.M.G., and Jungner, G. (1968). Principles and practice of screening for disease. Geneva: World Health Organization.(Accessed online October 25, 2011 from: http://www.who.int/bulletin/volumes/86/4/07-050112BP.pdf).

Winawer, S.J., Zauber, A.G., Ho, M.N., O'Brien, M.J., Gottlieb, L.S., Sternberg, S.S., Waye, J.D., Schapiro, M., Bond, J.H., and Panish,J.F. (1993). Prevention of colorectal cancer by colonoscopic polypectomy. The National Polyp Study Workgroup, *New England Journal of Medicine. Vol. 329(27)*:1977-1981.

Young, G.P., St John, D.J., Winawer, S.J., Rozen, P. WHO (World Health Organization) & OMED (World Organization for Digestive Endoscopy). (2002). Choice of faecal occult blood tests for colorectal cancer screening: recommendations based on performance characteristics in population studies: a WHO (World Health Organization) and OMED (World Organization for Digestive Endoscopy) report. *Am J Gastroenterol. Vol 97(10)*:2499-507.

10.2 Internet resources

American Cancer Society (ACS) Guidelines for the early detection of cancer: Colorectal cancer and polyps.

(Accessed online September 19, 2011: http://www.cancer.org/Healthy/FindCancerEarly/CancerScreeningGuidelines/american-cancer-society-guidelines-for-the-early-detection-of-cancer).

Australian Government Department of Health and Ageing. (2008). *Clinical Practice Guidelines for the Prevention, Early Detection and Management of Colorectal Cancer – A Guide for General Practitioners.* (3rd ed.).
(Accessed online August 11, 2011:
http://www.health.gov.au/internet/screening/publishing.nsf/Content/bw-gp-crc-guide).

Australian Government Department of Health and Ageing. (2005) *A Qualitative Evaluation of Opinions, Attitudes and Behaviours Influencing the Bowel Cancer Screening Pilot Program.* Final Report. Screening Monograph: 2/2005.
(Accessed online September 16, 2011:
http://www.health.gov.au/internet/screening/publishing.nsf/Content/qual-eval-cnt).

Australian Population Health Development Principal Committee. (2008). *Population-Based Screening.*
(Accessed online September 16, 2011:
http://www.cancerscreening.gov.au/internet/screening/publishing.nsf/Content/other-pop-health#framework).

Cancer Research UK. Bowel cancer – screening and prevention.
(Accessed online September 15, 2011:
http://info.cancerresearchuk.org/cancerstats/types/bowel/screeningandpreventi on/).

Centers for Diseases Control and Prevention (US) MMWR. Vital Signs: Colorectal Cancer Screening, Incidence, and Mortality: United States, 2002−2010.
(Accessed online September 15, 2011:
http://www.cdc.gov/mmwr/preview/mmwrhtml/mm6026a4.htm?s_cid=mm602 6a4_w).

National Institute for Health and Clinical Excellence, (2011). NICE publishes new guidelines on colonoscopic surveillance for the prevention of colorectal cancer in people with ulcerative colitis, Crohn's disease or adenomas.
(Accessed online August 9, 2011:
http://www.nice.org.uk/newsroom/pressreleases/2011045colonoscopicsurveillan ce.jsp).

International Agency for Research on Cancer. Early detection and Prevention - Quality Assurance Group Resources.
(Accessed online August 11, 2011:
http://www.iarc.fr/en/researchs-groups/QAS/current-topics.php).

Patient-Centered Outcomes Research Institute. (2011-ongoing) Review and Synthesis of Evidence for Eliciting the Patient's Perspective in Patient-Centered Outcomes Research. Literature review and interviews.
(Accessed online September 19, 2011:
http://www.pcori.org/patient-centered-outcomes-research/ and
http://www.pcori.org/committee-charters/).

U.S. Preventive Services Task Force. (2008). *Screening for Colorectal Cancer.*
(Accessed online August 8, 2011:

http://www.uspreventiveservicestaskforce.org/uspstf/uspscolo.htm).
World Health Organization. (2011). *Screening for Colorectal Cancer.*
        (Accessed online August 1, 2011:
        http://www.who.int/cancer/detection/colorectalcancer/en/).

3

Colorectal Carcinoma in the Young

Shahana Gupta[1]* and Anadi Nath Acharya[2]
[1]Department of Surgery, Medical College & Hospitals Kolkata,
[2]Department of Surgery,
Institute of Post Graduate Medical Education and Research, Kolkata,
India

1. Introduction

Colorectal cancer (CRC) is the most common malignancy of the gastrointestinal tract. In the United States, it is the third most commonly diagnosed cancer, next only to breast and lung. It is the second most common cause of cancer-related death both in the USA and in the UK. (www. cancer. org, O'Connell et. al. 2004a, Leff et. al. 2007). Its incidence has risen rapidly in Asia to pose a problem (Yuen et. al. 1997, Huang et. al. 1999, Mohandas et. al. 1999, Yiu et. al. 2004, Goh et. al. 2005,Gupta et. al. 2010). Sung et. al. (2005) in a review on CRC in Asia stated that many Asian countries, e. g., China, Japan, South Korea, Singapore have experienced an increase of two to four times in CRC incidence during the past few decades. In Hong-Kong CRC is the second most common cancer and the third most common cause of cancer death (Yuen et. al. 1997). Tamura et. al. (1996) in a Japanese study reported that age adjusted incidence for CRC per 100,000 population were 12. 6 and 8. 7 for males and females respectively in 1974, 20 and 13. 6 in 1980, 42. 5 and 25. 6 in 1991. Bae et. al. (2002) estimated on the basis of Korean data, that the expected number of cancer deaths in Korea showed an increasing trend for CRC, although the same did not hold for all cancers. In Iran, age adjusted CRC incidence per 100,000 population per year increased from 1. 61 in 1970-80 to 4. 2 in 1990-2000 in men and 2. 35 to 2. 72 for women (Hosseini et. al. 2004). The rising trend is more striking in affluent than in poorer societies and differs substantially amongst ethnic groups. Changes in dietary habits and lifestyle are recognized causes. Genetic characteristics of a population mediate the effect of life style change into disease propensity (Lin et. al. 2010).

Although the common perception is that it is a disease of an older person, there have been many reports from different parts of the world on CRC in the young adults (Bulow 1980, Denmark; Ohman 1982, Sweden;Jarvinen and Turunen 1984, Finland; Ibrahim and Karim 1986, Lebanon; Adloff et. al. 1986, France; Isbister and Fraser 1990, New Zealand; Yuen et. al. 1997, Hong-Kong; Fante et. al. 1997, Italy; Ashenafi 2000, Ethiopia; deSilva et. al. 2000, Srilanka; Paraf and Jothy 2000, Canada; Turkiewicz et. al. , 2001, Australia; Singh et. al. 2002a, Nepal; Kam et. al. 2004, Malaysia; Frizis et. al. 2004, Greece; Guraya and Eltinay2006, Saudi Arabia; Fazeli et. al. 2007, Iran; Karsten et. al. 2008, USA; Gupta et. al. 2010, India). O'Connell et. al. (2004a) have reviewed the literature. The proportion of patients in the young group in a population of CRC patients was significantly larger in reports from Asia and Africa, as compared to the Western reports.

---

* Corresponding Author

The definition of 'Young adults' varies, to a small extent, in the literature. Majority of articles defined 'young' as <40 years, although upper limits of 50 years, 35 years and 30 years have also been used. O'Connell et. al. (2004a) estimated the average value of incidence of CRC in the young adults (<40 years) in the population of all CRC patients as 7% and adjusted it to 6%, when outliers were removed. It has been suggested (Hamilton 2005) that the adjustment was 'too small' and a more realistic estimate was an average of 2. 2%. Leff et. al. (2007) gave an estimate of 2-3%. About 0. 1% of all CRC patients were diagnosed <20 years of age, ~1% between 20-34 years, ~4% between 35-44 years and a further ~12% between 45-54 years. These average figures reflect the extent of the problem in the West. The figures from Asian and African countries are considerably higher, a quarter or a half of a study group of CRC patients may belong to the under-40 group (Ashenafi 2000, Ethiopia; deSilva et. al. 2000, SriLanka; Singh et. al. 2002a, Nepal; Guraya and Eltinay 2006, Saudi Arabia; Gupta et. al. 2010, India). Numerical values given later will establish that the problem of CRC in the young adult in the developing world is alarming.

We now cite reports, from the West (USA, France, Scotland) and from Asia (Iran, Hong Kong), in which the incidence of the disease amongst the young adults has been studied in the same population over a period of time. O'Connell et. al. (2003) noted that in the USA, colon cancer incidence in older patients (60 + years) remained stable in the period 1973-1999 while rectal cancer incidence decreased by 11%. In the group of younger patients (20-40 years) colon cancer incidence increased by 17%, while rectal cancer incidence rose by 75% in the period 1973-1999. The improvement in the older age group is a reflection of more efficient cancer screening in the USA, a result of improved awareness of the disease. It is possible that relative ignorance about the problem of CRC in the young adult is responsible for the fact that the problem has worsened over the years. Other issues namely difference in molecular genetics, may also be present. In Iran, Hosseini et. al. (2004) defined the younger group as <60 years, compared figures in two 10 year periods 1970-1980 and 1990-2000 and found an increased proportion of < 60 years CRC patients (in a population of all CRC patients) in the latter decade, 37. 5% as against 70%. An increase in proportion of the young CRC patients was noted over a prolonged time span. Mitry et. al. (2001) from France reported that below-45 age standardized incidence rates doubled in the period 1976-1982 and then again in the period 1983-1989, in both genders and stabilized thereafter. In Hong-Kong, the overall incidence in > 50 years group increased at a rate of 4% a year during 1978-87, whereas in Scotland a higher overall incidence remained stable during this period (Yuen et. al. 1997).

O'Connell et. al. (2004b) in a study of American patients found that young (20-40 years) colon cancer patients tend to have later-stage and higher-grade tumours. However they have equivalent or better 5 year cancer-specific survival compared to 60+ older group, an apparently paradoxical result. Although most reports agree on a more severe advanced disease at presentation in the young (Adloff et. al. 1986, Cusack et. al. 1996, Nath et. al. , 2009) and many also agree with the opinion that prognosis is not poorer in the young (Jarvinen and Turunen 1984, Turkiewicz et. al. 2001, Karsten et. al. 2008) some reports (Moore et. al. 1984, Adkins et. al. 1987, Okuno et. al. 1987, Singh et. al. 2002a) do not share the view that prognosis is 'equivalent or better'. Inspite of this difference in assessment, a favourable prognosis in many studies should inspire more aggressive detection and treatment for the young.

The genetic basis of CRC has been investigated in recent years. A satisfactory understanding of the disease, tumour characteristics, relationship of disease susceptibility with age and issues related to survival rely on an understanding of the link between molecular genetics and disease. A complete resolution of this relation is a tall order, but a modest beginning is being made. Intelligent choice of treatment protocol, surgical as well as chemotherapeutic is also influenced by research on molecular genetics of CRC (Liang and Church 2010). Hereditary CRC usually occurs at a relatively young age, between 25 and 55 years in individuals with family history of CRC. Individuals who inherit the predisposing cancer gene have a greater chance of developing the disease (Murday and Slock 1989, Lynch et. al. 1991, Lynch and de la Chapelle 2003, Ewart Toland, 2012). The importance of family history in determining susceptibility to CRC in the young has been stressed in the literature (St. John et. al. 1993, Fuchs et. al. 1994, Turkiewicz et. al. 2001). There exist literature reports that identify genetic factors in younger CRC patients which differ from those in older patients and may be responsible for greater cancer susceptibility of the younger patients (Farrington et. al. 1998, Chan et. al. 1999, Morris et. al. 2007, Berg et. al. 2010, Lin et. al. 2010).

In this essay, we focus on the issue of CRC in young age, with particular reference to developing countries. The relative incidence figures of CRC in the young patients as compared to older patients in different parts of the world are given. These figures, in greater detail are given in the Indian context (section 2). Disease stage at presentation and tumour characteristics of younger patients, often in comparison with the older ones in different countries are then summarized (section 3). A brief reference to de novo cancer in Asians (section 4) is followed by a discussion of some recent genetic studies in the young (section 5). Section 6 contains a discussion on prediosposing factors and section 7 has focus on prognosis in the young. The paper concludes (section 8) with a brief reference to the effect of recent molecular genetic research on treatment protocol.

2. Incidence amongst young adults

The relative incidence of CRC in the younger group varies significantly from one country to another. As cited above, it is typically 2-3% in the West. Other European figures are: Fante et. al. (Italy): 1%; Endreseth et. al. (Norway):6%; Ohman (Sweden): 4%; Adloff et. al. (France): 3%; Yilmazlar et. al. (Turkey): 20%. The corresponding figures are much higher from several Asian and African countries: Nath et. al. (India): 35. 6%, <40 yrs; Gupta et. al. (India): 39%,<40 years; Singh et. al. (South Asia): 23%,<40 years (with a maximum incidence in 40-60 years, a decade earlier than Western figures): study period 1975-1981; Soliman et. al. (Egypt): 35. 6%,<40 yrs; Ashenafi (Ethiopia): mean age 47 years (61. 4% <50years, 36% <40 yrs,16% <30 yrs) in two 5 year periods with a 10 year gap; Guraya and Eltinay (Saudi Arabia): study period 1999-2004,63% <40 yrs, mean age 44years, peak incidence 30-39 years; Hosseini et. al. (Iran): 70% (<60 years):study period 1990-2000; Chew et. al. (Singapore):25% <40 years; Singh et. al. (Nepal): 28. 6% <40 years; de Silva et. al. (Sri Lanka): 19. 7% <40 years. Some of these references are detailed in Table 1. In Egypt, more than half of all CRC patients are below-50, patients under-30 constitute 22% of the population of all CRC patients (Soliman et. al. 1997). Qing et.al. (2003) in a comparative study of American and Chinese patients (1990-2000) reported that the mean age at diagnosis of 690 American patients was 69 years (20-91 years) and that of 870 Chinese patients was 48. 3 years (13-84 years); peak incidence was 70-79 years in Whites and 50-59 years in Orientals. The conclusion is that the Orientals are affected by the disease at a younger age. The same theme emerges from recent data from several Indian hospitals which includes our own recent work (Gupta et. al. 2010). In a period spanning 8 years (2000-2008), we found the ratio of under-40 to above- 40 years age group to be 0. 64. The study group comprised of 305 patients in SSKM Hospital, Kolkata, India, a premier referral Hospital. The values reported by three premier Oncology centers located in two cities in India and in another report by Pal (2006), based on work done

Sr. No.	Reference, Period of study	Age profile	Disease stage	Tumour characteristics
1	Lee 1968-91	62 patients, <40yrs	Dukes' A:8%, B:20%, C:23%, D:48%.	Half of stage D patients and 20% of lower stage patients (p=0. 037) had high grade lesions.
2	Minardi, 1976-97	37 patients, <40yrs	Dukes' C:37%, D: 22%.	Mucinous tumour : 42%; moderate and poor differentiation : 84%
3	Cusack	186 patients, <40yrs	Dukes' C & D: 65. 6%.	Poorly differentiated tumour in 41%, signet-ring cell tumours in 11. 1%, infiltrating tumour leading edges in 69% of young patients. Aggressive tumour biology with higher frequency in <40yr patients (p<0. 001), potentially metastatic.
4	Bedikian, 1944-1977	2609 patients,<50yrs age; 183 aged<40 yrs. Comparison between<30yr and 30-39yr age group and with yet older age group	96% of < 40 years group had carcinoma extending beyond colonic wall.	Moderate and poorly differentiated neoplasms (80%) and mucinous variety (33%) in young.
5	Beckman 1943-1977	69 patients: 20-39yrs	67% Dukes' C and D	Mucinous variety (28%).
6	Varma	A review: all age groups	Advanced stage more frequent in the young.	Greater frequency of mucinous tumour in the young.
7	Cozart, Unusual Case Registry 1992-93	55 patients, <30yrs	62% Dukes' C and D	Poorly differentiated /mucinous variety: 33%
8	Howard	801 patients including <40yrs group	Advanced signs and stages more frequent in the young.	Greater frequency of mucinous variety in the young

9	Adkins, 1973-1984	705 patients; 45 patients, <35yrs	In the younger group: Dukes' A:2,B:8, C: 28, D: 7 patients.	19: poorly differentiated,19: well or moderately differentiated tumour
10	Moore, 1967-1981	3. 2% of 1909 patients <40yrs	Higher incidence of advanced disease, especially in second or third decades.	Greater incidence of mucinous variety (32. 3% in young vs. 8. 6% in the whole study group). Poorly differentiated tumour: 98%; distant metastases in one-third patients. Vascular (24%) and perineural (11%) invasion in the young.
11	Karsten. , 1998-2005	Younger group: 41 patients <40yrs Older group : >60 yrs	Advanced stage: T-3/4 lesion in 87. 8% of young/63% in older group (p=0. 002).	Poorly differentiated, (p=0. 003), mucin secreting/ signet ring (p=0. 005), more common in the young
12	Fairley, 1998-2001 Cancer Registry (NPCR,SEER)*	All age groups Young:20-49yrs	Less localized, more aggressive disease in terms of stage in the young (20-49yrs)	Incidence of poorly differentiated tumour in young (<50yrs) (i) twice as high as well differentiated ones in the young (ii)60% higher than that for well differentiated cancers in the old
13	Lichtman 1987-1991	57. 2% <70yrs	Dukes' C and D more frequent at a lower age (p=0. 03). Mean Age A/B-1 67. 7 yrs, B-2 70. 1yrs, C/D 63. 9yrs	Grade not related to age

| 14 | Dozois, 1976-2002 | 1025 patients,<50yrs; Mean age 42. 4±6. 4 years 51% colon, 49% rectal (largest cohort of young-onset patients without genetic predisposition) | 70% colon, 60% rectal: stage C&D | Colon Cancer: Mucinous(11%) & Signet cell (2%) Grade 2+3 for both rectum & colon cancer: ~87% |
| 15 | Behbehani 11 yrs period pre-1980 | <40 years group: 56 patients | Advanced stage C&D: ~90% in young ~50% in general population | Poor differentiation: 21% in young, 8% in general population |

*NPCR: National Program of Cancer Registries; SEER: Surveillance, Epidemiology and End Results

Table 1. Summary of references in the literature on stage and tumour characteristics in the USA

in the same referral hospital where Gupta et. al. (2010) worked are 0. 58, 0. 63, 0. 45, 0. 62. Average of these five ratios is 0. 52, which is equivalent to ~34% of < 40 years CRC patients amongst all CRC patients. This figure is of the same order as the values from several Asian and African countries cited above. They are also substantially larger than values recorded in National Cancer Registry (PBCR) in four Indian metropolises. The PBCR ratio is 0. 20 and has remained stable over 16 years (1988-2004).

The difference between PBCR values and those reported by five premier hospitals in India, irrespective of their location and specialty, cited by Gupta et. al. (2010) has a clear message. The concern and facilities for cancer detection in the premier hospitals is greater than those in district hospitals. The data of the district hospitals are reflected in the PBCR values. This is the reason for the larger proportion of under-40 patients reported by the premier hospitals. The reason for delay in diagnosis of a young patient in either the premier hospitals or the district hospitals, particularly in the developing world, is that unless there is a family history these patients are not screened. So cancers are usually symptomatic at presentation. Even when symptoms occur, they may initially be misdiagnosed. Rectal bleeding for example is often put down to an anorectal cause. O'Connell et. al. (2004a) report an average delay in diagnosis of 6. 2 months, the reasons for which include a delay in presentation on the part of the patients, limited access to care and misdiagnosis on the part of the physician. This delay is larger in the developing world. Minimizing delay in diagnosis means not taking such symptoms lightly. Rectal bleeding usually has an anorectal cause, but when no such cause is obvious and the bleeding persists, colonoscopy is mandatory, regardless of patient's age. The same concern must apply to other less obvious symptoms.

In a review on CRC in Asia, Sung et. al. (2005) placed India at the bottom of the list amongst Asian countries, in order of decreasing CRC incidence. The data we provide does not contradict this assessment, but if relative incidence in the young is an indication, India has joined the rest of Asia.

3. Disease stage and tumour characteristics in the young adults

The most powerful predictor of outcome for young adults, as it is for older patients is disease stage. Two staging systems are in use and are cited in Table 1-3. One is the tumour-node-metastases (TNM) staging system of the American Joint Committee on Cancer (AJCC). Microscopic extent of tumour invasion (T stage) and nodal involvement (N stage) from histological assessment are combined with assessment for metastatic disease (M stage) to specify a tumour stage. Brief description of TNM stages are: Tumour stages (T): Tumour in T1, invades submucosa, T2: invades muscularis propria, T3 and T4 are more extensive, T3 indicates invasion through muscularis propria into subserosa or into nonperitonealised pericolic or perirectal tissues while T-4 invades adjacent organs. Regional Lymph node stages: N1: 1-3 positive nodes, N2:4 or more positive nodes. Distant metastases stages (M): M1: Distant metastases present. The other classification system known as Dukes' system is: A: limited to bowel wall, B: penetration of bowel wall, C: lymph node involvement, D: distant metastatic disease present (Fry et. al. 2008).

Mucinous adenocarcinoma is one of the histological subtypes of colorectal cancers. It accounts for 5-15% of all primary CRC and is defined as a tumour with >50% of its body showing a mucinous pattern on histological examination and with a large amount of extra cellular mucin produced by secreting acini. This is distinct from signet ring adenocarcinoma, a rare variant in which mucin remains inside the cell, which is well known for its aggressiveness. It has been suggested that mucinous adenocarcinoma behaves differently from more common histological subtypes of CRC. However, its clinical implications remain unclear. According to published series, mucinous adenocarcinoma affects younger patients, is more frequent in proximal part of the colon and tends to present at a more advanced stage (Negri et. al. 2005).

In Table 1, 2 and 3 we tabulate data on disease stage and tumour characteristics, in particular its mucinous nature, of CRC patients in the USA (Table 1), in Europe, inclusive of Turkey and the UK and Australia (Table 2) and in Asia and Africa (Table 3).

Several reports cited in Table 1 (Sr No 1,2,3,5,7,9,14) were entirely on features of CRC in the younger patients. In several other reports (Sr No. 4,6,8,10-13,15), both the younger and the older patient groups were studied and comparative features were assessed. The size of the younger group was mostly ~50, was ~200 in two reports (Sr No 3 and 4) and was 1025 in the work of Dozois et. al. (2005) (Sr no 14), the largest cohort of young CRC patients. In reports that included older and younger patients, older patients were much larger in number (Sr No 4,8-10). In all studies that were on younger patients alone, a high incidence of advanced stage (C+D: >70%)was reported. In studies that included both groups, the frequency of advanced disease in the young was as high or higher (Sr No. 4,11,15). In all of them, advanced disease stages were found to be more frequent in the young than in the old. In studies on younger patients alone, a significant proportion of patients had aggressive lesions, namely mucinous, poorly differentiated tumours with infiltrating leading edge. The frequency of aggressive tumour biology varied from one study to another but remained significant in all of them. In the comparative studies (Sr No. 6,8,10-12,15), the younger patients showed a higher frequency of aggressive tumour biology. Only one report (Sr No. 13) concluded that grade was not related to age.

Country	Sr No.	Reference, Period of study	Age profile	Disease stage	Tumour characteristics
France	1	Adloff 1973-1980	1037 patients; 3% <40yrs	No significant difference in stage between <40 and >40 Yrs group.	Greater frequency of mucinous and poorly differentiated carcinoma in the young
Finland	2	Jarvinen 1970-1979	249 patients, <40yrs	53% Dukes' C and D.	Premalignant condition more common in young
Greece	3	Frizis 1994-2003	Two groups: 11 young <40yrs; 45 old > 80 yrs.	Dukes' C 54. 5% in the young and 44. 4% in the elderly group.	Undifferentiated tumour: 36. 3% of the young and 8. 8% of elderly.
Sweden	4	Ohman 1950-1979	48/1061 patients are <40 years (21-39 years)	Dukes' A same proportion in young and old, Dukes' B fewer, Dukes' C more in young	
Norway	5	Endreseth 1993-1999	2283 patients with rectal cancer <70 years, <45 yrs: 132, 45-49 yrs: 153 50-69 yrs:1998	Dukes' C&D : under 45: 73/132(~55%) 45-69yrs: 998/2152(~46%)	Higher frequency of poorly differentiated tumours (27 vs. 15%) & N-2 stage (37 vs. 15%) with distant metastases (38 vs. 20%); 56% of under-40 years: developed metastases (20-26% of older group) after tumour resection
	6	Berg 2010	181 patients, 45 of them < 50 yrs	Dukes' C &D 54% in < 50 yrs group 46% in 51-70 yrs 36% in > 70 yrs	

Country	Sr No.	Reference, Period of study	Age profile	Disease stage	Tumour characteristics
UK	7	Leff 1982-1992	49 patients all < 40 yrs: 67% in 31-40 yrs, 2 in their teens	Among all patients: 60% Dukes' C&D. Among patients at risk (family history /predisposing factor): 56% Dukes' C	Among all patients: 59% moderately & 22% poorly differentiated . Among patients at risk: 53% moderately & 20% poorly differentiated
Italy	8	Fante 1984-1992	Three groups <40, 41-50, 51-55 years: ~1%, 6%, 6% of 1298 patients	Stage did not differ	Histological features did not differ
Turkey	9	Yilmazlar 1986-1993	237 patients; 46 below 40yrs	76%of the young: Dukes C&D	48% tumours are poorly differentiated or mucinous in young.
Australia	10	Turkiewitz 1971-1999	61/2384 below 40 years	Distribution of stage not significantly different in younger and older group	35%tumours in the young are poorly differentiated

Table 2. Summary of references in the literature on stage and tumour characteristics from Europe (inclusive of UK & Turkey) and Australia

Two of the reports from Europe listed in Table 2 (Sr.No.2,7) are entirely on young patients. One of these (Sr No. 2) has the largest study group of young onset patients (~250), while the other reports have ~100-150 (Sr Nos. 5,6,8) or less ~50 (Sr No. 1,4,7,10)young patients. The report, Sr No. 3 is on a much smaller population of 11 patients. A significant frequency of more advanced (C+D) tumour in the young (50-60%) was reported in several studies (Sr No. 2,3,5-7). This frequency was larger (76%) in a study from Turkey (Sr No. 9). Comparative assessment showed a higher frequency of advanced stages in the young as compared to that in the older patients (Sr No. 3-6). Significant frequency (~ ≤50%) of high grade tumours were reported in the young in several publications (Sr Nos. 3,5,7,9,10). Higher frequency of high grade tumours in the young as compared to the older group were cited in several other papers (Sr No. 1,3,5,7). Three studies (Sr No. 1,8,10) however, reported no difference in disease stage and one report (Sr No. 8) found no difference in tumour grade, between the younger and older patient groups. A significant occurrence of premalignant conditions in the young was reported in only one paper (Sr No. 2).

Country	Sr No	Reference, Period of Study	Age profile	Disease Stage	Tumour Characteristics
ASIA Iran	1	Fazeli 1995-2001	403 patients in two age groups, <40yrs and >40yrs	Older group: 53. 2% in stage II; younger group: 45%in stage III.	Poorly differentiated tumours found in larger proportion in younger patients (22% vs. 5. 9%)
Singapore	2	Kam 1989-2001	39 patients <30yrs, mean age 25yrs	Advanced disease stage in 70% patients.	Mucinous histology: 18%; differentiation: moderate 61%, poor 36%
	3	Chew 1997-2005	523 Asian cohorts 19-50 years Of them <40 yrs:134; >40yrs:389	63% Advanced stage (III-IV) <40yr group: 89/134;66% >40yr group: 245/389;63%	Predominantly poorly differentiated: (30% in <40 years 12% in > 40 years) mucinous, signet ring cell histological subtypes (16% vs. 9%).
Malaysia	4	Shahruddin 1990-94	21 patients <30yrs	Extensive disease	Mucinous histology
Israel	5	Shemesh-Bar, 1997-2007	406 patients, 203 in < 50 years	More advanced stage III-IV at diagnosis (56 vs. 41%) higher rate of N-2 disease (29 vs. 16%)	No difference in other features
	6	Neufeld 1999-2005	<50 years 90; 190 > 50 years	40% Advanced stage (III-IV) <40yrs:47/90;52% >40yrs:61/190;32%	Mucinous tumour in 11% in early onset group, 7% in late onset group

Country	Sr No	Reference, Period of Study	Age profile	Disease Stage	Tumour Characteristics
Taiwan	7	Chiang 7 year period	5436 patients 7% <40 years	Dukes' stage improves with age (A & B 31% < 30 years, 49% > 80 years)	Poorly differentiated tumours tended to decrease with age, 16. 9% < 30 years. 6. 2% > 80 years. Similar trend in Mucin producing characteristics (36% vs7. 5%)
India	8	Nath 2003-2007	287 patients 35. 6% < 40 yrs	Advanced T stage (T 0-2: 18. 9% T -3: 62. 3% T-4: 19. 7% vs. 34. 5%, 56. 0%, 9. 5%) and N-stage (N 0: 31. 1%, N1: 41%, N2: 27. 8% vs. 53. 9%, 26. 7%, 17. 2%)	Poorly differentiated and / or mucinous or signet cell carcinoma (52% vs. 20. 5%)
	9	Gupta 2000-2008	305 patients 40% < 40 yrs	60% presented in Dukes' stage III & IV	Mucinous tumour 80% Poor differentiation 50%
Nepal	10	Singh 2002[a]	91 patients 28. 6% < 40 yrs	92. 3% present in Dukes' stage III-IV vs. 61. 5% in older patients	Significantly higher poorly differentiated and mucinous carcinoma in the young.
SriLanka	11	de Silva 15 yr period	305 patients 19. 7% < 40 yrs	No significant difference in Dukes' stage with older group	Significant presence of mucinous (13. 3%) or signet ring type (5%) tumours.

Country	Sr No	Reference, Period of Study	Age profile	Disease Stage	Tumour Characteristics
AFRICA Egypt	12	Soliman* 1982-1996	1608 patients; 35. 6% <40 yrs	Dukes' stage is worse in > 40 years group (72% vs. 57%)	Tumour grade comparable in two groups; mucin producing tumours: 31% in younger group, 14% in older group

*Soliman et. al. (1997)

Table 3. Summary of references in the literature on stage and tumour characteristics from Asia and Africa.

Reports from Asia and Africa are listed in Table 3. Features of only the younger patients were assessed in four reports (Sr. No. 2-4,9). The younger groups were larger in several studies (523:Sr No. 3; 203:Sr No 5; 370: Sr No. 7and 576 : Sr No. 12) from Asia and Africa as compared to ones from the USA (Table 1) and Europe (Table 2). Higher incidence of CRC in the young in Asia and Africa was found to be consistent with these figures. In two studies (Sr No. 11,12) the disease in the young was assessed as less advanced at presentation and less aggressive. In one report (Sr No. 5),a more advanced disease stage was noted but no difference in tumour grade was found. A more advanced disease and tumour grade was reported in the young as compared to the older patients (which is usually the case in Table 1 & 2) in 5 of 12 reports (Sr No. 1,6-8,10). In a report by Chew et. al (2009, Sr No. 3) the same conclusion was reached; 'older' patients were however in the age group 40-50years. The frequency of advanced disease and high tumour grade in the young in these reports were similar to that in reports restricted to only the young patients (Sr No. 2,4,9).

Irrespective of the country, the size of the study group, time span and the year of study, the dominant result is the same. Young CRC patients present at a more advanced clinical stage, the tumours are mucinous and poorly differentiated, more so in comparison with the older patient group. The features in India and neighbouring Nepal and Sri Lanka are the same as in the rest of the world. We have noticed some difference in disease pattern in Asia and Africa as compared to the West in our discussions of the data in Tables 1-3. The issue of ethnic differences in determining the difference in disease characteristics is important. This issue, without specific reference to the disease in the young, received attention in several papers, e. g., Isbister (1992; New Zealand and Saudi Arabia), Soliman et. al. (2001; Egypt and the West), Fireman et. al. (2001;Arab and Jewish neighbours in Israel),Qing et. al. (2003;USA and China), Sung et. al. (2005;Asia and the West),Goh et. al. (2005;Asian patients of different races in Malaysia) and Fairley et. al. (2006;Blacks,Asians/Pacific Islanders and Whites).

The advanced stage at presentation of many colorectal cancers in young patients is not just a result of a delay in diagnosis. It may also be that the cancer in younger patients is more virulent by nature. This feature is rooted in subtleties of genetic differences. More aggressive' tumour characteristics, as evidenced by its mucinous nature and poor differentiation have also been linked to molecular genetic differences. Recent molecular biology studies have shown characteristic features of mucinous carcinoma, e. g., lower expression of p53, more frequent DNA replication errors expressed as microsatellite instability and specific codon 12 K-ras mutations and, when ploidy has been determined, a higher index if diploidy was found than for non-mucinous carcinoma (Negri 2005).

Tumour subsite: The issue of subsite location is important in screening strategies and in choice of treatment protocols. In the literature (e. g. , Breivik et. al. 1997) preference for subsite location has been associated with molecular genetic roots of CRC. Molecular genetic findings classify CRC into two groups. The first class of tumours show microsatellite instability (MSI), occur more frequently in the right colon, have diploid DNA, behave indolently, of which Hereditary Non polyposis Colorectal Cancer Syndrome (HNPCC) is an example. The larger incidence of proximal colon cancer in patients with HNPCC syndrome highlights the importance of genetics in preference for subsite location in colon cancer. In the other group belong tumours which tend to be left sided, show aneuploid DNA, behave aggressively, of which Familial Adenomatous Polyposis (FAP) is an example. Each group has its own characteristic gene mutations (Lynch and de la Chapelle, 1999).

Breivik et. al. (1997)in a study of 282 patients from 7 hospitals in Norway in the period 1987-9 concluded that proximal and distal CRC evolve by different genetic pathways and that these pathways are influenced by sex-related factors. Their results, analyzed by statistical models, pointed to hormonal mechanisms with important clinical implications. They found that presence of TP 53 mutations was dependent on tumour location only, with a positive association to cancers occurring distally (p=0. 002). Microsatellite instability was found almost exclusively in proximal colon cancers.

Stigliano et. al. (2008) compared a cohort of 40 HNPCC cases with 573 sporadic CRC cases in the period 1970-1993. Median age of diagnosis was 46. 8 years in HNPCC cases and 61 years in sporadic CRC cases. 85% had right sided lesion in HNPCC group as opposed to 57% in sporadic cancer group.

Slattery et. al. (1996) studied age, sex and tumour sub-site distribution in 1709 CRC patients from three geographic areas in the USA. Approximately 50% of CRC in men and greater than 50% of CRC in women were in the proximal segment of the colon. Men who were diagnosed prior to age 50 and both men and women diagnosed at age 70 or older had predominantly proximal cancers. People with proximal cancers and those diagnosed prior to age 50 were likely to have more advanced disease. In general, both men and women had more proximal cancers with advancing age, which were associated with more advanced disease.

Ionov et. al. (1993) showed that 12% of CRC patients carried ubiquitous somatic deletions in poly (dA. dT) sequences and other simple repeats. Tumours with these mutations showed distinctive genotypic and phenotypic features. Patients with these deletions showed a predominance of right sided tumours while those without deletions had a predominance of left sided lesions.

Thibodeau et. al. (1993)studied the association of microsatellite alterations with preference for tumour subsite. All four sites of alteration studied showed a dramatic change in preference from distal to proximal colon in the mutated form (typical values: proximal/distal; (26,49), (11,1 in the mutated form)).

Fancher et. al. (2011) studied 45 young patients, 20 males and 25 females,mean age 43. 6 years, in the USA and found preference for left sided lesions in females (16/8)and a preference for right sided lesions (12/10)in men (p=0. 35; small sample size);right sided cancers had a higher stage at presentation.

Kaw et. al. (2002) studied 1277 Filipino patients of whom 218 (17%)were <40 years, a mean age of 31. 3 years. Cancers of the right colon were noted to be more common in females (55%)and rectal tumours were seen more frequently in males (55%;p=0. 014),but when analysed in relation to age, right colon cancers were actually more common in men <40 years of age (p=0. 013);the incidence in women was higher only above the age of 50 years. The proportion of CRCs located on the right side was 28% for <40 years patients and 20% for the 40+ group. On the other hand, left colon cancers were seen in 30% of the older age group compared with 18% in the younger population (p=0. 001). For rectal cancer, there was no significant difference in proportion between the young and the old (p=0. 414).

Elsaleh et. al. (2000) in an older patient group (mean age 66. 7 ±12. 9 years) in Australia reported that MSI positive tumours were slightly more frequent in women than in men (10 vs 7%). Right sided tumours were more frequently MSI positive than left sided tumours (20 vs 1%). Men with right sided tumours benefited from chemotherapy (37 vs 12%) but men with left sided tumours did not.

Mahdavinia et. al. (2005), Fazeli et. al. (2007) and Malekzadeh et. al (2009) found that in Iranian patients with positive family history of CRC, the most frequently affected site of colon was the right side. Malekzadeh et. al. (2009) found that MSI was more frequent in early-onset patients and in proximal tumours. They reported that proximal and distal tumours harbor different p53 mutational spectra;distal CRCs showed a higher frequency of G to A transitions at CpG whereas G to A transitions at non-CpGs were more frequent in proximal tumours. Fazeli et. al. (2007) found that 62. 5% of patients with proximal colon tumours were males.

Nelson et. al. (1997) and Saltzstein et. al. (1997) showed that there was an increase in the relative proportion of proximal colon cancers with increasing age 'a shift to the right'. Thus with increasing age, full length colonoscopy will be a better screening tool. The exact age at which the shift occurs will vary with gender and ethnicity. There is a predominance of African-Americans amongst those at risk for proximal colon carcinoma and predominance of white males amongst those at risk for distal CRC.

Goh et. al. (2005) in a study of different races in Malaysia observed that demographic differences between Asia and the West may exist. No difference in anatomic distribution was found in Malay, Chinese and Indian races. They noted that in general CRC tends to be located distally in areas with a lower incidence of disease (parts of Asia) and migrated proximally with increasing incidence, as in Japan or Korea. They suggested that this may be related to a decrease in rectal cancer and an increasing proportion of elderly patients in the population. Young patients had a higher probability of having distal lesions as compared to the older patients.

Qing et. al. (2003) in a comparative study on Chinese and American patients, noted that the proportion of left sided lesions in Oriental patients (74%) was significantly higher than that in Whites (63. 7%) and that rectal cancers were significantly more common among Orientals (p<0. 001).

O'Connell et. al. (2004[a]) in their review quoted average values of subsite location in <40 years young patients as follows: ascending 22%, transverse 11%, descending colon 13%, rectum and sigmoid (including rectosigmoid junction) 54%,a dominance of left sided tumour in the young.

We summarize reports on preference for tumour sub-site from different countries in Table 4. Some of these are cited in Table 1-3 where patient groups are detailed. The others are detailed in Table 4.

	Sr. No.	Author, Country	Sub-site
Asia & Africa	1	Gupta, India	69. 7% distal tumours in < 40 yr group (rectal 57. 9%,left colon 11. 8%). Of patients with colon cancer proximal tumours constitute 72%.
	2	Singh, South Asia*	Rectum: commonest (83%) site of the lesion in young patients (21-30 yrs). No comparison with older patient group.
	3	Singh, Nepal	Rectum: most frequent site of tumor (76. 9% vs. 36. 9% in older age group)
	4	de Silva, Sri Lanka	No significant difference in tumour distribution between the young and the old.
	5	Shahruddin, Malaysia	Rectosigmoid region:most common (29%)' Left colon 19%,Splenic flexure 4%,Transverse colon 9%,Hepatic flexure 4%, Cecum 24% ;all patients<30yrs
	6	Goh, Asian patients of different races in Malaysia	No significant difference between <and > 65 years group; predominance (~90%)of left sided lesion in both age groups.
	7	Kam, Singapore	46% rectal and rectosigmoid; right-sided tumour:20%; patient group, all young <30yrs
	8	Ashenafi, Ethiopia	66. 7%rectal lesions; younger patients; mean age 47 years (61. 4% <50years, 36% <40 yrs,16% <30 yrs)
	9	Shemesh-Bar, Israel	Higher proportion of left side tumour in the young (82% vs. 71%)
	10	Chew, Singapore (Asian patients)	Predominantly left sided tumour (~80%)in <40 years and 41-50 years age group; no effect of age.
	11	Malekzadeh, Iran	Predominantly right sided tumour, general population
	12	Ibrahim, Lebanon	Rectosigmoid most common site in general population (553 patients),70. 7%;also in 32,<29 years younger group: 84. 4%
	13	Fazeli , Iran	Subsite distribution nearly independent of age group (< & > 40 years), distal ~ 80% in both groups.
	14	Chiang, Taiwan	No change in subsite preference from < 30 years to > 80 years
	15	Soliman**, Egypt	No change in subsite preference in < 40 years vs. > 40 years group, larger proportion of distal tumours (~65%) in both age groups

	Sr. No.	Author, Country	Sub-site
U. S. A.	16	Bedekian, USA	Increase in primary lesions in the right colon with increasing age at diagnosis; <40 yrs group compared with general population.
	17	Cozart, USA	Dominance of left sided lesions (12 right colon, 24 left colon,11 rectum) and left colon amongst colon cancer patients; study group comprises of only young patients<30yrs. No comparison with older group.
	18	Nelson, USA & Saltzstein, USA	Significant shift to right sided lesion with increasing age;<50 vs. >50yrs.
	19	Slattery, USA	Proximal cancers more frequent (>50%) in men<50 years and in both men and women >70 years(details in text).
	20	Fairley, USA	Rectal cancers more frequent in <50yrs group (37% vs. 26%); proximal colon cancer more frequent in >50 age group (42. 6% vs. 32. 1%),remaining <50%in both groups.
	21	Lichtman, USA	Older patients: more transverse/right sided lesions (p=0. 003). 138 patients;mean age of patients with different sites of tumour: Right colon 72 yrs,left colon 66. 1 yrs, rectum 61. 6 yrs
	22	Karsten, USA	Right sided lesion more frequent (44%)in young compared to 21% in older group, p=0. 004.
	23	Minardi, USA	Tumours evenly distributed in colon and rectum (under-40 group). Older group not compared.
	24	O'Connell[a] (International Review)	Rectum and sigmoid colon most frequent sites (54%) in the young <40 yrs patient group.
	25	Dozois, USA	Predominantly rectum (49. 1%) or left colon (29. 1%) than proximal colon (21. 9%). All young patients <50yrs. No comparison with older patient group.
	26	Behbehani, USA	Colon: Right 21%,Transverse 21%, Left 14% Sigmoid & Rectum 44% in the <40 yrs group; these figures are 34%,4%,8%,54% respectively in the older group.
Europe	27	Leff, UK	Only 12% right-sided colon cancer,<40 yrs patients, no comparison with older group.
	28	Fante, Italy	Majority of tumours in left colon and rectum in the whole patient group <40 – 55 years. Right colon: 37% in <40 years, 18% in 41-50 years, 14% in 51-55 years group.

*Singh et. al. 1984; **Soliman et. al. (1997)

Table 4. Tumour Sub-site in the young in different countries

In some of these papers, (Sr. No. 1, 2, 5, 7, 8, 10, 17, 23-25, 27), a preference for distal lesions in the young patients were cited, but were not compared with the older patient groups. In some others (Sr. No. 3, 9, 12, 16, 18-21) this comparison was made and a change in preference for tumour sub-site with increasing age was noticed. Shemesh-Bar et.al. (2010, Sr. No. 9) and Ibrahim et. al. (1986, Sr. No. 12) found that although left sided lesions formed the majority of tumours, their proportion decreased in the older group. Singh et. al (2002a, Sr. No. 3) and Fairley et. al. (2006, Sr. No. 20)found that the proportion of rectal cancers decreased with increasing age. In several reports preference for right sided lesions showed an increase with increasing age (Sr. No. 16, 18, 20-21). Slattery et. al. (1996, Sr. No. 19)reported an increase in proportion of proximal tumours with increasing age for women, exceeding 50% (62. 3%), only in the age group 70-79 years. Amongst men, proportion of proximal tumours exceeded 50%in the <50 yr groups (62. 5%, 30-39 yrs; 51. 1%, 40-49 yrs), falls below 50%in the 50-59 and 60-69 yrs groups and then rises again to 54% in the 70-79 yrs group. A decrease in proximal tumours with increasing age was reported by Karsten et. al. (2008, Sr. No. 22) and Fante et. al. (1997, Sr. No. 28). Both studies reported a dominance of distal tumours in different age groups (two in Sr. No. 22, three in Sr. No. 28), but proximal tumours decreased with increasing age. In a few papers (Sr. No 4, 6, 10, 13-15, 26) sub-site preference was found not to depend on age. Fazeli et.al. (2007, Sr. No. 13) reported that~ 80% of the tumours were distal in the young (<40 years) and also in the older age group. In these reports which did not find any effect of age on subsite preference, distal tumours were >50% in the young and in the older group. A preference for proximal tumours in a population of colon cancer patients were reported in several papers (Sr. No. 11 and Mahdavinia et. al. (2005) in general population of colon cancer patients from Iran, where incidence is lower than in the West and in Sr. No. 1 in young colon cancer patients < 40 years in India). Cozart et. al. (1993, Sr. No. 17) found tumour sub-site preference for left colon (24/12) in a small population of colon cancer patients; Dozois et. al. (2005, Sr. No 25) found the same preference in a much larger (1025 patients) young (<50yrs)population. We cite several prospective reports on change in relative preference of tumour sub-site over a long time period. Fazeli et. al. (2007, Sr. No. 13) reported that the nearly equal preference for distal tumours (~80%) in the <40 years and in the >40 years group in Iran, remained unchanged for two decades (1970-80, 1990-2000). In contrast, it was reported in a study on patients from New Zealand, in the period 1974-83 (Jass 1991), that the incidence of right colon cancers remained stable in younger patients (<50 years), that in older patients showed an increase and a marked reduction in left colon and rectal colon cancer in <50 years group was observed. An increase in proximal CRC relative to distal tumours was reported in another retrospective study in the period 1940-79 in the US (Beart et. al. 1983).

4. de novo CRC in Asia

The problem arising from inability to detect cancer early because of hospital infrastructure and relative lack of awareness of the disease may not be the only problem peculiar to the developing world in Asia and Africa. Sung et. al. (2005) pointed out that non-polypoidal (flat or depressed) lesions and colorectal neoplasm arising without preceding adenoma (de novo cancer) seemed to be more common in Asian than in other populations. Although most cases of colorectal cancer are thought to arise from a sequence of adenoma to carcinoma, evidence from Asia, in particular Japan suggests another mechanism. Clinicopathological studies have shown that there are two groups of colorectal cancer, polypoid and non-polypoid (superficial) tumours. The latter are flat lesions with a raised or depressed surface. Since these tumours are small (<1cm in diameter) and there are no adenomatous elements in their vicinity, they were proposed not to have originated from any precursor lesion and were termed de-novo carcinomas. These non-polypoid tumours are less likely to have K-ras mutations than are CRC arising from the adenoma-carcinoma sequence. Non-polypoid tumours of the colorectal regions tend to reach deeper layers of the intestinal wall in the early stage of the disease and with a higher degree of dysplasia. They are therefore more invasive than the polypoid adenomas (Sung et. al., 2005). Reports on de novo cancer have been published from Japan (Goto et. al 2004) and from Taiwan (Chen et. al 2003). About one-third of CRC patients in both countries have de-novo cancer. One study from UK also reported this feature (Rembacken et. al., 2000). Whether this feature is unique to Asia or whether it shows any preference for the younger or the older group of patients is not reported. Because of their flat appearance they are harder to identify by conventional colonoscopy. Chromoendoscopy and the use of magnifying colonoscopy may be necessary. The absence of polypoid growth preceding malignancy has posed difficulties in screening for early CRC by radiological imaging or even endoscopic techniques.

5. Early onset CRC and genetics

Colorectal tumours provide an excellent model system for understanding the molecular events that control the process of initiation and progression of human tumours. Rate of random mutational events alone cannot account for the number of genetic alterations found in most human cancers and it has been suggested that destabilization of the genome may be a prerequisite early in carcinogenesis. In CRC there are two separate destabilizing pathways. The more common involves chromosomal instability (CNI). The second mutational pathway in CRC displays increased rate of intragenic mutation characterized by generalized instability in microsatellites (MSI). Defects in mismatch repair genes (MMR) lead to high frequency MSI in CRC. National Cancer Institute definitions of MSI-L (L=low), MSI-H (H=high) and MSS (microsatellite stable) in CRC are given in Boland et. al. (1998). A recently recognized molecular alteration found frequently in MSI cancers is the CpG island methylator phenotype (CIMP). Colon cancer is usually observed in one of three specific patterns: sporadic, inherited or familial. Fewer than 10% of patients have an inherited predisposition to colon cancer. Sporadic cancer is common in persons older than 50 years of age, probably as a result of dietary and environmental factors as well as normal aging. Patients with inherited disease have CRC at a younger age, 10-20 years earlier than general population and are of interest in this essay. The area of hereditary CRC has been reviewed by Lynch and de la Chapelle (2003)and earlier by Lynch et. al (1991). Different aspects of molecular genetics of CRC have been discussed in this series (Ewart Toland, 2012) and elsewhere (Fearon and Volgenstein 1990; Loeb 1994; Jass 1995; Lynch 1996; Baba 1997; Gryfe et. al. 1997; Lengauer et. al. 1998; Lynch and Smyrk 1998; Lynch and de la Chapelle 1999; Yang 1999; Potter 1999; Jass et. al. 2002; Calvert and Frucht 2002; Zbuk 2009). In this section we discuss several recent papers which highlight the difference in genetic characteristics of younger CRC patients and those of the older group.

Morris et. al. (2007) showed that the incidence of tumours with microsattelite instability was significantly higher in patients aged ≤ 40 years, 18. 3% compared to 6. 6% in those aged 41 – 60 yrs (p<0. 0001). TP53 mutations were also more frequent (p=0. 002). However K-ras mutations were less common (p=0. 0001) when comparing the same age groups. They concluded that major age related differences in the clinical and molecular features of CRC exist.

Farrington et. al. (1998) pointed out that germ-line mutations in DNA mismatch-repair (MMR) genes impart a markedly elevated cancer risk, often presenting as autosomal dominant HNPCC. Not all gene carriers have a family history. Young probands with early onset CRC irrespective of family history were genetically tested and it was found that an appreciable proportion of young colon cancer probands carry a germline mutation in a DNA MMR gene.

Losi et. al. (2005) evaluated clinical features and molecular pathways, chromosomal instability (CNI) and MSI in early onset CRC. Of 71 patients (<45 years), 14 showed both MSI and altered expressions of MMR proteins. In the 57 MSI -negative (-) lesions, altered expression of APC, β-catenin and p53 genes were found more frequently than in MSI-positive (+) tumours. 7/14 MSI (+) tumours were associated with clinical features of HNPCC and in all but one, constitutional mutations in MLH-1 and MSH-2 genes could be detected. The same mutations were found in other family members. Involvement of chromosomal instability was demonstrated in a majority of early onset CRC.

Chan et. al. (1999)studied 59 Chinese patients <45 yrs and 58, >45 yrs in Hong Kong. The incidence of MSI-H varied statistically significantly with age, being observed in >60% of those <31 years at diagnosis and in <15% of those ≥46 years. More than 80% of Chinese CRC patients <31 years had germline mutations in MMR genes. In a novel case, mutation in hMSH-6 was present but MSI was absent.

Ho et. al. (2000) in a study on 124 young (<50yrs) Hong Kong Chinese CRC patients concluded that MSI occurs in a significant proportion of the subjects. Young age at CRC diagnosis, proximal tumour location, increasing number of first degree relatives with CRC and a personal history of metachronous cancer were independent predictors of MSI status in the patient group. In patients <30 years, MSI tumours were more likely to be located in distal large bowel. In a proportion of patients with MSI tumours, germline mutation in the two MMR genes hMSH2 and hMLH1 was identified. The authors opined that this observation suggests a differential activity of the MMR pathway in colorectal carcinogenesis in different age groups. They observed that the inconsistency between MSI-H and a family history in the early onset patients deserves further attention.

Liang et. al. (2003) studied 138 below-40 CRC patients and 339 patients who were 60+. They found a higher percentage of normal p53 expression (61. 1 vs. 46. 8%, p=0. 023) and high frequency microsatellite instability (MSI-H) (29. 4 vs. 6. 3% p<0. 001) in the young. The family history of the two groups was similar.

Durno et. al. (2005, 2006) found evidence of MSI in 73% cancers from individuals in 9-24 years of age, 50% of whom had features of HNPCC. Other reports found MSI in 46% of under- 21 patients with only 1/3 having a clear family history.

Sanchez et. al. (2009) performed a molecular classification of CRC based on microsattellite instability (MSI), CpG-island methylator phenotype (CIMP) and mutations in the K-ras and BRAF oncogenes. There were four classes, combinations of MSI-H and MSS with CIMP–H or CIMP (-). 69. 8% of tumours (391 subjects) were MSS-CIMP(-) and less likely to be poorly differentiated (p=0. 009). CIMP-H tumours were more common in older patients (p<0. 001). MSI-H/CIMP-H tumours had a high frequency of BRAF mutation and a low rate of K-ras mutation, the opposite was true for MSS-CIMP(-) tumours (p<0. 001). The four molecular phenotypes tended towards divergent survival. MSI-H cancers were associated with better disease free survival.

Alsop et. al. (2006) investigated association of young age in below-45 patients with somatic mutation of K-ras gene, a common event in CRC tumorigenesis. The role of these mutations was found to be comparatively minor in the younger group, in contrast to its significant role in CRC of older age of onset.

Soliman et. al. (2001) compared molecular pathology of CRC in Egyptian (44% <40 years) and Western patients. They found MSI-H carcinoma in 17% (2/12) of under-40 and 46% (12/26) of 40+ Egyptian patients; K-ras gene mutation in 0% (0/18) of under-40 group and in 17% (5/29) of 40+ group; p-53 overexpression in 57% (13/23) of under-40 group and 39% (13/33) of 40+ group. These data show that molecular pathology of CRC in young Egyptians differed from that in the old; in particular, K-ras mutation played a distinctly minor role in the younger group. Unique differences in molecular pathology of CRC between the Egyptian and Western patients were also discussed.

Breivik et. al. (1997) found that the presence of K-ras mutation was dependent on age and gender of the patient, with an especially low frequency amongst young males. Microsatellite instability was rare in tumours with K-ras and TP53 mutations.

Berg et. al. (2010) focused on the somatic tumour development in young patients with no known inherited syndromes. They studied mutations in oncogenes K-ras, BRAF, PIK3CA and the tumour suppressor gene PTEN and in TP53, in three age groups in 181 patients (45, < 50 yrs; 67, 51-70 yrs; 69, >70 yrs). Distinct genetic differences were found in tumours in the young and the elderly patients, who were comparable for known clinical and pathological variables. This result indicated that young patients had a different genetic risk profile for CRC development than older patients. Clinical implications of these differences were discussed by the authors. The total gene mutation index was lowest in tumours from the younger patients. In contrast the genome complexity assessed as copy number aberrations was highest in tumours from the youngest patients.

Casper et. al. (1994) showed in a study on 225 FAP patients that deletion of 5 base pairs at codon 1309 within exon 15 (the most common mutation) was identified in 20 families. Other mutations within exons 7-15 were found in 49 families. The 1309 mutation leads to development of colonic polyps at a younger age thus giving rise to an earlier malignant transformation. In patients with 5 base pair deletion at codon 1309, gastrointestinal symptoms and death from CRC occurred about 10 years earlier than in patients with other mutations.

Khan et. al. (2008) studied 35 patients with CRC diagnosed at <30 years age. They found no mutations in exons 4-10 of the p53 gene. The frequencies of polymorphism in p53 and in MDM2SNP309 did not differ from rates previously reported for normal control populations and no polymorphism in either gene could be associated with early onset CRC.

Ahmed et. al. (2005) reported a study on 363 CRC patients of whom 18 were of Bangladeshi origin. 22% of Bangladeshi patients presented with a locally advanced or a metastatic CRC, whereas the same figure for non-Bangladeshi patients was 11%. Sixty one percent of the Bangladeshi patients were below 40 years of age and did not report any family history. Microarray profiling between these two groups demonstrated 1203 differentially expressed genes (p<0. 05). The patient groups studied by Nath et. al. (2005) and by our group, (Gupta et. al. 2010) (Table 3) and by Pal (2006) belong predominantly to West Bengal in India, which is adjacent to Bangladesh. These studies reported dominance of younger patients in their study groups, advanced disease stage and aggressive tumour characteristics.

Liu et. al. (1995) studied the prevalence of DNA replication errors (RER) associated with genetic instability in relation to age among patients without HNPCC. RER was found in cancers of several different types, particularly in HNPCC. CRC in majority of <35 years group (58% of 31 patients) exhibited instability whereas CRC in > 35 years group uncommonly did (12% of 158). In 12 of <35 years group, instability was evaluated for alterations of MMR genes and in 5, it was found to harbor germline mutations. These data suggested that the mechanisms underlying tumour development in young CRC patients differ from those in most older patients.

Lin et. al. (2010) showed in a study cohort of 950 patients (2000-2005) that carcinogenic effects of Western lifestyle might be mediated via insulin-like growth factor-1 (IGF-1). IGF-1 is a peptide growth factor that promotes cell proliferation and inhibits apoptosis. Both in vitro and in vivo studies suggested that IGF-1 could promote CRC growth. Further, circulating levels of IGF-1 were associated with various cancers including CRC. It was shown that genetic variation controls variability of circulating IGF-1. The expression of IGF-1 was reported to vary in different ethnicities. In turn it was speculated that polymorphisms of the genes involved in the IGF axis might affect IGF-1 expression and possible cancer risk. The age at onset of CRC varied considerably. Extreme age at the CRC onset, very young or very old seemed to be associated with different carcinogenesis. It was shown that some genetic polymorphism affects age of onset of cancers. For example IGF-1 polymorphism plays a significant role in affecting disease onset in Lynch syndrome. These authors showed that older patients have a higher frequency of AA genotype of IGF-1 (-2995C/A), significantly higher (12. 7%) than that in younger patients (4. 2%). Mucinous differentiation, but not other clinicopathological factors was associated with the CA /AA genotype of IGF-1. The authors concluded that the genotype of the IGF-1 promoter was different in young CRC patients compared to older CRC patients and that IGF-1 SNP was associated with mucinous adenocarcinoma.

Yantis et. al. (2009) provided data to show that post translational regulation of mRNA and subsequent protein expression may be particularly important to the development of CRC in young patients. They compared 24 patients <40 yrs of age with 45 patients ≥ 40 yrs of age, who served as controls. Cases were evaluated for clinical risk factors of malignancy and pathologic feature predictive of outcome. More aggressive features in tumours of young patients, namely more frequent lymphovascular (81%) and venous (48%) invasion, an infiltrative growth pattern (81%) were reported. Significantly increased expression of miR-21, miR-20a, miR-145, miR-181b, and miR-203 was noted in the younger group.

6. Predisposing factors

Family history of CRC at a young age is a significant risk factor. Johns and Houlston (2001) performed a meta-analysis of 27 case-control and cohort studies of colorectal cancer risk and found that a family history of one affected first degree relative diagnosed before the age of 45 carried a 3. 87 fold (95% confidence interval 2. 40 – 6. 22) increased risk for the disease. Fuchs et. al. (1994) concluded that a family history of CRC is associated with an increased risk of disease, especially amongst the young. The relative risk factor of an under-45 yrs person with one or more affected first degree relative as compared with those without a family history was 3. St. John et. al. (1993) performed a case-control study of relatives of CRC patients and of matched control patients. They concluded that first degree relatives of patients with CRC have an increased risk of colorectal cancer. The risk was greater if diagnosed at an early age and when other first degree relatives were affected. Winawer et. al. (1996) observed that siblings and parents of patients with adenomatous polyps were at an increased risk for CRC particularly when adenoma was diagnosed at < 60 yrs age. Despite limited accuracy and compliance, family history is still the most easily obtainable risk factor for colorectal cancer.

Deficiency in host response to carcinogenesis is less easily recognized and treated. A personal history of other cancers, especially chronic immunosensitive cancers such as melanoma, if occurring at a young age, may indicate an increased susceptibility to CRC. Chronic immune suppression or clinical suggestions of impaired immunity may also mean the same.

FAP and HNPCC patients have a lifetime risk of 100 and 80 percent respectively, of developing CRC. In FAP, the affected persons develop hundreds to thousands of colonic polyps. Although the rate of transition to cancer is slow, the vast number of polyps virtually assures colon cancer development at a young age. Average age of developing cancer is 39 years, with 7% diagnosed by the age of 20 and 15% by 25. In HNPCC, the affected persons have a very high risk for CRC but do not develop the hundreds of polyps seen in FAP. These polyps are very likely to make a transition to cancer. Although sporadic colon cancer usually arises in colon polyps after a 5-10 years period of growth and transformation, in HNPCC this progression can occur within 1 -2 years. HNPCC occurs at a relatively young age, median 42-45 years, with 35%-40% diagnosed before 40 years of age. The proportion of HNPCC or familial colorectal cancer among all CRC varies by country from 1-10% with a median of 2-5% (Mecklin and Ponz de Leon 1994). HNPCC has been reported from many different populations, Europeans, white and Indian Americans, Asians, Australasians, South Americans and Egyptians (Sarroca et. al. 1978; Bamezai et. al. 1984; Ushio 1985; Lynch et. al. 1985; Mecklin 1987; Vasen et. al. 1990; Mecklin and Jarvinen 1991; Jass and Stewart 1992; Soliman et. al. 1998).

Ulcerative colitis (UC) is another important predisposing factor. The most important risk factors for development of CRC in UC patients are prolonged duration of disease, pancolonic disease, continuously active disease and severity of inflammation. Eaden et. al. (2001) performed a meta-analysis of the risk of CRC in UC. 116 of 194 reported studies were included in this analysis. Overall prevalence of CRC in UC patients was 3. 7%. The risk of CRC in UC patients was determined by decade of disease and a non significant increase in risk over time was observed.

7. Prognosis and survival of young patients

Opinion on the issue of survival of younger patients is not unanimous. We have divided literature reports on this issue, pre-2000 and post-2000, in two separate sections. The reports in which prognosis for the young is shown to be poorer and the ones in which they are not so, are separately grouped.

Pre-2000, poor prognosis: Moore et. al. (1984) concluded that poorer survival in younger (<40 years) patients was a result of an inherently more virulent lesion, a conclusion supported by a greater incidence of mucinous tumours, an indicator of poor prognosis and a higher incidence of advanced disease, especially in the second and third decades. They did not find delay in diagnosis as an important factor in determination of survival. Adkins et. al. (1987) ascribed poorer prognosis in the young (<35 years) to unfavourable histological features of the tumours and advanced disease at the time of presentation in these patients. Of 45 under-35 patients, 19 patients with poorly differentiated tumours survived for an average of 1 year, whereas 19 with well or moderately differentiated tumours survived for an average of 4. 5 years. Those few patients who presented early in the course of their disease responded well to radical resection. Okuno et. al. (1987) reported frequent occurrence of mucinous carcinoma, lymph node involvement and advanced stage according to Dukes' classification in the younger group (<39 years). The overall survival rate was poorer in the younger group (41% vs. 55. 9%), whereas the difference between the two groups in rates of curative resection was not statistically significant.

Pre-2000, favourable prognosis: Howard et. al. (1975) found that younger patients had a greater frequency of advanced signs, later stages of cancer and mucoid carcinoma, but when compared by clinical stage, they did as well or better than older patients. 5-year survival rates were 31% in <40 years group and 32% in>40 years group. Clinical staging was the most important prognostic factor irrespective of age. No inherent difference was found in the virulence of cancer in the young, survival rate being essentially the same. Adloff et. al. (1986) in a paper published much later reached identical conclusion. Walton et. al. (1976) in a study on 70 under-40 patients reported that survival time was shorter in patients with mucinous and anaplastic tumours and their incidences increased in this age group. Overall survival rates, however, did not significantly depend on age. Early diagnosis and prompt aggressive surgical treatment produced survival equivalent to that in patients of other age groups. Scarpa et. al. (1976) in a study on 47 adults in the age group 20-40 years found smaller tumours and depth of invasion as important prognostic factors but tumour grade had no correlation with survival. They concluded that there was no difference in survival rate between the young and the old. Bulow (1980) found, in an extensive study spread over 25 years (951 <40 patients, all <40 patients in Denmark in the period 1943-1967) that stage according to Dukes' classification and presence of intestinal obstruction and/or perforation and not age, determined prognosis. Ahlberg et. al. (1980) in a study group of 27 patients, aged <30 years, in 1969-70 in Scandinavia, concluded that prognosis was good, if predisposing factors were absent (9/15 survived 5 years), but not so otherwise. Ohman (1982) in a study group of 1061 patients, of whom 48 were below 40, in Sweden reported a five year survival rate in the overall population and in curable cases. Both rates were equal in the two age groups. Age factor had no impact. Five year survival was 100% in stage A, 50% in B, 33% in C. Proportion of Dukes' A lesion was equal in the two groups; there were fewer B and more C lesions amongst the young. Survival was not altered if ulcerative colitis was superimposed on carcinoma. Beckman et. al. (1984) studied 69 patients, 20-39 years and reported good prognosis. Neither age, sex, tumour size, location, mere presence of lymph node metastases, depth of tumour invasion nor predisposing disease of the colon was a strong prognostic factor. Metastases of six or more lymph nodes and distant spread of the tumour at the time of initial surgery were ominous findings; so was mucinous carcinoma, a relatively frequent occurrence. Jarvinen and Turunen (1984) in a study on 249 under-40 year patients between 1970 and 1979 found no difference in their 5 year survival rate from that of the general population. A premalignant condition was more common as age decreased. Family cancer syndrome, FAP and other predisposing diseases were observed in a significant proportion of study group. It was suggested that more emphasis should be placed on identification, family screening and treatment of conditions predisposing to colorectal cancer. LaQuaglia et. al. (1992) analysed their experience with 29 histologically verified cases of whom 20 were resected for cure. The predictors for survival were resectability, regional nodal involvement, depth of invasion, grade (Signet ring (45%) or anaplastic lesions (24%) were considered high grade) and interval from symptom onset to diagnosis. Median age at diagnosis was 19 years (10-21 years), median survival was 16 months, that for those undergoing complete resection was 33 months. In those undergoing resection for cure, tumour grade, regional nodal involvement and depth of invasion were the only factors that affected prognosis. Hidalgo (1995) in Spain studied 26, under-45 CRC patients (17. 2% of the whole group) whose potential risk factors were no different from those of the general population. Clinical presentation, tumour site and Dukes' stage were similar in the younger group and in the general population, but morbidity, mortality and post operative complications were lower. There were no differences in resection or survival rates. Chung et.al. (1998) in a study on 101 under 40 patients and 2064 older patients found no difference in tumour characteristics, Dukes' stage and overall 5 year survival, but reported a higher adjusted hazard ratio and adverse outcome in the <40 years group compared to 40-59 years group. They noted that a significant family history and predisposing conditions in the young warrants aggressive screening, surveillance and treatment. Heys et. al. (1994) in a review reported histological evaluations of the cancers in the younger age group patients and found that approximately four times as many tumours were of the mucinous type. This was associated with an increased risk of local recurrence. Dukes' staging and vascular invasion by tumour were prognostic indicators for overall patient survival. However survival rates for young patients with CRC were comparable to those of older patients, when equivalent Dukes' stage was considered.

Post-2000, favourable prognosis: O'Connell et. al. (2004b) used SEER (Surveillance, Epidemiology and End Results) database in the period 1991-1999 in the USA (1334 younger patients, 20-40 years; 46,457 older patients 60-80 years) to conclude that 5-year stage-specific survival was similar for stage I and III patients and better for younger patients in stage II and IV (p<0. 01). The same patient group showed later stage (more of stage III and IV) and higher grade tumours for younger patients. The authors noted that their population-based finding contradicts earlier single institution reports. Stigliano et. al. (2008) compared a cohort of 40 HNPCC cases with 573 sporadic CRC cases in the period 1970-1993. Median age of diagnosis was 46. 8 years in HNPCC cases and 61 years in sporadic CRC cases. Early stage cancer (Dukes' A & B) was 70% in HNPCC group and 61. 6% in sporadic group. The crude 5-year cumulative survival for primary CRC was 94. 2% in HNPCC vs. 75. 3% in sporadic cancer patients (p < 0. 0001). The influence of age on prognosis is apparent.

Berg et. al. (2010) studied 181 patients (45, < 50 yr; 67 (51-70 yr); 69, > 70 yr) and found no difference in survival while comparing age groups, even when adjustment for tumour stage at diagnosis had been made. Younger patients however presented at a more advanced disease stage (54, 46, and 36% in three groups). Tumour stage was the most powerful prognostic variable (p < 0. 001). Turkiewicz et.al. (2001) in a study spanning 29 years in Australia concluded that young patients with CRC had the potential to do just as well. The overall 5-years survival among younger patients in Stage A and B (53%) was found to be better than their counterparts in the older group. With influence of a family history of CRC being very apparent in this group, the authors conclude that emphasis must be on screening. Makela et. al. (2002) in a study of 102 under-50 patients in Finland over a 20 years period (1980-1999) concluded that young age is not a poor prognostic marker in colorectal cancer. Radical operation, venous invasion and tumour grade were good predictors of survival in patients below 50 years. Kam et.al. (2004) in a study in Singapore on 39 under-30 years patients inferred that age did not affect survival and recommended early endoscopy for all with persistent symptoms. They concluded that early diagnosis, radical resection and adjuvant therapy still form the cornerstone in management of colorectal cancer in this age group. Karsten et.al.

(2008) in the USA performed a comparative study of two groups, < 40 years and > 60 years of age, ethnically diverse, between 1998 and 2005. Fifty one percent of 41 young patients were Hispanic. Young patients were more likely to have a family history. Aggressive nature of tumour in the young was noted, but operative intervention and survival was similar in the two groups. Tohme et. al. (2008) in a study of 325 patients, 13. 2% of whom were below 45 concluded that age by itself was not a significant prognostic factor. The independent prognostic factors were delay in consultation, which was more frequent in younger patients (29. 7 vs. 18. 6 weeks, p=0. 01), positive family history in the young (44. 1% vs. 18. 2%), right sided tumour and peritoneal carcinomatosis. Leff et. al. (2010) in a British study of 49, <40 patients reported a 5-year and overall survival of 58% and 46% respectively. They concluded that prognosis in the young was not worse than that for CRC in the population as a whole. Mitry et. al. (2001) reported, in both overall and stage for stage comparisons that patients below the age of 45 years had a better survival rate than older patients, mortality rate was lower in the younger group (2. 1% vs. 8. 4%) although advanced stage presentation was more frequent and predisposing conditions were significantly higher in the below 45 group (11. 7 vs. 0. 4%, p<0. 001). Lin et. al. (2005) studied 45 histologically confirmed under-40 patients, 90% of whom reported with advanced (C+D) stage, between 1992-2002 in Taiwan. They reported that disease stage was an important prognostic factor, 5 year survival in B, C and D stage patients being 25, 16, and 0% respectively. Karnofsky performance status (KPS ≥ 70%), lymph node involvement and preoperative LDH levels were major determinants of survival. Surgical resection and adjuvant chemotherapy improved survival of advanced stage patients, but the improvement achieved does reach the level of a patient who reports early. Liang et. al. (2003) reported that although the younger patients with colorectal cancer had more mucin producing (14. 7 vs. 4. 7%, p<0. 001) tumours and a more advanced tumour stage at presentation (p<0. 001) than older patients, the operative mortality rate was lower (0. 7 vs. 5%) and cancer specific survival was similar (p<0. 05) in stage I, II, III disease or better in stage IV disease (22-28 vs. 12-17 months, p< 0. 001).

Post-2000, poor prognosis: Endreseth et. al. (2006) in a study on 2283 rectal cancer patients found overall 5-year survival to be 54% for patients younger than 40 years compared to 71-88% for the older patients (p=0. 029). Among those treated for cure, 56% of <40 group developed distant metastasis compared to 20-26% in the older group. Age younger than 40 years was a significant prognostic factor in this group and increased the risk of metastasis and death. A study from Nepal by Singh et. al. (2002[a]) reported a more aggressive disease in the younger group (<40 years) and a significantly lower 2 years survival rate (4% vs. 55%). Singh et. al. (2002[b])in a study on 18 under 40 patients in India found that the tumor was unresectable in 5 patients (28%). Fourteen patients (78%) had advanced cancer indicated by TNM stage III or IV disease. Among the 13 patients subjected to surgical treatment followed by adjuvant chemotherapy, only 3 had long term disease free survival beyond 2 years.

Prognosis and Genetics: There have been reports in the literature that suggest that the survival of MSI-H CRC patients is longer than that of patients with MSS CRC. This latter group constitutes the majority. In some studies however no survival advantage was detected and a National Cancer Institute workshop held in 1998 (Boland et. al. 1998) concluded that MSI had not been shown to be an independent predictor of prognosis (Gryfe et. al., 2000). We cite a number of mostly post-2000 papers that link prognosis to MSI tumour pathway.

Gryfe et. al. (2000), in a study on 607 under-50 patients found MSI in 17% of patients and concluded that MSI was associated with a significant survival advantage independent of all standard prognostic factors including tumour stage. Regardless of depth of tumour invasion, MSI-H CRC had a decreased likelihood of metastasis to regional lymph nodes. Elsaleh et. al. (2000) (mean age 66. 7±12. 9 years) in Australia report striking survival benefits for patients with MSI tumours (90 vs 35%, p=0. 0007) and also for patients with right sided lesions, who received adjuvant chemotherapy as compared to those who did not (48 vs 27% alive at end of study, p<0. 0001) and for women (53 vs 33%, p<0. 0001). Suh et. al. (2002) in a comparative study of MSI(+) and MSI(-) sporadic young (<40years) CRC patients showed that the former had better prognosis (p=0. 051). Their results suggested that sporadic MSI(+) CRC in the young had different histomorphologic features as compared to MSI(-) CRC and HNPCC cancers. Samowitz et. al. (2009)in a study of 990 rectal cancer patients in the US showed that even though MSI-H has been associated in many studies with improved prognosis of colon cancer, the effect of MSI-H and K-ras mutations posed significantly higher risk of death for rectal cancers. Liang et. al. (2003) reported that there was a higher percentage of normal p53 expression (61 vs. 48%) and high frequency microsatellite instability (MSI-H) (29. 4 vs. 6. 3%, p, 0. 001) in the young. Lukish et. al. (1998) in a study group of 36 patients in the <40 year age group determined their DNA replication error (RER) status (expressed as MSI) and compared the clinical and pathologic characteristics of RER(+) and RER(-) cases. They concluded that RER(+) tumours were common (47%) in young patients and patients with RER(+) tumours had a significantly improved prognosis:5 year survival probability 68% in RER(+), 32% in RER (-) tumours (p<0. 05). Knowledge of RER status therefore could affect initial therapy, postoperative chemotherapy and follow up.

The paradoxical good survival after surgery for patients with young age at diagnosis of CRC supports the idea that many cancers in the young are microsatellite unstable. A number of studies linked high frequency MSI to poor tumour differentiation or mucinous histology, a signature of many tumours in the young (Sanchez et. al. 2009; Kim et. al. 1994, Lin et. al 2010, Suh et. al., 2002). Ionov et. al. (1993) in their study of mutations involving poly (dA. dT) sequences (Section 5 for details) found that the presence of mutations was accompanied by an increase in the proportion of poorly differentiated lesions (6/9 vs 17/90, poor/well, moderate)and also in an increase in proportion of Stage A +B disease (2/14 vs 53/68; C+D/A+B). Crude survival was expected to be better than usual in young patients because of their youth and the improved tolerance to surgery and complications that youth confers (Liang and Church 2010).

Berg et. al. (2010) in a study of patients in different age groups (Section 5 for details), found that patients with TP53 mutated tumours had poorer survival rates than patients with wild type TP53 (938 vs. 1016 days, p =0. 04); however the difference was not significant when corrected for tumour stage. TP53 mutation were of higher prognostic significance in right sided tumours (883, 1051 days; mutated, wild type; p = 0. 005). Among patients in the younger age group, those with K-ras mutation had significantly shorter survival than patients with K-ras wild type samples (841, 1033 days, p=0. 02).

Barnetson et. al. (2006) studied a group of 870 below-55 years CRC patients for germline mutations in DNA MMR genes, proposed a model for prediction of the presence of mutations in these genes and validated the model in an independent group of 155 patients. Survival in carriers and non carriers was similar.

8. Molecular genetics and treatment protocol

Chemotherapeutic treatment protocol will progressively become more specific as the genetic basis of CRC gets better understood and the heterogeneity of the disease is better characterized. There are several literature reports that show these connections.

Fallik et. al. (2003) studied response to irinotecan in 72 patients, of whom 1 responded completely and 11 partially. Among the 7 tumours that displayed MSI-H phenotype, 4 responded to irinotecan whereas only 7 out of 65 MSI-L tumours did (p=0. 009). A better response to irinotecan was observed in the patients whose tumours have lost BAX expression (p<0. 001). 7 of 72 tumours had inactivating mutations in the coding repeat of the target genes. Amongst these seven, five responded to irinotecan, whereas only 6 of the other 65 tumours did (p<0. 001) indicating that MSI-driven inactivation of target genes modifies tumour sensitivity. It has been shown that tumours with mucinous histology, a common feature of many tumours in the young(section 7) and whose molecular genetic signatures have been referred to earlier (section 3), show poor response to fluorouracil-based first line chemotherapy (Negri et. al. 2005) and first-line oxaliplatin /irinotecan based combination chemotherapy (Catalano et. al. 2009).

9. Acknowledgement

We thank Mr. Anil Kumar Verma and Dr. Nilanjana Bose.

10. References

Adkins RB Jr., DeLozier JB, McKnight WG, et. al. Carcinoma of the colon in patients 35 years of age and younger. Am Surg 1987; 53: 141-5.

Adloff M, Arnaud JP, Schloegel M et. al. Colorectal cancer in patients under 40 years of age. Dis Colon Rectum 1986; 29:322-5.

Ahlberg J, Bergstrand O, Holmstrom B, et. al. Malignant tumours of the colon and rectum in patients aged 30 and younger. Acta Chir Scand suppl 1980; 500:29-31.

Ahmed S, Banerjea A., Hands RE et. al.; Microarray profiling of colorectal cancer in Bangladeshi patients. Colorectal Dis. 2005; 7:571-5.

Alsop K, Mead L, Smith LD, et. al.; Low somatic K-ras mutation frequency in colorectal cancer diagnosed under the age of 45 years. European Journal of Cancer 2006; 42: 1357-61.

Ashenafi, S. The frequency of large bowel cancer as seen in Addis Ababa University, Pathology Department. Ethiop. Med. J. 2000; 38:277-82.

Baba S. Recent advances in molecular genetics of colorectal cancer. World J. Surg. 1997; 21: 678-87.

Bae JM, Jung KW, Won YJ. Estimation of cancer deaths in Korea for the upcoming years; J. Korean Med. Sci. 2002, 17:611-5.

Bamezai R, Singh G, Khanna NN et. al. Genetics of site specific colon cancer: a family study. Clin. Genet., 1984; 26: 129–32.

Barnetson RA, Tenesa A, Farrington SM. Identification and survival of carriers of mutations in DNA mismatch repair genes in colon cancer. N. Engl. J. Med. 2006; 354: 2751-3.

Beckman EN, Gathright JB, Ray JE. A potentially brighter prognosis for colon carcinoma in the third and fourth decades. Cancer 1984; 54:1478-81.

Bedikian AY, Kantarjian H, Nelson RS, et al. Colorectal cancer in young adults. South Med J 1981;74:920–4.

Behbehani A, Sakwa M, Ehrlichman R, et. al. Colorectal carcinoma in patients under age 40. Ann. Surg. , 1985; 202: 610-4.

Berg M, Danielsen SA, Ahlquist T, et. al. ; DNA sequence profiles of the colorectal cancer critical gene set KRAS-BRAF-PIK3CA-PTEN-TP53 Related to Age at Disease Onset. PLoS ONE 2010; 5:e13978.

Beart RW Jr, Melton LJ, Maruta et. al. ; Trends in right and left sided colon cancer. Dis Colon Rectum 1983;26: 393-8.

Boland CR, Thibodeau SN , Hamilton SR et. al. A National Cancer Institute Workshop on Microsatellite Instability for cancer detection and familial predisposition: Development of International Criteria for the determination of Microsatellite Instability in colorectal cancer. Cancer Res 1998;58:5248-57.

Breivik J, Ragnhild AL, Gunn IM et. al. ; Different genetic pathways to proximal and distal colorectal cancer influenced by sex-related factors. Int. J. Cancer (Pred. Oncol.), 1997; 74: 664-9.

Bulow S. Colorectal cancer in patients less than 40 years of age in Denmark, 1943-1967. Dis Colon Rectum 1980; 23: 327-36.

Calvert PM, Frucht H. The Genetics of Colorectal Cancer. Annals of Internal Medicine 2002; 137: 603-12.

Caspari R, Friedi W, Mandil M et. al. ; Familial adenomatous polyposis: mutation at codon 1309 and early onset of colon cancer. Lancet 1994; 343: 629-32 (Erratum in Lancet 1994; 343: 863).

Catalano V, Loupakis F, Graziano F. , et. al. Mucinous histology predicts for poor response rate and overall survival of patients with colorectal cancer and treated with first-line oxaliplatin- and/or irinotecan-based chemotherapy. Br J Cancer 2009; 100: 881-7.

Chan TL, Yuen ST, Chung LP, et. al. Frequent Microsatellite Instability and mismatch repair gene mutations in Young Chinese patients with Colorectal cancer. J. Natl. Cancer Inst. 1999; 91:1221-6.

Chen CD, Yen MF, Wang WM et. al. A case-control study for the disease natural history of adenoma-carcinoma and de novo carcinoma and surveillance of colon and rectum after polypectomy: implication for efficacy of colonoscopy. Br J Cancer 2003; 88:1866-73.

Chew MH, Koh PK, Ng KH. et. al.; Improved survival in an Asian cohort of young colorectal cancer patients. Ins. J. Colorectal Dis. 2009; 24: 1075-83.

Chiang JM, Chan MC, Changchien CR, et. al. Favorable influence of age on tumour characteristics of sporadx colorectal adenocarcinoma. Dis. Col. Rectum 2003; 46: 904-10.

Chung YFA, Eu KW, Machin D et. al. Young age is not a poor prognostic marker in colorectal cancer. British J. Surg. 1998; 85:1255-9.

Cozart DT, Lang NP, Hauer-Jensen M. ; Colorectal cancer in patients under 30 years of age. Contributors to the Southwestern Surgical Congress Unusual Case Registry. Am J Surg 1993;166:764–7.

Cusack JC, Giacco GG, Cleary K, et al. ; Survival factors in 186 patients younger than 40 years old with colorectal adenocarcinoma. J Am Coll Surg 1996;183:105–12.

deSilva MV, Fernando MS, Fernando D. Comparison of some clinical and histological features of colorectal carcinoma occurring in patients below and above 40 years. Ceylon Med J 2000;45:166–8.

Dozois EJ, Boardman LA, Suwanthawna W. et. al. Young-Onset colorectal cancer in patients with no known genetic predisposition. Medicine 2008; 87: 259-63.

Durno C, Arnoson M, Bapat B, et. al. ; Family history and molecular features of children adolescents, and young adults with colorectal carcinoma. Gut. 2005; 54: 1146-50.

Durno CA, Gallinger S. Genetic predisposition to colorectal cancer: new pieces in the pediatric puzzle. J Pediatr Gastroenterol Nutr 2006; 43: 5-15.

Eaden JA, Abrams KR, Mayberry JT. The risk of colorectal cancer in ulcerative colitis: a metaanalysis. Gut 2001; 48: 526-35.

Elsaleh H, Joseph D, Grieu F. et. al. Association of tumour site and sex with survival benefit from adjuvant chemotherapy in colorectal cancer. The Lancet 2000; 355: 1745-50.

Endreseth BH, Romundstad P. Myrvold HE, et. al. ; Rectal Cancer in the young patient. Dis. Colon Rectum 2006; 49:993-1001.

Ewart Toland, A., Germline Genetics in Colorectal Cancer Susceptibility and Prognosis, Colorectal Cancer Biology - From Genes to Tumor, 2012.

Fairley TL, Cardinez CJ, Martin J et. al. Colorectal cancer in US Adults younger than 50 years of age, 1998-2001. Cancer 2006; 107: 1153-61.

Fallik D, Borrini F, Boige V, et. al.; Microsatellite instability is a predictive factor of the tumour response to irinotecan in patients with advanced colorectal cancer. Cancer Res. 2003; 63: 5738-44.

Fancher TT,Palesty JA,Rashidi L et. al.; Is Gender Related to the Stage of Colorectal Cancer at Initial Presentation in Young Patients? Journal of Surgical Reserch 2011;165,15-18

Fante R, Benatti P, diGregorio C. , et. al.; Colorectal carcinoma in different age groups: a population Fancher tbased investigation. Am. J. Gastroenterol 1997; 92: 1505-9.

Farrington SM, Lin-Goerke J, Ling J. et. al.; Systematic Analysis of hMSH2 and hMLH1 in young colon cancer patients and controls. Am. J. Hum. Genet. 1998; 63:749-59.

Fazeli MS, Adel MG, Lebaschi AH. Colorectal carcinoma: A retrospective, descriptive study of Age, Gender, sub site, stage and differentiation in Iran from 1995 to 2001 as observed in Tehran University. Dis. Colon Rectum, 2007; 50:990-5.

Fearon ER and Vogelstein B. A Genetic Model for Colorectal Tumorigenesis. Cell 1990; 61:759-67.

Fireman Z, Sandler E, Kopelman Y et. al. Ethnic differences in Colorectal Cancer among Arab and Jewish neighbours in Israel. Am. J. Gastroenterol, 2001;96:204-7.

Frizis A, Papadopoulos A, Akriditis G et. al. Are there any differences in colorectal cancer between young and older patients. Tech. Colorectal, 2004; 8 Supplement 1: s147-8.

Fry, R. D. , Mahmoud, N; Maron, D. J. et. al. (2008,18th Ed;vol 2) in Sabiston Textbook of Surgery, Townsend CM, Beauchamp RD, Evers BM et. al. ; Elsevier, p 1404-5.

Fuchs CS, Guovannucci EL, Coldetz GA, et. al. A prospective study of family history and the risk of colorectal cancer. New England J. Of Medicine 1994; 331: 1669-74.

Goh KL, Quek KF, Yeo GTS et. al. Colorectal cancer in Asians: a demographic and anatomic survey in Malaysian patients undergoing colonoscopy. Aliment Pharmacol Ther 2005; 22: 859–64.

Goto H, Oda Y, Tanaka T, et. al. ; Estimated incidence of colorectal de novo cancer in Japan. Gut 2004: 53 (suppl 36): A30.

Gryfe R, Swallow C, Bapat B et. al. Molecular biology of colorectal cancer. Curr Probl Cancer. 1997; 21: 23-300.

Gryfe R, Kim H, Hsieh ETK et. al. Tumour microsatellite instability and clinical outcome in young patients with colorectal cancer. New England J. of Medicine 2000; 342:69-77.

Gupta S, Bhattacharya D, Acharya AN et. al. Colorectal carcinoma in young adults: a retrospective study on Indian patients: 2000-2008. Colorectal Disease 2010; 12, e182-9.

Guraya SY, Eltinay OE. Higher prevalence in young population and rightward shift of colorectal carcinoma. Saudi Med J 2006; 27:1391-3.

Hamilton W. Letter to the Editor, Am. J. Surg. 2005; 189: 504.

Heys SD, O'Hanrahan TJ, Briltenden J, et. al. ; Colorectal cancer in young patients: a review of the literature. Eur. J. Surg. Oncol. 1994; 20: 225-31.

Hidalgo PM, Moreno SC, Moreno Gonzale E et. al. The incidence, prognostic factors and survival in young adults with colorectal adenocarcinoma. Rev. Esp Enfrm Dig. 1995; 87: 431-6.

Ho JWC,Yuen S,Chung L et. al. ,Distinct Clinical Features Associated With Microsattelite Instability In Clorectal Cancers Of Young Patients. Int. J. Cancer(Pred Oncol):2000;89:356-60

Hosseini SV, Izadpanah A, Yarmohammadi H. Epidemiological changes in colorectal cancer in Shiraz, Iran: 1980-2000. ANZ J Surg, 2004; 74: 547-9.

Howard E. W, Cavallo C, Hovey LM et. al. Colon Rectal cancer in the young adult; 1975; Am. Surg. 41:260-5.

Huang J, Seow A, Shi CY et. al. Colorectal Carcinoma among Ethnic Chinese in Singapore. Trends in Incidence Rate by Anatomic Sub site from 1968 to 1992. Cancer. 1999;85: 2519-25.

Ibrahim NK and Abdul Karim FW. Colorectal Adenocarcinoma in Young Lebanese adults. Cancer 1986; 58:816-20.

Isbister WH, Fraser J. Large-Bowel cancer in the young: a national survival study. Dis. Col. Rectum 1990; 33: 363-6.

Isbister WH. Colorectal cancer below age 40 in the Kingdom of Saudi Arabia. Aust NZJ. Surg. 1992; 62: 468-72.

Ionov Y,Peinado MA,Malkhosyan S. Ubiquitous somatic mutations in simple repeated sequences reveal a new mechanism for colonic carcinogenesis. Nature 1993; 363:558-61.

Jarvinen HJ, Turunen MJ. Colorectal carcinoma before 40 years of age: prognosis and predisposing conditions . Scand J Gastroenterol 1984; 19: 634–8.

Jass JR. Subsite distribution and incidence of colorectal cancer in New Zealand, 1974-1983. Dis Colon Rectum 1991; 34:56-9.

Jass, JR and Stewart, S. M. , Evolution of hereditary non-polyposis colorectal cancer. Gut, 1992; 33, 783–6.

Jass JR. Colorectal adenoma progression and genetic change: is there a link? Ann Med. 1995; 27: 301-6.

Johns LE & Houlston RS; A systematic review and metaanalysis of familial colorectal cancer risk. Am. J. Gastroenterol 2001, 96, 2992-3003.

Kam MH, Eu KW, Barben CP et. al. Colorectal Cancer in the young: a 12 year review of patients 30 years or less. Colorectal Disease 2004; 6: 191-4.

Karsten B, Kim J, King J et. al. Characteristics of colorectal cancer in young patients at an urban county hospital. Am Surg. 2008; 74: 973-6.

Kaw LL,Punzalan CK,Crisostomo AC et. al. Surgical Pathology of Colorectal Cancer in Filipinos:Implications for Clinical Practice. J. Am. Coll Surg 2002;195:188-95.

Khan SA, Idrees K, Forslund A, et. al. ; Genetic variants in germline TP53 and MDM2 SNP309 are not associated with early onset colorectal cancer. J Surg Oncol 2008; 97:621-5.

Kim H,Jen J,Vogelstein B et. al. Clinical and pathological characteristics of sporadic colorectal carcinomas with DNA replication errors in microsatellite sequences. Am. J Pathol. 1994;145:148-56.

LaQuaglia MP, Heller G, Filippa DA, et. al. ; Prognostic factors and outcome in patients 21 years and under with colorectal carcinoma. J. Pediatr. Surg. 1992; 27: 1085-90.

Lee PY, Fletcher WS, Sullivan ES, et al. Colorectal cancer in young patients: characteristics and outcome. Am Surg 1994; 60: 607–12.

Leff D. R. , Chen, A. , Roberts D. et. al. ; Colorectal cancer in the young patient. Am. Surg 2007; 73:42-7.

Lengauer C,Kinzler KW,Vogelstein B . Genetic instabilities in human cancers. Nature 1998;396:643-9.

Liang JT, Huang KC, Chen AL et. al. ; Clinicopathological and molecular biological features of colorectal cancer in patients less than 40 years of age. Br J Surg 2003; 19:205-14.

Liang J and Church J; How to Manage the patient with Early-Age-of-Onset (<50 years) Colorectal Cancer? Surg. Oncol Clin N Am 2010; 19:725-31.

Lichtman SM, Mandel F, Hoexter B et. al. Prospective Analysis of colorectal carcinoma. Dis. Colon. Rectum, 1994; 37:1286-90.

Lin JT, Wang WS, Yen CC, et. al. ; Outcome of colorectal carcinoma in patients under-40 years of age. J. Gastroenterol-Hepatol 2005; 20: 900-5.

Lin J-K, Shen M-Y, Lin T-C, et. al. Distribution of a single nucleotide polymorphism of insulin-like growth factor-1 in colorectal cancer patients and its association with mucinous adeno carcinoma. Int. J. Biol. Markers 2010; 25: 195-9.

Liu B,Farrington SM,Peterson GM et. al. Genetic instability occurs in the majority of young patients with colorectal cancer. Nature Medicine 1995,1:348-52.

Loeb LA. Microsatellite Instability:Marker of a mutated phenotype in cancer. Cancer Research 1994;54:5059-63.

Losi L, Di Gregorio C, Pedroni M, et. al. ; Molecular genetic alterations and clinical features in early-onset colorectal carcinomas and their role for the recognition of hereditary cancer syndromes. Am J. Gastroenterol,2005;100:2280-7.

Lukish JR,Muro K,De Nobile J et. al. Prognostic significance of DNA Replication Errors in Young patients with Colorectal cancer. Annals of Surgery,1998,227:51-6.

Lynch, H. T. , Drouhard, T. J. , Schuelke, G. S. et. al. Hereditary nonpolyposis colorectal cancer in Navajo Indian family. Cancer Genet. Cytogenet. , 1985;15: 209–13.

Lynch, H. T. , Smyrk, T. C. ,Watson, P. et. al. ; Hereditary colorectal cancer. Semin. Oncol. , 1991; 18:337–66.

Lynch, H. T. Desmoid tumours:Genotype-Phenotype differences in familial adenomatous polyposis-A nosological dilemma. Am. J. Hum. Genet. ,1996;59:1184-5.

Lynch, H. T. , Smyrk, T. C. Classification of familial adenomatous polyposis:A diagnostic nightmare. Am. J. Hum. Genet. , 1998; 62: 1288-9.

Lynch HT, and de la Chapelle A; Genetic susceptibility to non-polyposis colorectal cancer. J. Med. Genet; 1999; 36: 801-18.

Lynch HT and de la Chapelle; Hereditary Colorectal Cancer. N. Engl J Med 2003;348:919-932.

Mahadavinia M, Bishehsari F, Ansari R, et. al. ; Family history of colorectal cancer in Iran. BMC Cancer 2005; 5:112.

Makela J, Kiviniemi H, Laitinen S. Prognostic factors after surgery in patients younger than 50 years old with colorectal adenocarcinoma. Hepatogastroenterology. 2002; 49: 971-5.

Malekzadeh R, Bishehswin F, Mahdavinia M. et. al. Epidemiology and Molecular Genetics of Colorectal Cancer in Iran :A review. Arch. Iranian Mediane 2009; 12: 161-9.

Mecklin, J. P. , Frequency of hereditary colorectal carcinoma. Gastroenterology, 1987; 93, 1021-5.

Mecklin, J. P. and Jarvinen, H. J. , Tumor spectrum in cancer family syndrome (hereditary nonpolyposis colorectal cancer). Cancer, 1991; 68, 1109-12.

Mecklin, J. P. and Ponz de Leon, M. , Epidemiology of HNPCC. Anticancer Res. , 1994; 14, 1625-9.

Minardi AJ Jr, Sittig KM, Zibari GB, et al. Colorectal cancer in the young patient. Am Surg 1998;64:849-53.

Mitry E, Benhamiche AM, Jouve JL. Colorectal adenocarcinoma in patients under 45 years of age: comparison with older patients in a well-defined French population. Dis. Colon. Rectum 2001; 44: 380-87.

Mohandas KM, Desai DC. Epidemiology of digestive tract cancer in India. V. Large and small bowel. Indian J of Gastroenterol 1999; 18: 118-21.

Moore PA, Dilawari RA, Fidler WJ. Adenocarcinoma of the colon and rectum in patients less than 40 years of age. Am Surg 1984; 50: 10-4.

Morris M, Platell C, Iacopetta B. A population-based study of age-related variation in clinicopathological features, molecular markers and outcome from colorectal cancer. Anticancer Research 2007; 27:2833-8.

Murday V, and Slack J. , Inherited disorders associated with colorectal cancer. Cancer Surv. , 1989; 8, 139-57.

Nath J. , Wigley C. , Keighley MRB et. al. Rectal cancer in young adults: a series of 102 patients at a tertiary care centre in India. Colorectal Disease, 2009; 11:475-9.

National Cancer Registry Programme, Indian Council of Medical Research, NewDelhi. aConsolidated report of population based cancer registries(PBCR), 2001-4. December 2006, (supplement to Consolidated Report of Population Based Cancer Registries 1990-96:August 2001) www. icmr. nic. in bAtlas of Cancer in India (Chapter 7 of First All India Report 2001-02) National Cancer Registry Programme ICMR, www. canceratlasindia. org

Negri FV, Wotherspoon A, Cunnigham D, et. al. ; Mucinous histology predicts for reduced fluorouracil responsiveness and survival in advanced colorectal cancer. Annals of oncology 2005, 16: 1305-10.

Nelson RL, Dollear T, Freels S et. al. The relation of age, race, and gender to the subsite location of colorectal carcinoma. Cancer 1997;80:193-7.

Neufeld D, Shpitz B. Bugaev N. et. al. Young age onset of colorectal cancer in Israel. Tech. Coloproctal 2009; 13: 201-4.

O'Connell JB, Maggard MA, Liu JH et. al. Rates of Colon and Rectal Cancers are increasing in young adults. Am. Surg. 2003; 69: 866-72.

O'Connell, J. B. , Maggard, M. A. , Livingston, E. H. et. al. Colorectal cancer in the young. The Am J Surg. 2004a;187:343-8.

O'Connell J. B. , Maggard M. A. , Liu J. H. et. al. , Do young colon cancer patients have worse outcome? World J. Surg. 2004b; 28: 558-62.

Ohman U. Colorectal carcinoma in patients less than 40 years of age. Dis Colon Rectum 1982; 25:209-14.

Okuno M, Ikehara T, Nagayama M, et. al. Colorectal carcinoma in young adults. Am J Surg 1987; 154:264-8.

Pal, M. Proportionate increased in incidence of colorectal cancer at an age below 40 years: An observation. J. Can. Res. Ther. 2006; 2: 97-9.

Paraf F, Jothy S. Colorectal cancer before the age of 40: a case-control study. Dis. Col. Rectum 2000, 43: 1222-6.

Popat S, Hubner R, Houlston RS. Systematic review of microsatellite instability and colorectal cancer prognosis. J Clin Oncol 2005; 23: 609-18.

Potter JD. Colorectal Cancer:Molecules and population. J Natl Cancer Inst 1999;91:916-32.

Qing SH, Rao KY, Jiang HY et. al. Racial differences in the anatomical distribution of colorectal cancer: a study of differences between American and Chinese patients. World J Gastroenterol 2003; 9:721-5.

Rembacken BJ, Fujii T, Cairns A, et. al. Flat and depressed colonic neoplasms: a prospective study of 1000 colonoscopies in the UK. Lancet 2000; 355:1211-4.

Saltzstein SL, Behling CA, Savides TJ. The relation of age, race, and gender to the subsite location of colorectal carcinoma. Cancer 1998; 82:1408–10.

Samowitz WS, Curtin K, Wolff RK et. al. Microsatellite instability and survival in rectal cancer. Cancer Causes Control. 2009; 20: 1763-8.

Sanchez JA, Krumroy L, Plummer S. et. al. Genetic and epigentic classifications define clinical pheotypes and determine patient outcomes in colorectal cancer. Br J Surg 2009; 96:1196-204.

Sarroca, C. , Quadrelli, R. and Praderi, R. , Cancer colique familial. (Article in French) Nouv. Presse Med. , 1978;7: 1412.

Scarpa JF, Hartmann WH, Sawyers JL. Adenocarcinoma of the colon and rectum in young adults. South Med J 1976; 69: 24-7.

Shahrudin MD, Noori SM. Cancer of the colon and rectum in the first three decades of life. Hepatogastroenterology 1997;44:441–4.

Shemesh-Bar L, Kundel Y, Idelevich E. et. al. Colorectal cancer in young patients in Israel. World J. Surg. 2010; 34:2701-9.

Singh JP, Maini VK and Bhatnagar A. Large Bowel Malignancy; Epidemiology and gut Motility Studies in South Asia. Dis. Colon. Rectum 1984; 27: 10-15.

Singh Y, Vaidya P, Hemandas AK et. al. Colorectal carcinoma in Nepalese young adults: presentation and outcome. Gan To Kagaku Ryoho. 2002a; 29 Suppl 1:223-9.

Singh LJ, Moirangthem GS, Debnath K. Colorectal cancer in younger patients. Trop Gastroenterol 2002b; 23:144-5.

Slattery ML, Friedman GD, Potter JD et. al. Description of age, sex and site distributions of colon carcinoma in three geographic areas. Cancer, 1996; 78: 1666-70.

Soliman AS, Bondy ML, Levin B. et. al. Colorectal cancer in Egyptian patients under 40 years of age. Int. J. Cancer 1997; 71: 26-30.

Soliman AS, Bondy ML, El-Badawy SA et. al. Contrasting molecular pathology of colorectal carcinoma in Egyptian and Western patients ,British Journal of Cancer 2001; 85(7): 1037–1046.

St. John DJB, McDermott FT, Hopper JL et. al. Cancer Risk in Relatives of Patients with Common colorectal cancer. Annals of internal Medicine 1993; 118: 785-90.

Stigliano V, Assisi D, Cosimelli M, et. al. ; Survival of hereditary non-polyposis colorectal cancer patients compared with sporadic colorectal cancer patients. J. Exp. Clin. Cancer Res 2008; 27: 39.

Suh JH, Lim SD, Kim JC, et. al. ; Comparison of clinicopathologic characteristics and genetic alterations between microsatellite instability-positive and microsatellite instability-negative sporadic colorectal carcinomas in patients younger than 40 years old. Dis. Colon Rectum 2002; 45: 219-28.

Sung JJY, Lau JY, Goh KL et. al. Increasing incidence of colorectal cancer in Asia: implications for screening. Lancet Oncol. 2005;6: 871-6.

Tamura K, Ishiguro S, Munakata A et. al. Annual changes in colorectal carcinoma incidence in Japan. Analysis of survey data on incidence in Aomori Prefecture. Cancer 1996; 78: 1187-94.

Thibodeau SN, Bren G, Schaid D . Microsatellite Instability in Cancer of the Proximal Colon. SCIENCE 1993;260:816-9

Tohme C, Labaki M, Hajj G, et. al. ; Colorectal cancer in young patients: presentation, clinicopathological characteristics and outcome. J. Med. Liban, 2008; 56: 208-14 (Article in French).

Turkiewich D, Miller B, Schache D et. al. Young patients with colorectal cancer: how to they fare. ANZ J. Surg 2001; 71: 707-10.

Ushio, K., Genetic and familial factors in colorectal cancer. J. clin. Oncol. , 1985; 15(Suppl. 1), 281–98.

Varma JR, Sample L. Colorectal cancer in patients aged less than 40 years. J Am Board Fam Pract 1990; 3: 54–9.

Vasen, H. F., Offerhaus, G. J. , Den Hartog Jager, F. C. et. al. The tumor spectrum in hereditary non-polyposis colorectal cancer: a study of 24 kindreds in the Netherlands. Int. J. Cancer, 1990; 46, 31–4.

Walton WW, Hagihara PG, Griffen WO. Colorectal Adenocarcinoma in Patients Less than 40 Years Old; Dis Colon and Rectum, 1976; 19: 529-34.

Winawer SJ, Zauber AG, Gerdes H, et. al. ; Risk of colorectal cancer in the families of patients with adenomatous polyps. National Polyp Study Workgroup. The N. England J. of Med 1996; 334:82-7.

www. Cancer. org

Yang VW. The Molecular Genetics of Colorectal Cancer; Current Gastroenterology Reports1999;1:449-54

Yantiss RK, Goodarzi M, Zhou XK et. al. ; Clinical pathologic and molecular features of early onset colorectal carcinoma. Am J Surg Pathol 2009; 33: 572-82.

Yilmazlar T, Zorluoglu A, Ozguc H, et. al. ; Colorectal cancer in young adults, 1995; 81:230-3.

Yiu HY, Whittemore AS, Shibata A. Increasing colorectal cancer incidence rates in Japan. International Journal of Cancer, 2004; 109: 777-81.

Yuen ST, Chung LP and Leung SY. Colorectal carcinoma in Hong Kong, epidemiology and genetic mutation. Brit. J. Cancer; 1997; 76: 1610-6.

Zbuk K, Sidebotham EL, Bleyer A. et. al. , Colorectal cancer in young adults. Seminars in Oncology 2009; 36: 439-50.

4

Turning Intention Into Behaviour: The Effect of Providing Cues to Action on Participation Rates for Colorectal Cancer Screening

Ingrid Flight[1], Carlene Wilson[2] and Jane McGillivray[3]
[1]CSIRO Preventative Health Flagship,
[2]Cancer Council South Australia and Flinders University,
Flinders Centre for Innovation in Cancer,
[3]School of Psychology, Deakin University,
Australia

1. Introduction

Colorectal cancer (CRC) is the third most commonly diagnosed cancer in males and second in females; throughout the world over 1.2 million new CRC cases and 608,7000 deaths are estimated to have occurred in 2008 (Jemal et al., 2011). The only developed country to have demonstrated a significantly decreasing incidence in both males and females is the United States, and this is largely due to the early detection and removal of pre-cancerous lesions through CRC screening (Jemal et al., 2011). Thus, an understanding of the variables that encourage people to participate in CRC screening is important because early detection and treatment of precancerous lesions and adenomas results in a significantly higher survival rate than if treatment is delayed until physical symptoms of the condition are apparent. Population screening using a Faecal Occult Blood Test (FOBT) can facilitate the detection of CRC at its early stages. FOBT is the collective term for a guiaic FOBT (gFOBT) or a faecal immunochemical test (FIT). Both are home-based tests which, although differing in the technology utilised, involve a stool sample being sent to a laboratory to be analysed for occult blood, ideally followed by colonoscopy for those with a positive result. The cost effectiveness of FOBTs for the screening of CRC, measured as Quality Adjusted Life Years gained, is comparable to other screening procedures (Frazier et al., 2000) and more cost-effective than treatment after physical symptoms are evident (Fisher et al., 2006). Randomised clinical trials have shown that both biennial and annual screening using FOBT screening reduces CRC incidence (Mandel et al., 2000) and mortality (Hardcastle et al., 1996; Kronborg et al., 2004; Mandel et al., 1993), and a systematic review concluded that FOBT screening is likely to avoid 1 in 6 colorectal cancer deaths (Hewitson et al., 2007). Effectiveness, however, depends upon yield and is critically dependent upon participation rates, which for population-based screening programs have been low, often despite high levels of intention to participate. For example, in Australia the National Bowel Cancer Screening Program, which provides people turning 50, 55 and 60 years with a free FOBT, had a participation rate in 2008 of 41% of the eligible population (AIHW, 2010). In England, the second round (2003–2005) of the pilot bowel cancer screening program had a significantly lower uptake than in the first round (52% vs 58%) (Weller et al., 2006) and reported participation rates in 2008 in other countries with an established or pilot population FOBT screening program ranged mostly from a moderate 45–50% (Italy and Denmark, respectively) to a low 16–18% (Korean Republic and Japan, respectively) level (International Cancer Screening Network, 2008). Understanding motivators to intention to participate and motivators to test completion are critical issues that need to be addressed.

The central question in research within health psychology is identifying and understanding the range of influences that prompt an individual to take up healthy behaviours or reject patterns of behaviour which compromise their health. Many social cognitive health behaviour models include a measure of intention to behave in a specific way as a precursor to action (e.g., Theory of Planned Behaviour; (Ajzen, 1985). Stage models focus specifically on the importance of addressing intention as a core component of public health interventions. For example, the Transtheoretical, or Stages of Change, Model (Prochaska, 2008; Prochaska et al., 1988) suggests that people can be characterised in terms of their readiness to make a change. Stages include precontemplation (benefits of lifestyle change are not being considered), contemplation (starting to consider change but not yet begun to act on this intention), preparation (ready to change the behaviour and preparing to act), action (making the initial steps toward behaviour change), and maintenance of the behaviour over time; with both contemplation and preparation measuring aspects of intention.

One of the most difficult questions for researchers examining screening participation has been the question of how to move people along these stages to the performance of the actual behaviour and, ideally, maintenance of the behaviour. A range of social cognitive models of health behaviour have proven effective in describing individual motivation to perform a variety of health behaviours, including screening, by identifying a range of attitudinal predictors (Conner & Norman, 2005). Each of these deliberative models can successfully map variables that describe individual differences in the intention to perform a behaviour. However, the relationship between behavioural intention and actual behaviour is less than perfect; it has been shown that around 50% of people with positive intentions to engage in health behaviours successfully translate those intentions into action (Sheeran, 2002), and a medium-to-large change in intention leads to only a small-to-medium change in behaviour (Webb & Sheeran, 2006).

This 'gap', the difference between an individual's commitment to act and initiation of the necessary processes to actually carry out the behaviour, needs to be bridged—in other words, research that influences 'intention to try' (Bagozzi & Warshaw, 1990) needs to also identify cues that will enable people to link to the means for achieving the intended behaviour. Some health behaviour models incorporate a stimulus to action in their operationalisations in an attempt to capture this intervening, or additive, influence that prompts individuals to actually implement behaviour. For example, Becker and colleagues (1977) incorporated 'cues to action' as additional, independent predictors of health behaviour, over and above attitudinal variables. Although incorporated in the earliest descriptions of the Health Belief Model, a cue to action, or strategy to initiate "readiness", is a variable that has received limited attention in the empirical literature. Nevertheless, research does suggest that certain acts may serve to stimulate health behaviour including physician advice, advertising campaigns, and postcard reminders (Sheeran & Orbell, 2000).

Research originating outside the health area has examined the notion of volitional control and how it might be used to explain the problematic nature of the relationship between

Turning Intention Into Behaviour: The Effect of Providing Cues to Action on Participation Rates for Colorectal
Cancer Screening

69

behavioural intention and behaviour (Gollwitzer, 1993). This model suggests that individuals achieve volitional control of their intention to act by the development of implementation intentions; the plans made to achieve a specific behavioural target (e.g., a statement describing when, where and how a specific behaviour will be carried out). These plans serve to provide the cue to action identified by the Health Belief Model but go beyond this by providing the plan for goal achievement.

Recent empirical work suggests that the approach of providing cues to action in the form of a specific implementation intention improves prediction of behaviour over and above the intention to act alone. Thus, Milne, Orbell and Sheeran (2002) reported improved exercise participation; Sheeran and Orbell (2000) reported beneficial effects on the uptake of cervical cancer screening; Verplanken and Faes (1999) described improved dietary regimens; and Orbell et al. (1997) cited improved rates of breast self-examination.

A study examining uptake in the National Health Service Breast Screening Program (NHSBSP) in the UK (Rutter et al., 2006) has highlighted the importance of providing guidance on how to plan for a behaviour in order to ensure that people move from intention to actual behaviour (i.e., from the preparation to the action stage of the Transtheoretical Model, TTM). In this study, women invited to screen for breast cancer were asked to make specific plans for attending. The plans consisted of organising their travel, arranging to take time off work if necessary and changing the appointment if it was inconvenient. The results indicated that when women produced a *written* plan, actual rate of compliance with the screening appointment was 15% greater than in the control condition (no intervention) and 7% greater than women who failed to write down a plan although instructed to do so. Moreover, the influence from the production of cues to action in the form of a written plan was greatest for those who initially had a high intention to comply but a weak sense of control over making the necessary arrangements to put that intention into effect. This research suggests that uptake of FOBT might be significantly improved by providing a cue to action that seeks to stimulate people to do more than simply express their intention to screen. An effective informational intervention that results in the development of implementation intentions in the form of a plan describing the when, where, and how of faecal occult blood testing, and which enables the individual to deal with their own personal and environmental constraints, should provide those with the intention to act the further resources necessary for achieving their goal.

One possible mechanism for explaining the effectiveness in previous studies of asking participants to form implementation intentions is that doing so forces people to think through the steps necessary for actually completing the screening. This 'thinking through', in turn, may serve to raise people's confidence about their ability to successfully carry out the screening behaviour. Confidence in one's own capacity to act is known in the literature as 'self efficacy' and is widely reported as predicting health behaviour participation (Schwarzer & Fuchs, 1995). People's feelings of self efficacy are likely to be a particular consideration in using the FOBT because the test is performed by the individual and not administered, like mammography or Pap smear, by a health care professional. Previous studies looking at consumer-initiated screening behaviours have shown that feelings of confidence in one's ability to correctly perform the behaviour bear a strong relationship to people's performance of these behaviours. This includes performance of breast self-examination (Luszczynska, 2004), testicular self-examination (Lechner et al., 2002), and FOBT (DeVellis et al., 1990).

2. Aims

This study was designed to investigate the effect of the formulation of implementation intentions upon people's participation in screening using FOBT. We chose to examine uptake of FOBT rather than colonoscopy because, in comparison to the United States, usual CRC screening practice in Australia is by FOBT followed by colonoscopy for those with a positive result—in other words, colonoscopy is regarded as a diagnostic test rather than a screening test.

An additional aim was to monitor the impact upon participation of differing levels of directedness in formulating these intentions and to determine the impact of self efficacy and prior levels of generalised intention upon both implementation intention formation and participation.

Consistent with prior research, it was anticipated that the formulation of implementation intentions (regardless of level of directedness) would increase participation in FOBT over levels of participation in the control group. Furthermore, previous work in the area of preventive health behaviour suggests that people's feelings of self efficacy, or confidence to use the test (the terms 'self efficacy' [SE] and 'confidence' will hereinafter be used interchangeably) can be increased in response to appropriate cues to action, and it was anticipated that the provision of directions for the formulation of implementation intentions would increase people's feelings of self efficacy. It was further hypothesised that those who were already strongly intending to use an FOBT were expected to differ in implementation intention formation and participation from those whose intentions to test were initially weaker.

We conducted two randomised controlled trials to test these hypotheses. Study 1 was a trial conducted amongst a group of eligible, randomly selected males and females who were approached and agreed to participate in the trial. Study 2 was also a randomised controlled trial to examine the generalisability of results to population settings and which differed from Study 1 in that prior commitment to trial participation was not obtained and eligibility was unknown.

3. Study 1

3.1 Methods
3.1.1 Study design

The study was a parallel, randomised, controlled trial, stratified by sex, comparing return of FOBT between three intervention groups and one control group. People in the intervention groups received an FOBT of the immunochemical type (FIT) in the mail together with instructions on how to construct a (1) participant-determined and retained plan, (2) participant-determined and shared plan, or (3) researcher-directed and shared plan. The control group received the FOBT only.

3.1.2 Sample size and selection

Previous studies of implementation intentions have demonstrated that the effect of their formation upon behaviour is medium to large (Gollwitzer & Sheeran, 2006). To achieve statistical power of .80 to detect a medium-sized effect (allowing for the possibility of self efficacy and generalised intention as co-variants) and an alpha of 0.05, we aimed to recruit a minimum of 80 participants in each of the four groups described above. Accordingly,

Turning Intention Into Behaviour: The Effect of Providing Cues to Action on Participation Rates for Colorectal
Cancer Screening

71

allowing for non-contactability by telephone, a subsequent rejection rate of 30% and ineligibility, we needed to recruit at least 1600 participants to achieve a final sample size of 320 (160 men and 160 women).

A random sample of 6000 (3000 males, 3000 females) potential invitees aged between 50 and 76 years and residing in southern urban Adelaide, South Australia, was provided by the Australian Electoral Commission (AEC). The Australian Government was conducting a pilot National Bowel Cancer Screening Program (NBCSP) at the same time (2004) so individuals with postcodes within the Federal screening program were deleted from the sample provided.

Telephone contact numbers for the remaining sample were obtained by comparing the list against information contained in the electronic White Pages telephone directory. Those persons for whom telephone contact details were not indicated were excluded from the list, as were those whose address indicated that they resided in a hostel or nursing home; such individuals were unlikely to be in the position of deciding for themselves whether they should screen for CRC. The remaining sample was randomized separately by sex using a random number generator (Microsoft ® Office Excel 2003) and 400 (200 m; 200 f) names were assigned sequentially to one of 4 groups. In total 1642 names were allocated.

3.1.3 Study conduct

The trial proceeded through a number of phases, as described below and illustrated in Table 1. Phase 1: All potential participants were mailed an advance notification letter and accompanying information, to the effect that an attempt would be made to contact them by telephone to invite them to participate in a study on how best to encourage people to participate in screening for colorectal cancer. Potential participants were advised that they were ineligible to participate if they had ever participated in CRC screening or been diagnosed with CRC or polyps. This exclusion criterion was because in Australia such diagnoses normally follow a positive FOBT and subsequent colonoscopy, and we wanted to target those who had not displayed overt symptoms but were of average risk (that is, based solely on the fact that they were aged 50 years or more) of developing CRC. An opportunity was provided at this point for individuals to decline participation or to indicate that they were ineligible.

Phase 2: One week after the advance notification letter, attempts were made (to a maximum of 3 occasions) to telephone individuals and recruit them to the study. A Computer Assisted Telephone Interview (CATI) format was used by trained interviewers to collect interview responses (Microsoft ® Office Access 2003). For those who were contactable and agreed to participate, informed consent was formally requested and recorded before commencement of the CATI. The recruiting interviewers were blinded to an individual's group allocation until they reached that part of the CATI (after having determined eligibility) that, as part of obtaining informed consent, provided details of the particular intervention to which the participant had been assigned. To those that agreed to participate, the interviewer briefly described what an FOBT was and asked whether they had heard of it: *"Before we contacted you, had you ever heard of a screening test for colorectal cancer, where you are given a set of cards to take home and asked to smear a part of your stool on the cards on two separate occasions, and then return the cards to be tested for blood? This is called a Faecal Occult Blood Test, or FOBT. This is the type of screening test we will be sending you"*. Baseline measures were obtained: background demographics, level of commitment to using an FOBT, and confidence to use the kit.

Phase 1	Recruitment Phase 2	Interventions Phase 3	Measures Phase 4	Measures Phase 5
N=1642 Potentially eligible participants randomised to study arm then notification of intention to contact by telephone + information sheet mailed	N=994 contactable. N=364 agreed to participate in CATI interview: *Baseline measures:* Demographics Commitment to screen Self efficacy to use FOBT	N=364 *Control* FOBT screening package only (n=91) *Aide to retain* FOBT screening package + implementation plan to be formulated and retained by participant (n=81) *Aide to return* FOBT screening package + implementation plan to be formulated and returned to researcher (n=95) *Checklist to return* FOBT screening package + implementation plan devised by researcher completed and returned to researcher (n=97)	N=350 after exclusions (All groups) *Measures:* Return of kit within 6 weeks Return of kit after 6 weeks	N=328 after exclusions (All groups) *CATI interview measures:* Commitment to rescreen Self efficacy to use FOBT Reasons for not screening (if applicable) Reasons for screening (if applicable)

Table 1. Study 1 interventions by phase and arm, with attrition rates

Phase 3: The day following the recruitment interview, all participants were mailed a screening package which included an immunochemical FOBT. Accompanying the package, intervention groups also received an implementation plan to serve as a 'cue to action' to provide a strategy for goal achievement (completion and return of the FOBT). Two intervention groups received a participant-directed plan in the form of an 'Aide' that *invited* participants to think about, and write down, how they were going to deal with potential barriers to using the FOBT. Suggestions were made as to how these barriers could be addressed. Participants in one of these two groups were asked to retain their completed plan ('*Aide to retain*'); the other group were sent two copies of the plan and requested to return one copy of the completed plan to CSIRO (*'Aide to return'*). The third intervention group received a plan in the form of a researcher-directed 'Checklist' (*'Checklist to return'*) which *directed* participants to think about how they were going to deal with potential barriers. This group was also provided with two copies of the checklist and asked to return one completed checklist to CSIRO. Thus, those in the intervention groups were invited to formulate implementation plans at differing levels of directedness, and the researchers, through their requirement that two of the intervention groups return a completed plan, were able to verify that in fact a plan had been completed. The control group received a screening package without any accompanying plan.

Phase 4: Receipt of completed FOBTs was recorded by the Bowel Health Service (Repatriation General Hospital, Bedford Park, South Australia) and participation data relayed to the researchers. People who did not return their test after six weeks were sent a reminder letter. Participation in screening was defined as receipt of kit within 6 weeks (before reminder) or after 6 weeks.

Phase 5: Approximately 7 weeks following FOBT despatch, participants were contacted by telephone. Confidence to use the FOBT was again measured, as was (for those who had returned their FOBT) commitment to screen every two years in the future, following recommended screening guidelines. Additionally, participants' reasons for screening or not screening were elicited, depending on whether a completed FOBT had been returned at the time of interview (data not included in these analyses).

3.2 Materials
3.2.1 Development of implementation plans

Two versions of implementation plan were designed; one as an 'aide' and the other as a more prescriptive 'checklist'. Each version was introduced to the participant with the words *"Many people find that they intend to complete the FOBT but then forget or 'never get around to it'. It has been found that if you form a definite plan of exactly when and where you will carry out an intended behaviour you are more likely to actually do so and less likely to forget or find that you don't get around to doing it. It would be useful for you to plan when, where and how you will complete the FOBT. To help you do this, we would like you to use the attached sheets we have provided"* (adapted from Milne et al., 2002). Both plans were designed to support confidence and addressed practical aspects of completing the test (reading the instructions; deciding the most convenient time to use the FOBT; deciding the most convenient location to use the FOBT; preparing for the test; using the FOBT; remembering to use the FOBT; sending the FOBT for analysis). Both versions commenced with the instruction: *"Using this plan, decide when you will use the screening kit, where you will use the kit, and the procedure you will use to carry out the screening test and obtain your result from the Bowel Health Service"*. They thereafter differed in their level of directedness in covering the practical aspects. For example, for 'remembering to use the kit' the aides contained the following instruction: *"It is easy to forget to do things unless we have a way to remind us. Decide now how you can make it easier for you to remember – for example, by leaving the kit or this plan in a prominent location, or writing yourself a note. Write below how you will remind yourself to use the kit on two separate occasions"*. In contrast, for the same instruction the checklist stated *"Place a reminder in a prominent place so that you do not forget to use the kit"* with two check boxes (1st sample done; 2nd sample done) to indicate that this instruction had been carried out. The complete documents are available from the first author on request.

3.2.2 Development of self efficacy scale

Self efficacy was measured using 4 items derived from terms developed by Vernon et al. (1997) and our clinical experience of the challenges and impediments surrounding FOBT use. Participants were asked to rate their degree of confidence in surmounting the barriers described. The items were scored on a 5-point Likert scale ranging from *strongly disagree* (1) to *strongly agree* (5). The items were: "I feel confident that I would be able to carry out an FOBT"; "I feel confident that the test will not be overly distasteful or embarrassing"; I feel confident that I would be able to find time in the day to complete the test"; "I feel confident that I could complete the test correctly". The scale had good internal consistency, with a Cronbach alpha coefficient of .86.

3.2.3 Commitment to screen

Commitment to screen was measured in Phase 2 by asking *"Right now, how strongly committed are you to doing this test, where 1 is undecided and 5 is very committed?"*. The follow-up interview measured commitment to screen again (for those who had returned their FOBT): *"Now that you have done this screening test once, do you think you'll go on doing it every two years?"* (yes/no answer) and *"Right now, how strongly committed are you to doing this test again, where 1 is undecided and 5 is very committed?"*

3.2.4 Screening offer

The screening package, or kit, included (a) a bowel cancer screening information pamphlet; (b) an immunochemical FOBT ((iFOBT also known as a faecal immunochemical test for haemoglobin [FIT], InSure™, Enterix Australia) that does not require dietary or drug restrictions; (c) a combined Participant Details and Consent Form confirming personal details, nominating a preferred doctor for follow-up, and consent to obtain clinical follow-up reports if required; and (d) a reply-paid return envelope.

3.3 Data analysis

Random missing values on pre- and post self efficacy (SE) variables (17/2800, 0.61%) were imputed using the expectation maximisation method, so that as many observations as possible were available for computing self efficacy total scores. The scores were split at the median baseline SE score of 17; scores ≤16 were designated 'low' and scores ≥17 'high' SE. Participation rates were viewed as 'early' or 'late' at a cut-off point of 6 weeks following despatch of FOBT, at which time a reminder was sent to non-responders. Chi-square analysis was conducted to assess FOBT awareness, FOBT participation and return of implementation plans between groups; Fishers exact test was utilised where cells contained <5. Paired samples t-tests and one-way ANOVAs compared score means for self efficacy and commitment to screen. A median split was not performed for commitment to screen as the majority of people had high intention to screen. Binary logistic regression was used to examine the ability of self efficacy and commitment to screen to predict return of FOBT, and Generalised linear models (GLM) were used to assess interactions between variables. All tests were conducted using a two-sided alpha level of 0.05.

3.4 Results

Recruitment and participation attrition rates are shown at Table 1. From a sampling frame of potential participants (3,000 men and 3,000 women), n=1642 were notified that they would

be contacted and invited to participate. Of n=994 able to be contacted and eligible, n=364
individuals (36.6%) agreed to participate in the study. Subsequently n=14 were excluded
from analysis because they didn't receive an FOBT (n=3); had undergone screening since
joining the study (n=4); reported symptoms that precluded them from using the FOBT
(n=4), or were unable to participate due to barriers unrelated to the study (n=3). Baseline
and screening participation data were therefore available for n=350/994 participants (35%).

	Control N=90 (%)	Aide to retain n=79 (%)	Aide to return n=91 (%)	Checklist to return n=90 (%)	Test of difference
Male	48 (53)	41 (52)	44 (48)	34 (38)	$X^2 (3)=5.270$,
Female	42	38	47	56	p=.153
Age, mean	61.1	60.5	61.2	61.7	NS
Age group**					$X^2 (6)=2.236$, p=.897
Age 50–59	43 (48)	38 (48)	45 (49)	37 (41)	
Age 60–69	31 (34)	29 (37)	32 (35)	39 (43)	
Age 70–76	15 (17)	11 (14)	14 (15)	13 (14)	
Highest level of education					$X^2 (6)=5.894$ p=.435
Some high school	46 (51)	35 (45)	39 (43)	52 (58)	
Completed high school/trade	32 (36)	27 (35)	36 (40)	26 (29)	
University qualification	12 (13)	16 (20)	16 (18)	12 (13)	
Country of birth: Australia	67 (74)	57 (72)	71 (78)	61 (68)	$X^2 (3)=2.539$, p=.468
Never heard of FOBT prior to participation	64 (71)	65 (82)	59 (65)≠	65 (72)	$X^2 (3)=5.618$ p=.132

*percentages have been rounded so may not be equivalent to 100%
** n=3 missing values for age group
≠n=2 missing values

Table 2. Study 1 Participant demographic characteristics*

At follow-up (post intervention and mailing of FOBT), n=13 participants declined or were
unable to be interviewed and n=9 were unable to be contacted; follow-up data were
therefore available for n=328/994 (33%) participants.

At recruitment, the groups (n=350 participants) were balanced for gender, mean age, age
group, level of education and Australian birth, and awareness of FOBT. The majority of
participants had never heard of an FOBT before they were approached, i.e. they were in pre-
contemplation stage (Table 2).

3.4.1 FOBT participation

Completed FOBTs were returned by n=286/350 (81.7%) of eligible participants over a period
of 15 weeks (mean = 3.12 weeks). Contrary to the hypothesis that formation of
implementation plans would improve FOBT uptake, there was no significant difference

between the groups in FOBT participation or return within 6 weeks (i.e., before and after reminder) (Table 3).

	Control N=90 (%)	Aide to retain n=79 (%)	Aide to return n=91 (%)	Checklist to return n=90 (%)	Test of difference
FOBTs returned	76 (84)	66 (84)	70 (77)	74 (82)	X^2 (3)=1.980, p=.577
Return of kits within 6 weeks	67 (74)	61 (77)	62 (68)	66 (73)	X^2 (3)=.869, p=.833
Plans returned*			62	66	X^2 (1)=.367, p=.545

*These numbers do not correspond with participants who returned FOBTs within 6 weeks

Table 3. Study 1 return of kits and implementation plans by group

3.4.2 Return of implementation plans
Most participants who returned a completed FOBT and were also required to return a completed implementation plan did so. There was no significant difference in rate of return between aide and checklist (Table 3), suggesting that differing levels of directedness had no impact on whether the plans were completed. There were no cases of a plan being returned without an accompanying completed kit.

3.4.3 Self Efficacy (SE)
A mixed between-within subjects analysis of variance was conducted to assess the impact of the different interventions on follow-up SE scores. There was no significant interaction between intervention group and time [$F(3, 324) = .874$, p=.455]. There was a substantial main effect for time [$F(1,324) = 46.424$, p=<.005], $\eta2 = .125$] with groups showing an increase in self efficacy (Time 1, M = 17.45, SD = 1.95; Time 2, M = 18.3, SD = 1.91). The main effect comparing the groups was not significant [$F(3,324) = .156$, p=.93], suggesting that provision of assistance with planning did not influence SE (Table 4).

	Control mean (SD)	Aide to retain mean (SD)	Aide to return mean (SD)	Checklist to return mean (SD)
Time 1	17.21 (1.81)	17.67 (2.03)	17.50 (1.73)	17.45 (2.22)
Time 2	18.39 (2.04)	18.26 (1.98)	18.32 (1.93)	18.36 (1.73)

Table 4. Study 1 group mean self efficacy scores pre- and post intervention

Subsequent analyses compared self-efficacy between those who returned FOBTs and those who did not. Table 5 shows that when we compared SE over time for FOBT non-returners using a paired samples t-test there was a decrease in confidence that approached significance (p=.08). In other words, the confidence of non-participants to screen was impacted negatively by the provision of the FOBT. By contrast, confidence among those who returned an FOBT increased significantly, regardless of group assignment. This result suggests that, in general, confidence to complete the test in the future is likely to decrease for those people who don't complete initial screening, regardless of initial level of confidence.

		M	SD	df	t
SE score non-returners (full sample)	Time 1	16.77	1.893	47	1.758
	Time 2	16.15	2.278		
SE score returners (full sample)	Time 1	17.57	1.944	279	8.674***
	Time 2	18.71	1.561		
Low baseline SE score non-returners	Time 1	15.46	1.208	25	0.220
	Time 2	15.35	2.279		
Low baseline SE score returners	Time 1	15.69	.978	116	15.388***
	Time 2	18.32	1.711		
High baseline SE score non-returners	Time 1	18.32	1.287	21	2.752**
	Time 2	17.09	1.925		
High baseline SE score returners	Time 1	18.92	1.202	162	0.489
	Time 2	18.99	1.383		

** $p < .01$
***$p < .001$

Table 5. Study 1 mean self efficacy scores pre- and post-intervention, overall and by return/non return of FOBTs

In order to determine whether confidence at baseline influenced reaction to the various interventions, participants were characterised as having a low or high SE score at baseline (determined by a median-split between 16 and 17), and change in confidence over time compared (See Table 5). Low SE non-returners did not significantly change their SE scores post intervention, whereas low SE returners' scores significantly increased post intervention. Similarly, for those with a high SE score at baseline, non-returners' scores significantly decreased post intervention but did not significantly change if they returned an FOBT. This latter result is likely to reflect ceiling effects given that the maximum score possible for SE was 20. These results suggest that self efficacy was increased when the test was completed but the initial level of confidence to complete the test was low, and conversely confidence was decreased when the initial level was high but the test was not completed.

3.4.4 Commitment to screen and maintain screening
At baseline, the majority of people (n=217/343, 63%) were committed or very committed to doing the test (M=4.39, SD=.924; median=5) and there were no group differences (Table 6). Those who returned an FOBT were asked their level of commitment to maintain screening, and just over half (n=137/239, 57.3%) were "very committed" to screening again (M=4.38, SD=.840, median=5, n=47 missing values), regardless of intervention assignment. For those that did return an FOBT, a paired-sample t-test indicated that for the sample as a whole there was a statistically significant decrease in commitment to screen from baseline, ie after exposure to the intervention and FOBT (Table 7). When we examined the relationship between commitment and self efficacy by comparing commitment level between those who had a low or high SE baseline score, it was apparent that the decrease in commitment came from those that had a high initial SE score (Table 7).

	Control mean (SD)	Aide to retain mean (SD)	Aide to return mean (SD)	Checklist to return mean (SD)	ANOVA	
					F, (df)	p
Time 1* (n=343)	4.48 (.844)	4.57 (.854)	4.33 (.974)	4.23 (.984)	2.21 (3, 339)	.087
Time 2** (n=239)	4.41 (.938)	4.33 (.816)	4.53 (.704)	4.24 (.878)	1.25 (3,235)	.294

*Includes non-returners and returners; 7/350 missing values
**Includes only those who returned an FOBT; 47/286 missing values

Table 6. Study 1 mean commitment to screen by group pre- and post intervention

		M	SD	df	t
Commitment to screen (full sample, n=233)	Time 1	4.52	0.804	232	2.15*
	Time 2	4.38	0.843		
Low baseline SE score commitment to screen (n=99)	Time 1	4.20	0.947	98	-1.522
	Time 2	4.36	0.814		
High baseline SE score commitment to screen (n=134)	Time 1	4.76	0.578	133	4.485***
	Time 2	4.39	0.866		

*<.05
***<.001

Table 7. Study 1 FOBT returners' commitment to screen pre- and post-intervention, overall and by SE level at baseline

3.4.5 Effect of self efficacy and commitment to screen on use of FOBT

Logistic regression was used to assess the independent and joint effects of baseline SE and baseline commitment to screen on return of FOBT. SE alone made a statistically significant contribution, X^2 (1, n=350)=11.535, p<.001, OR=1.27, CI 1.10-1.47), predicting 5.3% of the variance (Nagelkerke R squared) in screening uptake. Commitment to screen alone also made a statistically significant contribution X^2 (1, n=343)=13.837, p<001, OR=1.67, CI 1.28-2.18), and explained 6.4% of the variance. When these predictors were entered together into the logistic regression model, there was a statistically significant effect, X^2(2, n=343)=17.487, p<.001), but only commitment to screen displayed a unique and statistically significant contribution (p=.012, OR=1.46, CI 1.07-1.97); baseline self efficacy was marginally significant (p=.06, OR=1.17, CI.993-1.37). This suggests that those who are committed to using the FOBT will do so regardless of their level of confidence. The total variance explained by the combined model was R^2=8.0%, indicating that factors other than these also contribute to the likelihood of completing an FOBT.

4. Study 2

Study 2 was conducted to examine the generalisability of Study 1's results to the broader population. This approach more closely approximated that undertaken in current population screening programs utilising FOBTs.

4.1 Methods
4.1.1 Sample size and selection
Sample selection proceeded as described for Study 1. A separate sample of 6000 men and women aged between 50 and 76 years, randomly selected from four South Australian electoral divisions, was obtained from the AEC. People residing in postcodes included in the pilot NBCSP were omitted from the sample, as were those whose address indicated they resided in a hostel or nursing home. The remaining sample was randomised separately by sex and 400 men and women were assigned sequentially to one of 4 groups. In total 1600 names were allocated.

4.1.2 Study conduct
Phase 1: All potential participants were mailed an advance notification letter (which aligns with the protocol adopted by the NBCSP) and accompanying information as for Study 1, and were informed that they would shortly be receiving a screening package in the mail. Exclusion due to ineligibility was dependent upon self-identification and communication of this fact to the researchers before despatch of FOBT. Willingness to participate was not deliberately ascertained.

Phase 2: Three weeks after the advance notification letter, a screening kit including an immunochemical FOBT was sent to individuals. As for Study 1, intervention groups also received a discrete implementation plan. The nature of this approach precluded us from ascertaining willingness to participate and from obtaining pre- and post measures of self efficacy and commitment to screening.

Phase 3: Receipt of completed FOBTs was recorded by the Bowel Health Service and participation data relayed to the researchers.

4.1.3 Data analysis
Participation rates were viewed as 'early' or 'late' at a cut-off point of 6 weeks following despatch of FOBT, when a reminder was sent to non-responders. Chi-square analysis was conducted to assess FOBT participation between groups.

4.2 Results
N=1600 men and women were sent an advance warning letter. Those who did not identify themselves as ineligible or not wishing to participate were then mailed a screening kit and accompanying material according to intervention group. In total, n=225 were excluded from the study (n=118 identified themselves as ineligible; n=83 didn't wish to participate; n=24 packages were undeliverable). Analyses were therefore conducted for n=1375 men and women. Recruitment and participation attrition rates are shown at Table 8.

At baseline, the groups were balanced for gender (Table 9). It wasn't possible to ascertain age group breakdowns because the AEC supplied a random sample within an age range (50–74 years) which wasn't broken down into groups (for Study 1 we ascertained age from the participant). The study design also precluded us obtaining other demographic information (mean age, education, country of birth) as we did for Study 1. However, given that the underlying sampling mechanism was identical (i.e., supplied by the AEC), there is some confidence that the groups were balanced on these other factors.

Recruitment Phase 1	Interventions Phase 2	Measures Phase 3
N=1600 Potentially eligible participants randomised to study arm then mailed information sheet and notification that they would shortly receive an FOBT kit. Ineligibility was defined and dependent upon self-report	*Control* FOBT screening package only (n=400) *Aide to retain* FOBT screening package + implementation plan to be formulated and retained by participant (n=400) *Aide to return* FOBT screening package + implementation plan to be formulated and returned to researcher (n=400) *Checklist to return* FOBT screening package + implementation plan devised by researcher to be completed and returned to researcher (n=400)	(All groups, n=1375) Return of kit within and after 6 weeks

Table 8. Study 2 interventions by phase and arm, with attrition rates

	(Control) n=345 (%)	Aide to retain n=350 (%)	Aide to return n=334 (%)	Checklist to return n=346 (%)	Test of difference
Male	176 (51.0)	176 (50.3)	170 (50.9)	178 (51.4)	$X^2 (3)=0.96$,
Female	169	174	164	168	p=.992

Table 9. Study 2 participant demographic characteristics

4.2.1 FOBT participation

Completed FOBTs were returned by 548/1375 (39.9%) of participants over a period of 26 weeks (mean = 5.51 weeks). This rate is similar to that achieved in the NBCSP in 2008 (i.e., 41% (AIHW, 2010). As for Study 1, contrary to our hypothesis that the formation of implementation plans would improve FOBT uptake, there was no significant difference between the groups in FOBT participation or return within 6 weeks (before and after reminder) (Table 10).

	Control n=345 (%)	Aide to retain n=350 (%)	Aide to return n=334 (%)	Checklist to return n=346 (%)	Test of difference
FOBTs returned	144 (41.7)	131 (37.4)	131 (39.2)	142 (41.0)	$X^2(3)=1.633$, p=.652
Return of kits within 6 weeks	106 (30.7)	98 (28.0)	97 (29.0)	94 (27.2)	$X^2 (3)=3.269$, p=.352
Return of plans with FOBT			83/131 (58.4)	62/142 (43.6)	$X^2 (1)=9.389$, p=.001

Table 10. Study 2 overall return of kits and within 6 weeks (i.e. before reminder) by group

Turning Intention Into Behaviour: The Effect of Providing Cues to Action on Participation Rates for Colorectal
Cancer Screening

81

4.2.2 Return of implementation plans

A considerable proportion of those who returned an FOBT and were also required to return a completed implementation plan did not do so, and significantly fewer people returned the prescriptive plan (i.e., checklist) than the aide (Table 10), suggesting that level of directedness may have an effect on whether the plans were completed—those who were required to formulate their own plan based on suggestions for action were more likely to return a plan compared to those given a prescriptive checklist. Notwithstanding this result, given that the requirement for return was to act as an indicator of whether plans had actually been formulated, it appears that around half the participants used the FOBT without adhering to planning instructions, particularly those who received a prescriptive plan.

5. Discussion

We hypothesised that the formation of implementation plans would assist return of FOBT kits by providing a physical cue to action. In addition we hypothesised that the process of completing a plan would increase confidence in ability to complete the test and that those who were strongly committed to screening at baseline would differ in formation of implementation plans and participation to those with a less strong initial commitment.

Notwithstanding the difference in overall participation figures between Study 1 (81.7%) and Study 2 (39.9%), we found that for both studies provision of assistance with planning, regardless of directedness, had no influence on completion of an FOBT. The lack of influence of an implementation plan concurs with the conclusions of other researchers who have also found no effect of implementation planning on subsequent behaviour (Jackson et al., 2005; Michie et al., 2004; Rutter et al., 2006; Skar et al., 2011). Even so, this result goes against the large body of evidence suggesting that formulating action plans has a positive effect on the intention-behaviour gap. It has been suggested, however, that there exists sparse evidence for a positive effect of implementation intentions on behaviours outside student samples, who are more likely to comply with task demands (actually formulating the plan) (Jackson et al., 2005; Schweiger Gallo & Gollwitzer, 2007). It has also been argued that implementation plans are only effective where there is motivation to achieve a goal (Sniehotta, 2009) and that where goal intentions are positive, so will be the effects of implementation intentions (Gollwitzer, 1993; Oettingen et al., 2000). The majority of FOBT returners in Study 1 already had a high intention to screen, which may be attributable to the fact that that they had made a conscious decision to participate and were presumably more motivated to act, but in any case there was no evidence of a differential effect of combining high commitment with formation of implementation plans on FOBT return. Indeed, the high proportion of implementation plans returned by Study 1 participants (82%) may be indicative only of compliance with the study requirements (i.e., to return plans) rather than evidence of the use of these plans.

However, and in contrast to Study 1, it is evident that nearly half the FOBTs returned in Study 2 were completed without making a plan, a result which could reasonably be extrapolated to the group that was asked to retain their formulated plan. It has been suggested that non-completion may reflect ambiguity of study instructions (Michie et al., 2004) but, given that nearly all Study 1 participants returned identically-constructed implementation plans with a completed FOBT, this was not the case in our population. Rather, this outcome suggests that some felt they had no need to complete plans, perhaps because their intentions were sufficiently strong to make the use of plans unnecessary.

Indeed, we found from Study 1 that commitment had the most significant influence on FOBT use—because the majority of participants were strongly committed, we were unable to determine if having a weak level of commitment would influence formulation of an implementation plan or use of the FOBT. Of those Study 2 participants that did formulate and return plans, significantly fewer used the prescriptive 'checklist' format. Participants may have been "turned off" by the directedness of the checklist, particularly since they were a population sample and had not made a mindful decision to participate in a study. Study 1 demonstrated that provision of directions did not increase people's self efficacy. These results accord with a meta-analysis of 66 randomised controlled studies that concluded that forming implementation intentions had negligible effects on self efficacy and goal intentions (Webb & Sheeran, 2008).

For the group as a whole, baseline self efficacy did not have a strong influence on whether people used the test; rather, the act itself of completing the FOBT determined confidence—self efficacy was increased when the initial level of confidence to complete the FOBT was low, and conversely confidence was decreased when the initial level was high but the test was not completed. Rather than confidence to use the FOBT, from Study 1 it appears that being initially committed to screening had a more significant influence on whether people actually did use the FOBT, confirming the general consensus that intention to perform a behaviour is a necessary precursor of action. Even so, we found in Study 1 that commitment to screening, while a significant predictor of FOBT use, in conjunction with self efficacy explained only 8.0% of the variance, indicating that other factors exist which contribute to the likelihood of completing an FOBT. For example, Gregory et al. (2011) found that social-cognitive predictors of intention to screen for CRC and actual screening behaviour, although overlapping, were not the same, and Power and colleagues (2008) in their study of CRC screening found that life difficulty variables were better predictors of action than intention.

It is puzzling to note that there was a significant decrease in commitment to repeat screening by those that did use the FOBT and had a high initial level of confidence, in contrast to those with low confidence whose level of commitment to screening did not change. It may be that initial commitment was high for most because the participants were an 'interested' sample, and that those with high SE who screened reinforced their view that they were capable of completing an FOBT without necessarily moving from that conclusion and forming a commitment to rescreen. Conversely, those with low confidence but who did complete their test, thereby increasing their confidence, could have felt 'motivated' to repeat the experience again and so not changed their level of commitment. Interestingly, the same lessening of intention by those with high self efficacy was noted in a study examining the role of self efficacy in testicular self-examination (Umeh & Chadwick, 2010). The researchers found that those with high self efficacy appeared to have worsened attitudes toward self examination when both vulnerability and severity estimates were low. The same situation could well apply to CRC screening, particularly as perceived susceptibility is a Preventive Health Model (PHM) construct demonstrated to be associated with CRC screening ((Flight et al., 2010; Tiro et al., 2005). Commitment to future CRC screening in one or 2 years would perhaps, as Umeh and Chadwick (2010) have suggested, be temporarily rejected if the penalties of inaction are deemed insignificant, a viewpoint which may stem from a defensive reaction activated by anxiety. This view suggests that an emphasis on the development of messages designed to increase perceptions of personal risk of CRC without raising anxiety are warranted.

The low rate of participation in Study 2 may reflect a dissonance of messages appropriate to an individual's stage of readiness to screen (Prochaska, 2008). The differences in study design, particularly recruitment strategy, between studies 1 and 2 may have resulted in basic sample differences in stage of readiness to screen at baseline. Specifically, including only participants prepared to complete questionnaires in Study 1 resulted in a highly committed sample, likely to be in contemplation or preparation to act stage, characterised by a high participation rate. By contrast, Study 2 invitees were a population sample, most of who were probably in pre-contemplation on receipt of the FOBT, with participation rates comparable with those achieved by the national screening program (i.e. ~ 40%). Pre-contemplation is a stage where it could be argued that a person's knowledge, attitudes and intentions are in a more unstable state. People in this stage have been shown to have higher barriers, higher chance health locus of control, low powerful others health locus of control, lower perceived susceptibility and lower CRC knowledge (Gregory et al., 2011). It follows that these factors should be addressed to facilitate movement through contemplation to the action stage. However, our implementation plans as formulated were aimed at those with an intention to act and focused on the where, when and how of successful completion of the FOBT. It could be daunting for those who had never heard of FOBT screening to receive a test and accompanying material designed to assist with completing the test without first being given information aimed at overcoming barriers and lack of knowledge associated with the pre-contemplation stage.

6. Conclusion

The provision of assistance with the preparation of implementation plans, regardless of their level of directedness, had no influence on FOBT participation in the 2 studies conducted. One reason for their lack of effect may be that the majority of participants were likely to be in pre-contemplation stage in Study 2 and in the action stage in Study 1. Thus ceiling effects limited the potential for cues to impact behaviour among participants in Study 1, and Study 2 participants may have benefited from an intervention that tackled Contemplation as an intermediary to Action. This stage mismatch has implications for population-based screening programs and may contribute toward less than optimal screening uptake rates. Future research could usefully address the potential for the communication within a population setting of material targeted to specific decision stages, designed to progressively move an individual toward action and maintenance of action. Our research indicated that confidence to screen and commitment to screen separately and together exerted a greater influence on actual FOBT participation; however, these factors accounted for a small amount of variance and future research should address the contribution of other factors.

7. Acknowledgements

We would like to thank Ian Zajac, CSIRO, for timely statistical advice.

8. References

AIHW. (2010). *National Bowel Cancer Screening Program: Annual monitoring report 2009; Data supplement 2010.* Canberra: Australian Institute of Health and Welfare & Australian Department of Health and Ageing

Ajzen, I. (1985). From intentions to actions: A theory of planned behavior. In: *Action-Control: From cognition to behavior*, J. Kuhl & J. Beckman (Eds.), (pp. 11-39), ISBN 978-038-7134-451, Heidelberg, Germany: Springer

Bagozzi, R. & Warshaw, P. (1990). Trying to consume. *Journal of Consumer Research*, Vol. 17, pp. 127-140, ISSN 0093-5301

Becker, M.; Haefner, D. & Maiman, L. (1977). The health belief model in the prediction of dietary compliance: A field experiment. *Journal of Health and Social Behaviour*, Vol. 18, pp. 348-366, ISSN 0022-1465

Conner, M. & Norman, P. (Eds.). (2005). *Predicting Health Behaviour: Research and Practice with Social Cognition Models* (2nd ed.). ISBN 13 978 0335 21176 0, Maidenhead, UK: Open University Press

DeVellis, B., Blalock, S.J. & Sandler, R. (1990). Predicting participation in cancer screening: The role of perceived behavioural control. *Journal of Applied Social Psychology*, Vol. 20, pp. 639-660, ISSN 0021-9010

Fisher, J.; Fikry, C. & Troxel, A. (2006). Cutting Cost and Increasing Access to Colorectal Cancer Screening: Another Approach to Following the Guidelines. *Cancer Epidemiology Biomarkers & Prevention*, Vol. 15, No. 1, pp. 108-113, ISSN 1055-9965

Flight, I.; Wilson, C.; McGillivray, J. & Myers, R. (2010). Cross-cultural validation of the Preventive Health Model for colorectal cancer screening: An Australian study. *Health Education & Behavior*, Vol. 37, No. 5, pp. 724-736, ISSN 1090-1981

Frazier, A.; Colditz, G.; Fuchs, C. & Kuntz, K. (2000). Cost-effectiveness of screening for colorctal cancer in the general population. *JAMA*, Vol. 284, pp. 1954-1961, ISSN 0098-7484

Gollwitzer, P. (1993). Goal achievement: The role of intentions. *European Review of Social Psychology*, Vol. 4, pp. 141-185, ISSN 1046-3283

Gollwitzer, P. & Sheeran, P. (2006). Implementation intentions and goal achievement: A meta-analysis of effects and processes. *Advances in Experimental Social Psychology*, Vol. 38, pp. 69-119, ISSN 0065-2601

Gregory, T.; Wilson, C.; Duncan, A.; Turnbull, D.; Cole, S. & Young, G. (2011). Demographic, social cognitive and social ecological predictors of intention and participation in screening for colorectal cancer. *BMC Public Health*, Vol. 11, pp. 38, ISSN 1471-2458

Hardcastle, J.; Chamberlain, J.; Robinson, M.; Moss, S.; Amar, S.; Balfour, T.; James, P. & Mangham, C. (1996). Randomised controlled trial of faecal-occult-blood screening for colorectal cancer. *Lancet*, Vol. 348, pp. 1472-1477, ISSN 0099-5355

Hewitson, P.; Glasziou, P.; Irwig, L.; Towler, B. & Watson, E. (2007). *Screening for colorectal cancer using the faecal occult blood test, Hemoccult*: Cochrane Database of Systematic Reviews Issue 1. Art. No.: CD001216. DOI: 10.1002/14651858.CD001216.pub2

International Cancer Screening Network. (2008). Inventory of Colorectal Cancer Screening Activities in ICSN Countries, May 2008. Retrieved 22 June 2011, from http://www.appliedresearch.cancer.gov/icsn/colorectal/screening.html

Jackson, C.; Lawton, R.; Knapp, P.; Ranor, D.; Conner, M.; Lowe, C. & Closs, S. (2005). Beyond intention: do specific plans increase health behaviours in patients in primary care? A study of fruit and vegetable consumption. *Social Science & Medicine*, Vol. 60, pp. 2382-2391, ISSN 0037-7856

Jemal, A.; Bray, F.; Center, M.; Ferlay, J.; Ward, E. & Forman, D. (2011). Global Cancer Statistics. *CA: A Cancer Journal for Clinicians*, Vol. 61, pp. 69-90, ISSN 0007-9235

Kronborg, D.; Jorgensen, O.; Fenger, C. & Rasmussen, M. (2004). Randomized study of biennial screening with a faecal occult blood test: results after nine screening

rounds. *Scandinavian Journal of Gastroenterology,* Vol. 39, No. 9, pp. 846-851, ISSN
0036-5521

Lechner, L.; Oenema, A. & Nooijer, J. (2002). Testicular self-examination (TSE) among Dutch
young men aged 15-19: Determinants of the intention to practice TSE. *Health
Education Research,* Vol. 17, pp. 73-84, ISSN 0268-1153

Luszczynska, A. (2004). Change in breast self-examination behavior: Effects of intervention
on enhancing self-efficacy. *International Journal of Behavioral Medicine,* Vol. 11, No. 2,
pp. 95-103, ISSN 1070-5503

Mandel, J.; Bond, J.; Church, T.; Snover, D.; Bradley, G.; Schuman, L. & Ederer, F. (1993).
Reducing mortality from colorectal cancer by screening for fecal occult blood.
Minnesota Colon Cancer Control Study. *New England Journal of Medicine,* Vol. 328,
No. 19, pp. 1365-1371, ISSN 0028-4793

Mandel, J.; Church, T.; Bond, J.; Ederer, F.; Geisser, M.; Mongin, S.; Snover, D. & Schuman, L.
(2000). The effect of fecal occult-blood screening on the incidence of colorectal cancer.
New England Journal of Medicine, Vol. 343, No. 22, pp. 1603-1607, ISSN 0028-4793

Michie, S.; Dormandy, E. & Marteau, T. (2004). Increasing screening uptake amongst those
intending to be screened: the use of action plans. *Patient Education and Counseling,*
Vol. 55, pp. 218-222, ISSN 0738-3991

Milne, S.; Orbell, S. & Sheeran, P. (2002). Combining motivational and volitional interventions
to promote exercise participation: Protection motivation theory and implementation
intentions. *British Journal of Health Psychology,* Vol. 7, pp. 183-184, ISSN 1359-107X

Oettingen, G.; Honig, G. & Gollwitzer, P. (2000). Effective self-regulation of goal attainment.
International Journal of Educational Research, Vol. 33, pp. 705-732, ISSN:0883-0355

Orbell, S.; Hodgins, S. & Sheeran, P. (1997). Implementation intentions and the theory of
planned behaviour. *Personality and Social Psychology Bulletin,* Vol. 23, pp. 945-954,
ISSN 0146-1672

Power, E., Van Jaarsveld, C.H.M., McCaffery, K., Miles, A., Atkin, W. & Wardle, J. (2008).
Understanding intentions and action in colorectal cancer screening. *Annals of
Behavioral Medicine,* Vol. 35, pp. 285-294, ISSN 0883-6612

Prochaska, J. (2008). Decision making in the Transtheoretical Model of Behavior Change.
Medical Decision Making, Vol. 28, pp. 845-849, ISSN 0272-989X

Prochaska, J.; Velicer, W.; DiClemente, C. & Fava, J. (1988). Measuring processes of change:
applications to the cessation of smoking. *Journal of Consulting and Clinical
Psychology,* Vol. 56, No. 4, pp. 520-528, ISSN 0022-006X

Rutter, D.; Steadman, L. & Quine, L. (2006). An implementations intervention to increase
uptake of mammography. *Annals of Behavioural Medicine,* Vol. 32, No. 2, pp. 127-
134, ISSN 0883-6612

Schwarzer, R. & Fuchs, R. (1995). Self-efficacy and health behaviours. In:*Predicting health
behavior: Research and practice with social cognition models,* M. Conner & P. Norman
(Eds.), (pp. 163-196). ISBN 033519320X, Buckingham, UK: Open University Press

Schweiger Gallo, I. & Gollwitzer, P. (2007). Implementation intentions: A look back at fifteen
years of progress. *Psicothema,* Vol. 19, No. 1, pp. 37-42, ISSN 0214-9915

Sheeran, P. (2002). Intention-behavior relations: A conceptual and empirical review.
European Review of Social Psychology, Vol. 12, No. 1, pp. 1-36, ISSN 1046-3283

Sheeran, P. & Orbell, S. (2000). Using implementation intentions to increase attendance for
cervical cancer screening. *Health Psychology,* Vol. 19, pp. 283-289, ISSN 0278-6133

Skar, S.; Sniehotta, F.; Molloy, G.; Prestwich, A. & Araujo-Soares, V. (2011). Do brief online
planning intereventions increase physical activity amongst university students? A

randomised controlled trial. *Psychology and Health,* Vol. 26, No. 4, pp. 399-417, ISSN 0887-0446

Sniehotta, F. (2009). towards a theory of intentional behaviour change: Plans, planning, and self-regulation. *British Journal of Health Psychology,* Vol. 14, No., pp. 261-273, ISSN 1359-107X

Tiro, J.; Vernon, S.; Hyslop, T. & Myers, R. (2005). Factorial validity and invariance of a survey measuring psychosocial correlates of colorectal cancer screening among African Americans and Caucasians. *Cancer Epidemiology Biomarkers & Prevention,* Vol. 14, pp. 2855-286, ISSN 1573-3521

Umeh, K. & Chadwick, R. (2010). Early detection of testicular cancer: revsiting the role of self-efficacy in testicular self-examination among young asymptomatic males [Epub ahead of print]. *Journal of Behavioral Medicine,* published online 22 April 2010, ISSN 1573-3521

Vernon, S.; Myers, R. & Tilley, B. (1997). Development and validation of an instrument to measure factors related to colorectal cancer screening adherence. *Cancer Epidemiology Biomarkers & Prevention,* Vol. 12, pp. 339-349, ISSN 1573-3521

Verplanken, B. & Faes, S. (1999). Good intentions, bad habits, and effects of forming implementation intentions on healthy eating. *European Review of Social Psychology,* Vol. 29, pp. 592-604, ISSN 1046-3283

Webb, T. & Sheeran, P. (2006). Does changing behavioral intentions engender behavior change? A meta-analysis of the experimental evidence. *Psychological Bulletin,* Vol. 132, No. 2, pp. 249-268, ISSN 0033-2909

Webb, T. & Sheeran, P. (2008). Mechanisms of implementation intention effects: The role of goal intentions, self-efficacy, and accessibility of plan components. *British Journal of Social Psychology,* Vol. 47, pp. 373-395, ISSN 2044-8309

Weller, D.; Moss, S.; Butler, P.; Campbell, C.; Coleman, D.; Melia, J. & Robertson, R. (2006). *English Pilot of Bowel Cancer Screening: an evaluation of the second round. Final Report to the Department of Health.* Edinburgh: University of Edinburgh. UK.

5

Psychological Impact and Associated Factors After Disclosure of Genetic Test Results Concerning Hereditary Nonpolyposis Colorectal Cancer

Hitoshi Okamura
Hiroshima University,
Japan

1. Introduction

Advances in genetics in recent years have made major contributions to the development of medical genetics. The existence of "familial tumors" has been recognized, and genetic testing, with a potentially incalculable benefit to humanity, is being attempted (Offit, 1998). Numerous gene analyses related to the genesis and development of colorectal cancer have been conducted, and the existence of hereditary colorectal tumors in the form of hereditary nonpolyposis colorectal cancer (HNPCC) and familial adenomatous polyposis (FAP) has been identified.

HNPCC is caused by inherited germline mutations in mismatch repair genes and accounts for 2 -5% of colorectal cancers. The condition is characterized by young-onset, synchronous and metachronous tumors, and a predisposition to gynecologic, urinary tract, and extracolonic gastrointestinal cancers. Genetic testing usually begins with a family member who has been diagnosed with an HNPCC syndrome-related cancer (proband). If a deleterious mutation is identified, testing can be offered to the proband's family members, since they are at risk of carrying the mutation. Knowing one's genetic risk for hereditary cancers may facilitate the early detection or prevention of cancer.

However, in contrast to the advances in scientific techniques, a great deal of apprehension exists with regard to the psychological or ethical, legal, and social issues (ELSI) associated with the application of these techniques. Since important personal genetic information that does not change throughout one's lifetime is handled during genetic diagnosis and an individual's genetic information is partly shared with blood relatives, with the impact of such genetic information not being limited to the individual, we find ourselves in a situation where new life health-care norms that also take psychosocial aspects into consideration are required. For this reason, a variety of studies have been conducted regarding the psychosocial aspects involved in the screening-test-taking behavior of high-risk people, the psychological aspects of high-risk people, interest in genetic counseling and genetic testing, and the psychosocial effects of genetic counseling. Studies on psychosocial aspects after being informed of the test results have also been reported recently, but many of these studies are concerning hereditary breast and ovarian cancer, and very few studies examining the impact of genetic testing for hereditary colorectal tumors have been performed. ˙

In this article, the psychological consequences related to HNPCC are reviewed with regard to the following four points: (1) attitude toward genetic testing, (2) risk perception, (3) psychosocial effects of genetic counseling, and (4) psychosocial aspects after undergoing genetic testing and being informed of the test results. I have reviewed and selected nearly all the articles regarding these themes using the PubMed database.

2. Attitude toward genetic testing

Many subjects who undergo genetic counseling for HNPCC also wish to undergo genetic testing. However, some subjects refuse to undergo genetic testing, despite its potential benefits. Some previous studies investigated the relationships between the intention to undergo genetic testing and psychosocial variables.

Hadley et al. (2003) investigated attitudes, intention, and the completion of genetic testing among 111 newly identified family members (first-degree relatives) of individuals with HNPCC. Most (97%) stated their intention to pursue testing. Fifty-one percent reported that learning about their children's risks was the most important reason to consider testing. The participants' intentions to pursue genetic testing were significantly affected by concerns regarding their ability to handle the emotional aspects of testing and the psychosocial effect on family members. On the other hand, 39% identified the potential effect on their health insurance as the most important reason not to undergo testing.

Wakefield et al. (2007a) qualitatively assessed 22 individuals' attitudes toward genetic testing for HNPCC. The most frequently reported pros were "to help manage my risk of developing cancer", "to help my family", and "to know my cancer risk." The participants expressed concern about the potential psychological impact of genetic testing. The authors also found that some affected individuals may not fully comprehend the meaning of their potential test results.

Wakefield et al. (2008) conducted a randomized trial to measure the effectiveness of a tailored decision aid designed specifically to assist individuals to make informed decisions regarding genetic testing for HNPCC. The decision aid explains the evidence available regarding HNPCC-related cancer risks, the differences between a mutation search and predictive testing, and the potential benefits, risks, and limitations of testing (Wakefield et al., 2007b). One hundred and fifty-three individuals were randomly assigned to a group who received the decision aid or a group who received a control pamphlet. Evaluations were conducted 1 week after consultation and 6 months after the completion of the intervention using a questionnaire, and 95 subjects completed the 6-month follow-up questionnaire. Although the decision aid had no significant effect on the actual genetic testing decision, the participants who received the decision aid had significantly lower levels of decisional conflict regarding genetic testing and were more likely to be classified as having made an informed choice concerning genetic testing than participants who received a control pamphlet. Furthermore, men who received the decision aid had significantly higher knowledge levels regarding genetic testing than men who received a control pamphlet.

These reports suggest that most individuals pursue genetic testing to help manage their own risk of developing cancer and to learn about their children's risks. On the other hand, however, concerns about psychological and psychosocial issues may present barriers to undergoing genetic testing. The development of patient education tools, such as the decision aid, is needed.

3. Risk perception

HNPCC mutation carriers have a life-time risk of colorectal cancer of about 80%, while female carriers have a 40-60% risk of endometrial cancer and a 10-15% risk of ovarian cancer. Communicating cancer risk and assessing the perceived risk is very important for genetic counseling because of subsequent cancer prevention behavior or cancer-related distress. Four reports were extracted regarding risk perception among individuals at risk for HNPCC.

Codori et al. (2005) assessed the effect of genetic counseling on perceived lifetime risk and cancer-distress among 101 adult first-degree-relatives of colorectal cancer patients from families with known or suspected HNPCC. Most persons overestimated their cancer risk, and a higher perceived risk was associated with believing that colorectal cancer cannot be prevented. The individual perceived risk changed after counseling, although the mean perceived risk was unchanged.

Domanska et al. (2007) investigated the perceived cancer risk among 47 HNPCC mutation carriers and correlated the findings with individual characteristics. A perceived risk of colorectal cancer above 60% was reported by 49% individuals, and only one reported a perceived risk > 80%. Female mutation carriers, individuals under the age of 50 years, and individuals who received their counseling within 1 year prior to the study reported a higher perceived risk of colorectal cancer. Individuals who had lost a parent to HNPCC-related cancer at an early age also reported a higher perceived risk. Regarding gynecological cancer, 33% of the women reported a perceived risk of 40-60% for endometrial cancer, whereas the remaining 67% either underestimated or overestimated their risk.

van Oostrom et al. (2007) studied the difference in cancer risk perception among 271 individuals who opted for genetic cancer susceptibility testing for a known familial BRCA1/2 or HNPCC related germline mutation. The assessment was conducted before, 1 week after, and 6 months after disclosure of the test results. Individuals from BRCA1/2 and HNPCC mutation families did not differ with regard to their risk perceptions over time. Individuals from BRCA1/2 families perceived hereditary cancer as being more serious.

Grover et al. (2009) examined colorectal cancer risk perception among individuals tested for mismatch repair genes mutation and identified factors associated with an appropriate interpretation of their cancer risk. In this study, in particular, the authors paid attention to individuals with an indeterminate genetic test result. Pathogenic mutations in *MLH1* and *MSH2* have been identified in only 30% to 64% of families who meet the clinical criteria for HNPCC and have undergone testing. Genetic testing may not yield a definitive result because of the lack of an identifiable mutation in one of the known genes or a mutation of unclear pathogenic significance. In the absence of an identified family mutation, these results are considered indeterminate or uninformative. Patients remain at an increased risk for colorectal cancer, and intensive cancer screening recommendations are made based on their personal and family cancer histories. A total of 159 individuals who met the Revised Bethesda Guidelines and had previously undergone genetic testing participated in this study. Ninety individuals with a pathogenic mutation (true positive) correctly estimated their cancer risk. However, only 62% of individuals with an indeterminate genetic test result correctly estimated their risk. Individuals with a history of HNPCC-associated cancer or indeterminate genetic test results were significantly less likely to estimate their cancer risk as being increased.

These reports suggest that despite educational efforts and an increasing amount of data on the risk of cancer associated with HNPCC, few individuals report a perceived risk that is actually correct. In particular, individuals at risk for HNPCC who receive an indeterminate genetic test result may be falsely reassured. It is important that health care providers continue to device a counseling approach for promoting a correct understanding of cancer risk and for discussing the implications of uninformative results on the lifetime cancer risk.

4. Psychosocial effects of genetic counseling

Cancer genetic counseling has become popular as a result of the recent development of genetic tests that pinpoint familial cancer risk. Such counseling is composed of presymptomatic risk assessment and management (cancer risk counseling) and reproductive risk counseling. The former has two components: risk assessment and counseling regarding behavioral, medical, and surgical options to decrease risk. A basic goal of cancer risk counseling is to derive and explain an individual's cancer risk in clear terms, and the counselor's role is to educate and enumerate options for patients and clinicians, answer questions regarding what is known, and suggest appropriate referrals to help individuals reach difficult decisions.

A cancer risk counseling session is comprised of the following components: 1) baseline risk perception; 2) medical history and exposure history; 3) pedigree construction and pedigree documentation; 4) empiric risk assessment and genetic risk assessment; 5) options for early detection and prevention; 6) options, risks, and benefits of genetic testing; and 7) response to questions, support, and plans for follow-up. Throughout these discussions, a sensitivity to the psychological and ethical aspects of counseling is essential. Therefore, continued follow-up by the counselor after the session is the best way to limit the potential for adverse effects as a result of the knowledge of an inherited cancer risk, and ready access to liaison mental health professionals with experience in cancer genetics is thought to be a valued asset of cancer risk counseling.

Psychological research on aspects of cancer genetic counseling has focused on three broad areas: factors predicting interest in cancer genetic testing (Lerman et al., 1996), the psychological impact and effect of genetic counseling and testing for inherited cancer risk (Lerman et al., 1997), and the relationship between psychological distress and preventive behaviors (Kash et al., 1992). In each of these areas, the results have implications for the management of at-risk individuals. However, such data is unlikely to be applicable to every case because of cultural differences among study populations and the complexity of the instruments used in research studies, in addition to the fact that most of these studies have been performed for hereditary breast cancer. In this section, four studies on the psychological impacts of genetic counseling regarding HNPCC are reviewed.

Keller et al. (2002) explored distress before and after comprehensive interdisciplinary counseling in families at risk for HNPCC. Sixty-five individuals (31 patients with colorectal cancer and 34 unaffected at-risk persons) participated in this study. Data were collected from semi-structured questionnaires before, as well as 4-6 weeks after counseling. Distress declined after counseling, as did worries related to HNPCC. A trend toward a greater anticipated ability to cope with a positive gene test was also observed after counseling. Changes after counseling were generally more pronounced for persons at risk, compared with those for patients with cancer. A substantial minority, however, said that they experienced increased worry and physical symptoms after counseling.

Bleiker et al. (2007) examined: 1) levels of cancer-specific distress more than one year after genetic counseling for HNPCC; 2) associations between sociodemographic, clinical and psychosocial factors and levels of distress; 3) the impact of genetic counseling on family relationships; and 4) the social consequences of genetic counseling. One hundred and sixteen individuals who participated in this study completed a self-report questionnaire by mail an average of 4 years after the last counseling session. Among all the subjects, 6% had clinically significant levels of cancer-specific distress (Impact of Event Scale). Having had contact with a professional psychosocial worker for cancer risk in the past 10 years was significantly associated with higher levels of current cancer specific distress. Only a minority of the subjects reported any adverse effects of genetic counseling on communication regarding genetic counseling with their children, family relationships, obtaining life insurance, choice or change of jobs, and obtaining a mortgage.

Keller et al. (2008) conducted a prospective study that examined the impact of multidisciplinary risk counseling on the psychosocial outcome of 139 affected cancer patients and 233 family members without cancer but at risk for HNPCC. Participants completed questionnaires specific to HNPCC before and 8 weeks after attending the cancer clinic. The levels of distress among affected patients exceeded those of unaffected individuals, as did worry regarding their relatives' risk. A significant reduction in general anxiety (Hospital Anxiety and Depression Scale), distress specific to familial colorectal cancer (Impact of Events Scale), and general cancer worry (Distress due to Hereditary Disorder) was demonstrated after counseling among both the affected patients and unaffected individuals. The reduction in distress was more pronounced among affected patients given a high risk of HNPCC than among those with an intermediate risk.

Hasenbring et al. (2011) prospectively examined the impact of an initial interdisciplinary genetic counseling on feelings of anxiety with a special focus on subgroups related to personal cancer history, sex, age, and education. A significant interaction between time, sex, and age was identified for change in anxiety. While women in general and men older than 50 years revealed a significant reduction in anxiety, younger men did not show any change over time. A logistic regression analysis indicated that clinical Hospital Anxiety and Depression Scale-A cases could be predicted based on general distress (Brief Symptom Inventory) as well as by HNPCC-related cognitions of intrusion and avoidance (Impact of Event Scale) with a correct classification of 86%.

These studies indicate that anxiety and cancer-specific distress are reduced after genetic counseling, suggesting an overall beneficial impact of comprehensive counseling. On the other hand, a minority of individuals, such as cancer-affected younger men, exhibited adverse effects of genetic counseling on psychosocial variables. Thus, healthcare providers (genetic counselors, human geneticists, oncologists, and psycho-oncologists) should always be aware of psychosocial issues after genetic counseling. However, as little data is available on the psychosocial effects of genetic counseling regarding HNPCC, further data accumulation is needed.

5. Psychosocial aspects after being informed of genetic test results

Since 1991, when a gene for hereditary cancer was first identified, studies expressing concern about the psychosocial aspects of gene diagnosis began in Western countries, with the results starting to be reported in 1993. Although studies investigating psychosocial aspects after the subjects had undergone actual genetic testing and had been informed of the test results have been reported, many of these studies have concerned hereditary breast and ovarian cancer, and only a few studies have been performed for HNPCC. Furthermore, little is known about the factors associated with psychosocial aspects. However, HNPCC testing might offer more benefit than hereditary breast and ovarian cancer testing because of the differences in the risk management options available to mutation carriers. In HNPCC, a colonoscopy every 1–2 years is more effective for detecting and preventing adverse health outcomes than measures available to carriers of hereditary breast and ovarian cancer mutations. Therefore, identifying the psychosocial situations in which individuals at risk for colorectal cancer have lived after the disclosure of genetic information or the way in which healthcare providers are able to support the mental states of these individuals are important.

Ten original articles (review articles were not included) assessing psychosocial aspects after individuals had been informed of genetic test results regarding HNPCC were extracted. In this chapter, cross-sectional studies that assessed psychosocial aspects at one time point after disclosure and prospective studies that followed-up psychosocial aspects for 1 year or longer after disclosure are described separately. A summary is shown in Table 1.

5.1 Cross-sectional studies assessing psychosocial aspects after the subjects had been informed of the test results

Four articles were extracted. Esplen et al. (2001) investigated psychosocial function in 50 individuals who were engaged in the genetic test process for HNPCC (the period between the psychosocial assessment and the disclosure of the test results was 1 – 48 months). Twenty-three individuals were identified as carriers (13 had a previous history of CRC), seven were non-carriers and 20 individuals were still awaiting their test results. The psychosocial scores demonstrated that a subgroup of individuals exhibited distress, with greater distress for those individuals awaiting results or testing positive. A high level of satisfaction was associated with the experience of testing.

Claes et al. (2004) assessed the short-term impact (1month after test result disclosure) of genetic testing using a semi-structured interview and self-reported questionnaires. The subjects were 40 cancer-unaffected relatives who had undergone predictive testing for HNPCC. Distress was within the normal ranges. Distress decreased significantly from pre- to post-test in non-carriers but not in carriers.

Murakami et al. (2004) identified the prevalence rates and predictors of psychological distress and evaluated the feelings of guilt at one month after the disclosure of test results in Japanese probands and unaffected relatives. The prevalence of major and minor depression, acute stress disorder (ASD), posttraumatic stress disorder (PTSD), and posttraumatic stress symptoms (PTSS) were assessed using the Structured Clinical Interview based on the Diagnostic and Statistical Manual of Mental Disorders, 3rd edition revised (DSM-III-R) or the DSM-IV; feelings of guilt were investigated using a numeric scale and a semi-structured interview. Forty-two participants completed the 1-month follow-up interview. Although none of the participants met the criteria for major depression, ASD, or PTSD at the time of the follow-up interview, 7% of the participants met the criteria for minor depression and 5% had PTSS. The only predictor of psychological distress was the presence of a history of major or minor depression. Twelve percent of the participants had feelings of guilt.

Psychological Impact and Associated Factors After Disclosure of Genetic Test Results Concerning Hereditary Nonpolyposis Colorectal Cancer

93

Author, year	Subjects	Study design	Assessment period after disclosure	Study method / outcome measures	Main study findings	Associated factors
Esplen et al, 2001	50 affected and unaffected individuals	Cross-sectional	1 – 48 months	Questionnaires / CES-D, IES, STAI	The psychosocial scores demonstrated that a subgroup of individuals exhibited distress, with greater distress for those individuals awaiting results or testing positive.	Disclosure their test results to family and non-family members
Aktan-Collan et al, 2001	271 unaffected individuals	Prospective	1 and 12 months	Questionnaires / STAI	The mutation-positive subjects were more anxious than their counterparts immediately after the test disclosure, but the differences had disappeared at the follow-ups. In other variables, neither differences between the groups defined by mutation status nor changes with time were detected.	Not shown
Claes et al, 2004	40 unaffected individuals	Cross-sectional	1 month	Questionnaires / SCL-90, STAI	Distress was within normal ranges. Distress decreased significantly from pre- to post-test in non-carriers and did not in carriers.	Not shown
Murakami et al, 2004	42 affected and unaffected individuals	Cross-sectional	1 month	Semi-structured interview / major depression, minor depression, ASD, PTSD, PTSS, guilt	Although none of the participants met the criteria for major depression, ASD, or PTSD at the follow-up interview, 7% of participants met the criteria for minor depression and 5% had PTSS. Twelve percent of participants had feelings of guilt.	Presence of history a major depression

Table 1. (continued)

Meiser et al, 2004	40 unaffected individuals	Prospective	2 weeks, 4 months and 12 months	Questionnaires / HADS, IES, STAI	Carriers showed a significant increase in mean scores for intrusive and avoidant thoughts 2 weeks and a significant decrease in mean depression scores 2 weeks and 4 months. For non-carriers, significant decreases in mean scores for intrusive and avoidant thoughts, depression scores and mean state anxiety scores were observed at all follow-up assessment time points.	Not shown
Gritz et al, 2005	155 affected and unaffected individuals	Prospective	2 weeks, 6 months and 12 months	Questionnaires / CES-D, IES-R, QLI, STAI	Mean scores on all outcome measures remained stable and within normal limits for cancer-affected participants. Among unaffected carriers, mean depression and state anxiety scores increased from baseline to 2 weeks and decreased from 2 weeks to 6 months. Among unaffected non-carriers, mean depression and anxiety scores did not differ...	Baseline mood disturbance, lower quality of life, and lower social support
Claes et al, 2005	72 unaffected individuals	Prospective	1 month and 12 months	Questionnaires / IES, SCL-90, STAI	Mean levels of distress (cancer-specific distress, state anxiety, psychoneuroticism) were within normal ranges and none of the participants had an overall pattern (on all scales) of clinically elevated levels of distress.	Not shown

Table 1. (continued)

Psychological Impact and Associated Factors After Disclosure of Genetic Test Results Concerning Hereditary Nonpolyposis Colorectal Cancer

95

Study	Sample	Design	Time points	Questionnaires	Results	Associated factors
Collins et al, 2007	73 unaffected individuals	Prospective	2 weeks, 4 months, 1 year, and 3 years	Questionnaires / HADS, STAI, IES-R	Mean cancer-specific distress in carriers increased at 2 weeks with a return to baseline levels by 12 months. This level was maintained until 3 years. Non-carriers showed sustained decreases after testing with a lower level at 3 years compared with baseline. Mean depression and anxiety scores did not differ between carriers and non-carriers and, at 3 years, were similar to baseline.	Not shown
Yamashita et al, 2008	46 affected and unaffected individuals	Cross-sectional	1 month	Questionnaires / IES-R	Comparison of the IES-R scores showed that they tended to be higher in the mutation-positive group, but the differences were not statistically significant.	Personality tendency "nervousness", Verbal memory
Shiloh et al, 2008	253 affected and unaffected individuals	Prospective	6 months and 12 months	Questionnaires / CES-D, IES-R	Mean reductions were indicated in distress and depression levels within the first 6 months after testing. The interaction between time and mutation was neither significant for distress nor for depression.	Coping style (high monitors)

CES-D: Center for Epidemiological Studies-Depression, IES: Impact of Event Scale (IES-R: Impact of Event Scale-Revised), HADS: Hospital Anxiety and Depression Scale,
QLI: Quality of Life Index, SCL-90: Symptom Checklist, STAI: State-Trait Anxiety Inventory
ASD: acute stress disorder, PTSD: post-traumatic stress disorder, PTSS: post-traumatic stress symptoms

Table 1. Characteristics of studies on psychosocial aspects and associated factors after being informed of genetic test results regarding HNPCC

Yamashita et al. (2008) elucidated the psychological impact at one month after the disclosure of genetic test results regarding HNPCC and assessed the associated factors, focusing on memory function in particular. The subjects were persons who were suspected of having HNPCC and had been given the choice of undergoing genetic testing. .The post-genetic testing psychological impact was evaluated using the Impact of Event Scale-Revised (IES-R), and personality tendencies and memory function were evaluated. Final data were obtained from 46 Japanese probands and unaffected relatives (mutation-positive in 18 subjects, uninformative in 18 subjects, and mutation-negative in 10 subjects). A comparison of the IES-R scores showed that they tended to be higher in the mutation-positive group, but the differences were not statistically significant. The personality tendency "nervousness" and the verbal memory assessed prior to disclosure were significantly associated with the total IES-R score.

5.2 Prospective studies assessing psychosocial aspects after the subjects had been informed of the test results

Six articles were extracted. Aktan-Collan et al. (2001) assessed general anxiety, fear of cancer and death, satisfaction with life, and attitude regarding the future using a questionnaire survey in 271 individuals with no personal cancer history who were tested for HNPCC. Measurements were made before the first counseling (baseline), at the test disclosure session, and 1 and 12 months after disclosure. Although the mutation-positive individuals were more afraid of cancer than those who were mutation negative at every measurement point, the fear of cancer decreased significantly from the baseline until after disclosure in both groups. The mutation-positive subjects were more anxious than their counterparts immediately after the test disclosure, but the differences had disappeared at the follow-up examinations. Regarding the other variables, no differences among the groups defined according to mutation status or changes over time were detected.

Meiser et al. (2004) assessed the psychological impact of predictive genetic testing for HNPCC in 114 individuals with no personal cancer history (32 carriers and 82 non-carriers) using mailed self-administered questionnaires prior to and 2 weeks, 4 months and 12 months after the disclosure of the test results. Compared with the baseline results, carriers showed a significant increase in the mean scores for intrusive and avoidant thoughts regarding colorectal cancer at 2 weeks after test result disclosure and a significant decrease in the mean depression scores at 2 weeks and 4 months after test result disclosure. For non-carriers, significant decreases in the mean scores for intrusive and avoidant thoughts regarding colorectal cancer were observed at all follow-up assessment time points relative to the baseline. Non-carriers also showed significant decreases from the baseline in the mean depression scores at 2 weeks, 4 months and 12 months after test result disclosure. Significant decreases in the mean state anxiety scores from the baseline were also observed for non-carriers at 2 weeks after test result disclosure.

Gritz et al. (2005) examined the impact of HNPCC genetic test results on the psychological outcomes of cancer-affected and -unaffected participants up to 1 year after test result disclosure. A total of 155 persons completed the study measures before HNPCC genetic testing and at 2 weeks and 6 and 12 months after the disclosure of the test results. The mean scores for all the outcome measures remained stable and within the normal limits for cancer-affected participants, regardless of the mutation status. Among unaffected carriers of HNPCC-predisposing mutations, the mean depression, state anxiety, and cancer worry scores increased from baseline to 2 weeks after test result disclosure and decreased from 2 weeks to 6 months after test result disclosure. Among unaffected non-carriers, the mean depression and anxiety scores did not differ, but the cancer worry scores decreased during the same time period. Affected and unaffected carriers had higher mean test-specific distress scores at 2 weeks after test result disclosure, compared with non-carriers, in their respective groups; the scores decreased for affected carriers and all unaffected participants from 2 weeks to 12 months after test result disclosure. Higher levels of baseline mood disturbance, a lower quality of life, and lower social support were associated with a risk for both short- and long-term increases in distress.

Claes et al. (2005) evaluated distress one year after the disclosure of a predictive genetic test result for HNPCC in 72 cancer-unaffected relatives (36 carriers and 36 non-carriers). The mean levels of distress (cancer-specific distress, state anxiety, and psychoneuroticism) were within the normal ranges and none of the participants had an overall pattern (on all scales) of clinically elevated levels of distress. Carriers had significantly higher cancer-related distress one year after test result disclosure than non-carriers. In both groups, colorectal cancer-related distress decreased. Non-carriers additionally showed decreased endometrial cancer-related distress and state anxiety.

Collins et al. (2007) conducted a 3-year study of individuals who received predictive genetic test results for previously identified familial mutations regarding HNPCC. Questionnaires were sent before attendance and 2 weeks, 4 months, 1 year, and 3 years after receiving the test results. Psychological measures were included each time. The study included 73 individuals with no personal cancer history (19 carriers and 54 non-carriers). The results showed an increase in mean cancer-specific distress in carriers at 2 weeks with a return to baseline levels by 12 months. This level was maintained until 3 years. Non-carriers showed sustained decreases after testing with a significantly lower level at 3 years compared with at baseline. These scores tended to be lower than those for carriers at 3 years. The mean depression and anxiety scores did not differ between carriers and non-carriers and, at 3 years, were similar to the baseline scores.

Shiloh et al. (2008) assessed the emotional effects of genetic testing for HNPCC at baseline before testing and again at 6 and 12 months after testing. The subjects were 253 cancer-affected and -unaffected individuals. Negative emotional reactions were evaluated using the Revised Impact of Event Scale and the Center for Epidemiological Studies-Depression Scale. Monitoring coping style was assessed at baseline using the Miller Behavioral Style Scale. Mean reductions were indicated in distress and depression levels within the first 6 months after testing. High monitors (individuals who vigilantly attended to threatening cues in their environment in an attempt to emotionally process the situation and who actively engaged in information seeking and cognitive problem solving with the intention of taking precautions) were generally more distressed than low monitors, specifically if they had indeterminate or positive results.

5.3 Summary

Many studies have shown that genetic testing does not result in short- or long-term significant adverse psychological outcomes, including depression, anxiety, and posttraumatic stress disorder (PTSD), in either carriers or non-carriers or in either cancer-affected or cancer–unaffected individuals. However, healthcare providers should assess psychological responses, such as minor depression, posttraumatic stress symptoms (PTSS), and feelings of guilt, particularly in individuals who have a history of major or minor depression, nervous personality tendencies, baseline mood disturbances, a lower quality of life, or lower social support.

Lastly, two cases that showed adverse psychological reactions after being informed of genetic test results will be presented. The first case is a man who was diagnosed as having acute stress disorder at a 1-month follow-up examination after the disclosure of a genetic test result, despite the fact that the test result had been negative. The second case is a man who felt guilty after hearing of the positive test results of family members of individuals belonging to his support group.

5.4 Cases exhibiting adverse psychological reactions

[Case 1] Mr. A was a 39-year-old married man without children who came for genetic counseling and testing because of a family history of colon cancer. He had no history of cancer, but his father had a history of colon cancer and his sister had died of the disease at an early age. To confirm the diagnosis of HNPCC, a blood sample was obtained and mutations in the hMSH2 and hMLH1 genes were analyzed. He then consented in writing to participate in our study, and a baseline interview was conducted. He did not meet any of the criteria for any psychiatric disorders.

Approximately two months after the blood test, he underwent post-test counseling and was informed that no mutations had been detected in either the hMSH2 or hMLH1 gene. Four weeks after the disclosure of the test result, at a 1-month follow-up examination, he was diagnosed as having acute stress disorder according to a structured clinical interview based on the DSM-IV. The total score of the Impact of Event Scale-Revised was high. The score for Total Mood Disturbance in the Profile of Mood States was higher than that at the baseline interview. He reported that although he felt emotional relief to learn the negative result, his worries regarding colon cancer had increased instead of disappearing.

Mutation-negative individuals often choose not to participate in follow-up counseling after genetic testing. However, this case suggests that it is important to evaluate the psychological outcome after genetic testing regardless of the test result, and that psychiatrists or psychologists should support the genetic counseling system.

[Case 2] Mr. B, a 59-year-old man, underwent a total colectomy for the resection of colorectal cancer. He and his 25-year old son requested predictive genetic testing 3 years later to reduce uncertainty and to help plan his son's future, since Mr. B's mother had died of colon cancer secondary to HNPCC. Mr. B and his son were provided with both an educational session explaining the genetics of hereditary diseases and counseling regarding the possible impact of positive test results. The tests revealed the presence of a mutation in the father but not in the son. Mr. B was relieved that his "bad blood" had not been passed on to his son. Later, however, he began to experience anhedonia and became depressed for several days. His primary care physician could not determine the reason for his feelings.

Mr. B was the chairperson of a hereditary cancer patient support group run by patients, their families, and health care providers. The group had been established to help families with hereditary cancer exchange information and experiences. Mr. B began to feel guilty because his son had tested negative while the family members of others in his support group had tested positive for the disease.

6. Conclusion

Cancer genetic counseling and genetic testing for HNPCC are now conducted in ordinary clinical settings. However, as mentioned above, few studies have examined the psychosocial aspects of genetic testing for HNPCC, and psychosocial assessments and long-term follow-up care for individuals who have undergone genetic counseling or testing and at-risk relatives with no personal history of cancer remain insufficient. To develop this field, the following problems should be examined: 1) the development of a cancer genetic counseling model, including psychosocial support; 2) the education of cancer genetic counselors; 3) the availability of appropriate information concerning cancer genetics; 4) the recruitment of subjects at risk for cancer susceptibility; and 5) the accumulation of further psycho-oncology research results. While it is by no means easy to deal with these problems, it is essential that medical oncologists, surgical oncologists, psycho-oncologists, medical geneticists, nurses, and all other health care providers involved in cancer care vigorously approach this new area in collaboration with one another.

7. References

Aktan-Collan K, Haukkala A, Mecklin JP, Uutela A, Kääriäinen H. (2001). Psychological consequences of predictive genetic testing for hereditary non-polyposis colorectal cancer (HNPCC): a prospective follow-up study. *International Journal of Cancer*, 93 (4), 608-611

Bleiker EM, Menko FH, Kluijt I, Taal BG, Gerritsma MA, Wever LD, Aaronson NK. (2007). Colorectal cancer in the family: psychosocial distress and social issues in the years following genetic counselling. *Hereditary Cancer in Clinical Practice*, 5 (2), 59-66

Claes E, Denayer L, Evers-Kiebooms G, Boogaerts A, Legius E. (2004). Predictive testing for hereditary non-polyposis colorectal cancer: motivation, illness representations and short-term psychological impact. *Patient Education and Counseling*, 55 (2), 265-274

Claes E, Denayer L, Evers-Kiebooms G, Boogaerts A, Philippe K, Tejpar S, Devriendt K, Legius E. (2005). Predictive testing for hereditary nonpolyposis colorectal cancer: subjective perception regarding colorectal and endometrial cancer, distress, and health-related behavior at one year post-test. *Genetic Testing*, 9 (1), 54-65

Collins VR, Meiser B, Ukoumunne OC, Gaff C, St John DJ, Halliday JL. (2007). The impact of predictive genetic testing for hereditary nonpolyposis colorectal cancer: three years after testing. *Genetics in Medicine*, 9 (5), 290-297

Codori AM, Waldeck T, Petersen GM, Miglioretti D, Trimbath JD, Tillery MA. (2005). Genetic counseling outcomes: perceived risk and distress after counseling for hereditary colorectal cancer. *Journal of Genetic Counseling*, 14 (2), 119-132

Domanska K, Nilbert M, Soller M, Silfverberg B, Carlsson C. (2007). Discrepancies between estimated and perceived risk of cancer among individuals with hereditary nonpolyposis colorectal cancer. *Genetic Testing*, 11 (2), 183-186

Esplen MJ, Madlensky L, Butler K, McKinnon W, Bapat B, Wong J, Aronson M, Gallinger S.(2001). Motivations and psychosocial impact of genetic testing for HNPCC. *American Journal of Medical Genetics*, 103 (1), 9-15

Gritz ER, Peterson SK, Vernon SW, Marani SK, Baile WF, Watts BG, Amos CI, Frazier ML, Lynch PM. (2005). Psychological impact of genetic testing for hereditary nonpolyposis colorectal cancer. *Journal of Clinical Oncology*, 23 (9), 1902-1910

Grover S, Stoffel EM, Mercado RC, Ford BM, Kohlman WK, Shannon KM, Conrad PG, Blanco AM, Terdiman JP, Gruber SB, Chung DC, Syngal S. (2009). Colorectal cancer risk perception on the basis of genetic test results in individuals at risk for Lynch syndrome. *Journal of Clinical Oncology*, 27 (24), 3981-3986

Hadley DW, Jenkins J, Dimond E, Nakahara K, Grogan L, Liewehr DJ, Steinberg SM, Kirsch I. (2003). Genetic counseling and testing in families with hereditary nonpolyposis colorectal cancer. *Archives of Internal Medicine*, 163 (5), 573-582

Hasenbring MI, Kreddig N, Deges G, Epplen JT, Kunstmann E, Stemmler S, Schulmann K, Willert J, Schmiegel W. (2011). Psychological impact of genetic counseling for hereditary nonpolyposis colorectal cancer: the role of cancer history, gender, age, and psychological distress. *Genetic Testing and Molecular Biomarkers*, 15 (4), 219-225

Kash KM, Holland JC, Halper MS, Miller DG. Psychological distress and surveillance behaviors of women with a family history of breast cancer. *Journal of the National Cancer Institute*, 84 (1), 24-30

Keller M, Jost R, Haunstetter CM, Kienle P, Knaebel HP, Gebert J, Sutter C, Knebel-Doeberitz M, Cremer F, Mazitschek U. (2002). Comprehensive genetic counseling for families at risk for HNPCC: impact on distress and perceptions. *Genetic Testing*, 6 (4), 291-302

Keller M, Jost R, Haunstetter CM, Sattel H, Schroeter C, Bertsch U, Cremer F, Kienle P, Tariverdian M, Kloor M, Gebert J, Brechtel A. (2008). Psychosocial outcome following genetic risk counselling for familial colorectal cancer. A comparison of affected patients and family members. *Clinical Genetics*, 74 (5), 414-424

Lerman C, Narod S, Schulman K, Hughes C, Gomez-Caminero A, Bonney G, Gold K, Trock B, Main D, Lynch J, Fulmore C, Snyder C, Lemon SJ, Conway T, Tonin P, Lenoir G, Lynch H. (1996). BRCA1 testing in families with hereditary breast-ovarian cancer. *JAMA*, 275 (24), 1885-1892

Lerman C, Biesecker B, Benkendorf JL, Kerner J, Gomez-Caminero A, Hughes C, Reed MM. (1997). Controlled trial of pretest education approaches to enhance informed decision-making for BRCA1 gene testing. *Journal of the National Cancer Institute*, 89 (2), 148-157

Meiser B, Collins V, Warren R, Gaff C, St John DJ, Young MA, Harrop K, Brown J, Halliday J. (2004). Psychological impact of genetic testing for hereditary non-polyposis colorectal cancer. *Clinical Genetics*, 66 (6), 502-511

Murakami Y, Okamura H, Sugano K, Yoshida T, Kazuma K, Akechi T, Uchitomi Y. (2004). Psychologic distress after disclosure of genetic test results regarding hereditary nonpolyposis colorectal carcinoma. *Cancer*, 101 (2), 395-403

Offit K. (1998). *Clinical Cancer Genetics: Risk Counseling & Management*. ISBN: 0-471-14655-2, Wiley-Liss, New York

Shiloh S, Koehly L, Jenkins J, Martin J, Hadley D. (2008). Monitoring coping style moderates emotional reactions to genetic testing for hereditary nonpolyposis colorectal cancer: a longitudinal study. *Psychooncology*, 17 (8), 746-755

van Oostrom I, Meijers-Heijboer H, Duivenvoorden HJ, Bröcker-Vriends AH, van Asperen CJ, Sijmons RH, Seynaeve C, Van Gool AR, Klijn JG, Tibben A. (2007). Comparison of individuals opting for BRCA1/2 or HNPCC genetic susceptibility testing with regard to coping, illness perceptions, illness experiences, family system characteristics and hereditary cancer distress. *Patient Education and Counseling*, 65 (1), 58-68

Wakefield CE, Kasparian NA, Meiser B, Homewood J, Kirk J, Tucker K. (2007a). Attitudes toward genetic testing for cancer risk after genetic counseling and decision support: a qualitative comparison between hereditary cancer types. *Genetic Testing*, 11 (4), 401-411

Wakefield CE, Meiser B, Homewood J, Peate M, Kirk J, Warner B, Lobb E, Gaff C, Tucker K. (2007b). Development and pilot testing of two decision aids for individuals considering genetic testing for cancer risk. *Journal of Genetic Counseling*, 16 (3), 325-339

Wakefield CE, Meiser B, Homewood J, Ward R, O'Donnell S, Kirk J; Australian GENetic testing Decision Aid Collaborative Group. (2008). Randomized trial of a decision aid for individuals considering genetic testing for hereditary nonpolyposis colorectal cancer risk. *Cancer*, 113 (5), 956-965

Yamashita M, Okamura H, Murakami Y, Sugano K, Yoshida T, Uchitomi Y. (2008). Psychological impact and associated factors after disclosure of genetic test results concerning hereditary nonpolyposis colorectal cancer. *Stress and Health*, 24, 407-412

Part 3

Nutrition

6

Physical Activity, Dietary Fat and Colorectal Cancer

Martina Perše

University of Ljubljana, Faculty of Medicine, Institute of Pathology, MEC,
Slovenia

1. Introduction

Colorectal cancer (CRC) is one of the most commonly diagnosed cancers worldwide, with over 1.2 million new cases being recorded in 2008. Global cancer statistics show that there is great (10-fold) variation in the occurrence of CRC worldwide, with the highest incidence rates in economically developed countries and regions, such as Australia, New Zealand, Europe and North America. The latest report shows that CRC incidence rates are rapidly increasing in countries within Eastern Europe and Eastern Asia, which were formerly considered low-risk areas. In some countries, e.g., the Czech Repubic and Japan, the incidence of CRC has already exceeded the peak observed in the high-risk areas. Epidemiological studies have demonstrated that the increasing incidence of CRC in these developing countries is mostly due to a higher incidence of CRC in younger age groups, which readily adopt new lifestyle habits (Jemal et al., 2011). In addition, reports have shown that persons who were born in Asia and later migrated to the United States have a higher risk of CRC than their counterparts who have remained in Asia (Flood et al., 2000).

Changes in worldwide variations in the incidence rates, together with the results of migrant studies, provide convincing evidence that the incidence rates depend largely on environmental (i.e., non-genetic) risk factors, including lifestyle. It is estimated that most cases of CRC occur sporadically (70-80%). Approximately 15% of CRC cases develop as a result of inherited factors and 5-10% of them result from known genetic syndroms, e.g., familial adenomatous polyposis (FAP) and hereditary non-polyposis colorectal carcinoma (HNPCC) (Souglakos, 2007).

There are different approaches and strategies concerning how to reduce the incidence of and mortality due to CRC. Those directed toward the treatment of CRC, i.e., surgical and therapeutic measures, are mostly costly, painful and the prognosis is not promisig. Efforts have also recently been directed toward the identification and removal of precancerous lesions (visible polypoid adenomas) through screening programs, which is a promising approach and is an important step in reducing mortality due to CRC (Orlando et al., 2008). On the other hand, efforts invested into strategies directed toward public health promotion campaigns for the prevention or reduction of risk factors in populations at high risk of CRC have been few and obviously ineffective. Recent studies have shown that there is low level of awareness of the role that physical activity plays in preventing CRC among adults in the USA and Europe (Coups et al., 2008; Keighley et al., 2004).

Epidemiological studies have shown that around 30-40% of CRC may be preventable by maintaining a healthy lifestyle and suitable diet. The available evidence suggests that the population attributable risk of physical inactivity is 13-14%, which is the same as the risk due to a Western eating pattern (Coups et al., 2008). These data, and all the aforementioned facts, show that the majority of sporadic CRC cases are preventable by adjustment of appropriate environmental and lifestyle factors (dietary habits, low body index, physical activity) and that there is a need to improve strategies of public health promotion campaigns in countries with increased risk of CRC. Public health promotion campaigns, if adopted, could have a major impact in the fight against sporadic CRC and would address many health and financial challenges.

This chapter is therefore an attempt in this direction and provides a current review of the literature on the relation between physical activity or dietary fat and CRC and the mechanisms of their interaction.

2. Physical activity and CRC

The first evidence of the preventive role of physical activity against cancer appeared in 1922, when two groups of investigators, independently of each other, observed that cancer mortality rates declined with increasing physical activity required for an occupation (Lee, 2003). In spite of these results, further investigations in this area were not undertaken until the 1980s, when investigators observed that men with sedentary jobs had a higher colon cancer risk than men with jobs requiring strenuous activity (Larsson et al., 2006). Since then, the link between physical activity and cancer risk has been examined extensively, not only for cancer of the colon and rectum but also for breast and prostate cancer and, to a lesser extent also for cancers of the endometrium, lung, ovary, testis, pancreas and kidney. Nevertheless, cancer of the large bowel is the most frequently investigated cancer in relation to physical activity in humans. There have today been over 60 epidemiological studies investigating effects of physical activity on CRC in humans. Studies have been conducted in different parts of the world (North America, Europe, Australia, New Zealand and Asia-Japan) and among different populations and races. The results of these publications are convincing and clearly indicate that physical activity protects against colon cancer in all age groups, in various racial and ethnic groups and in diverse geographic areas around the world (Friedenreich & Orenstein, 2002; Kruk & Aboul-Enein, 2006; Lee, 2003; Thune & Furberg, 2001).

2.1 Physical activity and rectal cancer

Although colon and rectal cancer share some environmental risk factors, evidence of an association between rectal cancer and physical activity is inconsistent. A meta-analysis of 19 cohort studies even estimated that physical activity provides no protection against rectal cancer (Samad et al., 2005). It is therefore currently suggested that there is no association between physical activity and rectal cancer (Friedenreich & Orenstein, 2002; Kruk & Aboul-Enein, 2006; Lee, 2003; Thune & Furberg, 2001).

2.2 Physical activity and colon cancer in humans

Summarized observational epidemiological evidence on the association between physical activity and cancer suggests that the average risk reduction for colon cancer is 30-40% (Lee,

2003) or even 40-50% (Friedenreich & Orenstein, 2002). However, estimates from meta-analyses are little lower. A meta-analysis of 19 cohort studies estimated that physical activity may reduce the risk of colon cancer on average by 20-30% (Samad et al., 2005). The World Health Organization conducted a meta-analysis using data from studies prior to 2000 and estimated that around 16% of the global colon cancer disease burden can be ascribed to physical inactivity (Bull, 2004, as cited in Wolin et al., 2009). The most reliable results are probably those from the most recent meta-analysis, which included all available case-control (24) or cohort studies (28) that had been published to June 2008, but only those that investigated the association between physical activity and colon cancer or colon and rectal cancer separately. Studies on the association between physical activity and rectal cancer or colorectal cancer combined were not included. However, this meta-analysis showed a 24% average risk reduction for colon cancer when comparing the most to the least active individuals across all studies (Wolin et al., 2009).

The results of some studies suggest that the beneficial effects of exercise may be attenuated or less consistent in women (Kruk & Aboul-Enein, 2006; Thune & Furberg, 2001). However, most studies have found no difference in colon cancer risk according to gender (Friedenreich et al., 2006), which is in agreement with the latest meta-analysis. It was estimated that the protective effect of physical activity on colon cancer is similar for men (24%) and women (21%). The risk appeared smaller in cohort studies (men=19%; women=11%) than in case-control studies (men=28%; women=32%) (Wolin et al., 2009). It has been suggested that surveys used to measure physical activity were developed mainly for men and are thus less precise in estimating household work. Women may spend between 30 minutes to 6 hours a day on household chores and family care activities and from 4 to 16 hours a day on occupational activities, which makes it challenging to assess their physical activity accurately (Howard et al., 2008).

2.2.1 Type, duration and intensity

Although it is clear that physical activity is associated with a decreased risk of developing colon cancer, details of the relationship are less clear. It is known that the frequency of muscle contraction (e.g., number of activities performed per day, week, month), duration (number of minutes or hours per day), intensity (how much energy is expended) and activity levels throughout the participant's entire lifetime, are important components of activity that can significantly affect the protective effects of physical activity on colon cancer risk (Friedenreich & Orenstein, 2002). Few studies have examined the type, intensity and duration of physical activity required. Since they used different criteria of physical activity in their tests for trends, meta-analyses of trends across these studies have not yet been conducted (Wolin et al., 2009).

Physical activity is often thought of as recreational activity or exercise but it is much more than this. Physical activity is any bodily movement produced by the skeletal muscles that results in a quantifiable expenditure of energy and thereby comprises all leisure-time activities as well as occupational activities. Leisure-time physical activity refers to sports, conditioning exercises (structured and planned activity in order to improve or maintain physical fitness), household activities, self-care activities (e.g., dressing, eating, talking, standing, walking, climbing stairs) etc. (Kruk & Aboul-Enein, 2006).

Evidence is consistent that both occupational and leisure-time physical activity can affect colon cancer risk (Wolin et al., 2009). A dose-response relationship has been noted. Higher activity has been related to a reduced risk of colon cancer for both leisure-time and occupational physical activities (Friedenreich & Orenstein, 2002; Kruk & Aboul-Enein, 2006; Thune & Furberg, 2001; Wolin et al., 2009). Since little information is available, conclusions cannot be made about the type, intensity, frequency and duration of physical activity that is most beneficial.

Based on the current level of knowledge, it is believed that 30-60 min/day of regular physical activity of moderate to vigorous intensity is sufficient to decrease the risk of colon cancer in the general population (Friedenreich & Orenstein, 2002; Lee, 2003; Thune & Furberg, 2001).

2.2.2 Other factors

More detailed investigations on the effects of physical activity in relation to colon cancer site have recently been conducted. A few studies have evaluated the association between physical activity and colon cancer risk by anatomic site (proximal versus distal) and produced contradictory results. One study found no significant difference in risk estimates among different parts of the colon (Mai et al., 2007), while other studies found a reduction of risk only in transverse or sigmoid segments of the colon (Nilsen et al., 2008) or predominantly in the proximal colon (Lee et al., 2007).

It is believed that physical activity is associated with a reduced risk of colon cancer independently of diet or other environmental risk factors. This is supported by studies that have found that adjustment for potentially confounding factors, such as age, diet and obesity or body mass index, does not diminish the observed protective association (Friedenreich & Orenstein, 2002; Thune & Furberg, 2001).

However, it has been suggested that determination of potentially confounding variables is not always easy. When there are multiple hypothesized mechanisms, some of which may be in the causal path, the determination of confounding variables may be especially difficult. "For instance, if physical activity is associated with colon cancer through its ability to help maintain body weight, adjustment for body mass index would be inappropriate. If physical activity acts through other mechanisms, body mass index may be an important confounding variable because it is associated both with physical activity and colon cancer." An understanding of the biological mechanisms involved in the association between physical activity and colon cancer is therefore fundamental to evaluating confounding factors. In order to identify and understand the modifying effects of physical activity on other risk factors, the use of effect modification is advised (Slattery & Potter, 2002).

Slattery et al. examined confounding effect modification and observed the relative importance of high-risk diet, body mass index, energy intake and glycemic index in colon cancer prevention, which were found to be dependent on the level of physical activity (Slattery & Potter, 2002). Some studies have suggested a greater protective effect of physical activity in lean than in obese persons (Friedenreich et al., 2006; Larsson et al., 2006; Thune & Furberg, 2001). The findings of one cohort study even indicated that sedentary behavior, in particular television or video watching, is associated with an increased risk of colon cancer, independent of the time spent participating in physical activity and body mass index (Howard et al., 2008). Little is actually known about how physical activity may modify or be modified by other dietary and lifestyle factors, so conclusions based on currently available evidence can be misleading. Additional research in this direction is needed to provide public health recommendations regarding physical activity as a means of primary prevention of CRC.

2.2.3 Physical activity may affect cancer treatment and outcome

As shown above, physical activity has an important role in the prevention of colon cancer. Does physical activity also have a beneficial effect in CRC patients and survivors, though? A literature search shows that most attention on the efficacy of physical activity in colon cancer has been paid to cancer prevention. There have been few studies investigating the efficacy of activity in CRC patients. Nevertheless, available evidence suggests that physical activity may affect cancer treatment and outcome. It has been proposed that exercise during the pretreatment period may increase (boost) physical and psychological functioning, resulting in better physical preparation for treatment (shown in detail in Friedenreich & Orenstein, 2002). A study evaluating the benefits of physical activity in cancer patients and survivors shows improved functional capacity and quality of life (Johnson et al., 2009).

2.3 Physical activity and CRC in animal models

The effect of physical activity on CRC has mainly been evaluated using two rodent models of CRC, i.e., DMH/AOM animal model and Apc^{Min} mice. The first model is a chemically induced animal model. Animals develop colon lesions after the application of a carcinogen (dimethylhydrazine (DMH) or azoxymethane (AOM)). Colorectal carcinogenesis in this model is a multistep process with molecular, morphological and histological features similar to those seen in human sporadic colon carcinogenesis (Perse & Cerar, 2011). The second model is a genetically predisposed model. Apc^{Min} mice carry a dominant heterozygous nonsense mutation at codon 850 of the mouse homologue of the human tumor suppressor gene, APC, which results in the development of multiple adenomas throughout the intestinal tract. This mutation is implicated in both sporadic and inherited human colorectal carcinogenesis.

The first studies on carcinogen treated rats were directed at evaluating the effects of different voluntary or forced exercise (swimming, treadmill running, voluntary wheel-running) on colorectal lesions in the later stages of development (tumors, adenomas, carcinomas). These studies found that exercise significantly reduced the incidence and multiplicity of tumors, as well as the incidence and multiplicity of adenocarcinomas but had little or no effect on the incidence and multiplicity of adenomas (Basterfield et al., 2005).

Various studies have recently evaluated the effects of exercise on aberrant crypt foci (ACF), which are the first microscopically visible precursor lesions of CRC. They found that moderate-intensity exercise reduced the number of ACF in colons of DMH–treated rats (Fuku et al., 2007), low intensity exercise had no significant effect on the incidence of ACF (Lunz et al., 2008), while excessive and exhausting exercise significantly increased the number of ACF and, consequently, also the risk of development of colon cancer (Demarzo & Garcia, 2004).

In contrast to the results obtained from the chemically induced model, the results of various studies on Apc^{Min} mice are inconsistent. Two studies reported that exercise (treadmill running) had no effect on the incidence of intestinal adenomas in females, while a tendency toward a reduced incidence in males was observed (Colbert et al., 2000; Colbert et al., 2003). It was then found that the beneficial effects of exercise may be related to the exercise mode (treadmill/wheel running), gender (Mehl et al., 2005) and energy balance (Colbert et al., 2006). A recent study found that voluntary wheel running exercise also inhibited tumor formation in female Apc^{Min} mice (Ju et al., 2008).

The reasons for the inconsistent results are not clear. In has been suggested that different types of exercise may elicit different physiological changes related to stress hormone release and may alter the inflammatory effects (Mehl et al., 2005). Another possible reason is the large variation in tumor yield among individual ApcMin mice, which may have resulted in false-negative or non-significant results when a small number of animals were used (Ju et al., 2008). Finally, it is likely that this model may be suitable for investigating and assessing the effect of physical activity on CRC development in organisms with an inherited mutation or genetic predisposition.

However, experimental studies investigating the modifying effect of other dietary and lifestyle factors in relation to the beneficial effect of exercise are scarce. One study investigated the effect of exercise in animal models maintained on different types of high-fat diet. It was found that a different type of high-fat diet (21 % coconut + 2% corn oil versus 23 % corn oil) may be associated with a different outcome of colon carcinogenesis in carcinogen treated rats exposed to exercise (Thorling et al., 1994). A second study reported that 6 weeks and 9 weeks of voluntary exercise (wheel running) successfully decreased the number of intestinal polyps in ApcMin mice on low and high fat diets, respectively (Ju et al., 2008). We recently found that exercise has a protective role in colon carcinogenesis in carcinogen treated rats, in the case of both low and high fat consumption diets. However, in terms of the combined effect of dietary fat and exercise, our results suggest that the protective role of exercise on colon carcinogenesis may be reduced in relation to the amount and type of fat in the diet (Perse, 2010). The lack of understanding of the biological mechanisms operating between physical activity and other risk factors warrants further research.

2.4 Mechanisms of physical activity modulation
A number of plausible biological mechanisms for the protective effect of physical activity against colon cancer have been suggested. They are mostly based on various experimental results. There are currently few empirical clinical data to support any of the hypothesized biological mechanisms for the protective effect of exercise on colon cancer.

2.4.1 Effects on gastrointestinal transit time and gut microbiota
The most frequently quoted explanation for reduced colon cancer among physically active people is that physical activity accelerates the movement of stool through the colon and shortens the gastrointestinal transit time, thereby reducing the contact of potential carcinogens and cancer promoters with colon mucosa (Kruk & Aboul-Enein, 2006). Although plausible, the epidemiological evidence of an association between gastrointestinal transit time and colon cancer risk has so far been inconsistent and this explanation has not yet been directly confirmed (Friedenreich et al., 2006).

The colon contains a vast population of many types of bacteria, which have potentially important functions and may contribute to cancer development (Tammariello & Milner, 2010). It was recently found that voluntary wheel running influnced the composition of cecal microbiota, which in turn produced higher concentrations of n-butyrate. Butyrate is a short-chain fatty acid end product of bacterial fermentation in the intestines, which has been related to intestinal motility and an inhibitory effect on tumor development (Matsumoto et al., 2008).

2.4.2 Effects on blood insulin, IGF-1 and body weight
Similarities in geographic patterns and dietary and lifestyle risk factors for CRC and type 2 diabetes have led to the suggestion that there is an association between the two diseases

(Giovannucci, 2001). Based on meta-analysis of case-control and cohort studies, individuals with diabetes have an approximately 30% increased relative risk of developing CRC compared to non-diabetic individuals, regardless of gender or the anatomical site of CRC (Larsson et al., 2005). Preliminary results have shown that CRC is more common in people with increased circulating levels of insulin and glucose. A long-term increase in circulating levels of insulin may influence every step of colon carcinogenesis by stimulating cell proliferation or inhibiting apoptosis (Pisani, 2008). In addition to type 2 diabetes, obesity may cause problems with insulin metabolism and an alteration in blood glucose (explained in Murthy et al., 2009).

Physical activity can contribute to increased insulin sensitivity in skeletal muscles, both directly and indirectly through its influence on body weight (Giovannucci, 2001). Regular physical activity significantly lowers insulin levels by stimulation of the signaling pathways that contribute to increased expression and translocation of GLUT 4, which is responsible for basal and insulin-stimulated glucose uptake into the cells (explained in detail in Kramer & Goodyear, 2007).

An increasing body of evidence suggests that variations not only in the levels of insulin but also in the levels of insulin-like growth factors (IGF) may account for colon cancer and for its high incidence in Western countries. The IGF family of proteins (peptide ligands, receptors, binding proteins and proteases) are involved in the regulation of somatic growth, cell proliferation, transformation and apoptosis. Among them, IGF-1 and IGFBP-3 have been most frequently investigated in relation to CRC. It has been hypothesized that IGF-1 is implicated in the etiology of CRC as a potent mediator of cell survival and growth (for more detail see Sandhu et al., 2002). In spite of this, current evidence does not support an association between the blood level of IGF-1 and CRC. Among exercise studies in humans, 50% have found no change in IGF-1, 37% an increase in IGF-1 and 13% a decrease in IGF-1 (Friedenreich & Orenstein, 2004). Likewise, no significant association between circulating levels of IGF-1 and exercise in animal models of CRC has been found (Colbert et al., 2000; Colbert et al., 2003; Colbert et al., 2006; Ju et al., 2008; Mehl et al., 2005).

2.4.3 Effects on inflammatory modulators

A number of studies have demonstrated that regular exercise has anti-inflammatory effects, which may play a significant role in the prevention of colon carcinogenesis, as well as many other diseases, such as atherosclerosis, type 2 diabetes and breast cancer. A marked increase in circulating levels of interleukin (IL)-6 after exercise, without any muscle damage, has been observed. It was found that the level of circulating IL-6 increases in an exponential fashion (up to 100-fold) in response to exercise and declines after exercise. It has been demonstrated that plasma IL-6 increase is related to exercise intensity, duration, the mass of muscle recruited and one's endurance capacity. Recent data demonstrate that IL-6 released from contracting human skeletal muscle has anti-inflammatory, immunosuppressive, metabolic and hypertrophic effects in humans (Petersen & Pedersen, 2005; Petersen & Pedersen, 2006).

Until recently, IL-6 was generally considered to be a pro-inflammatory cytokine released primarily from immune cells. However, dramatic increases in circulating IL-6 during exercise have led to the finding that skeletal muscles are a primary source of IL-6. Skeletal muscle has thus been found to be an immunogenic and an endocrine organ, which by contraction stimulates the production and release of cytokines, which can influence metabolism and modify cytokine production in tissues and organs (Mathur & Pedersen, 2008).

It has been found that IL-6 induces the production of cytokine inhibitors, such as IL-1 receptor antagonist (IL-1ra) and IL-10, which are anti-inflammatory molecules. IL-1ra inhibits signaling transduction through the IL-1 receptor complex, while IL-10 inhibits the production of cytokines (IL-1α, IL-1β, TNF-α) and chemokines (IL-8, protein α), which play a critical role in the activation of granulocytes, monocytes, natural killer cells and T and B cells and in their recruitment to sites of inflammation (Petersen & Pedersen, 2005; Petersen & Pedersen, 2006).

IL-6 may increase basal and insulin-stimulated glucose uptake via increased GLUT 4 translocation. IL-6 has been shown to enhance AMP-activated protein kinase (AMPK) in both skeletal muscle and adipose tissue, which stimulates fatty acid oxidation and increases glucose uptake (Nielsen & Pedersen, 2008). TNF-α has been implicated in the pathogenesis of insulin resistance related to obesity (Steinberg, 2007). Evidence exists that TNF-α blocks AMPK signaling. However, exercise may also suppress TNF-α production via IL-6 independent pathways (Petersen & Pedersen, 2006).

2.4.4 Effects on immune function

It has been suggested that the immune system plays a role in reducing cancer risk by recognition and elimination of abnormal cells through immune components. Increased inflammation and/or depressed immune function are important risk factors that may lead to several cancers, including CRC. This is in accordance with the finding of an increased incidence of cancers among patients with inflammatory bowel disease (IBD) or AIDS. AIDS patients show an increased risk not only of AIDS-related malignancies (e.g., Kaposi's sarcoma) but also other cancers, such as lung and colon. An intact immune system is usually able to destroy cancer cells as soon as they appear.

It has been demonstrated that lifestyle factors can significantly affect immune function. Regular physical activity can enhance both the functionality and number of innate immune cell components, such as cytotoxic T lymphocytes, natural killer cells, lymphokine-activated killer cells and macrophages. Moderate physical activity results in enhanced immune function, whereas exhausting exercise, overtraining or high-intensity exercise may lead to suppression of the immune function (Pedersen & Hoffman-Goetz, 2000).

2.4.5 Effects on arachidonic acid metabolism

There have been studies suggesting that exercise affects enzymes that are implicated in arachidonic acid metabolism. Arachidonic acid is part of the phospholipids in the membranes of cells and in its free form serves as a precursor in the production of eicosanoids. After liberation (by the enzyme phospholipase A2 (PLA_2)), arachidonic acid is available as a substrate for cyclooxygenases (COX) and lipoxygenases (LOX) to form prostaglandins (PG) and leukotriens (LT). Increased levels of COX-2 and PGE_2 have been found to promote the development of CRC by increasing proliferation and decreasing colonic motility and apoptosis and have been associated with aggressive tumor progression. A relationship between PG and CRC is also supported by studies showing a reduced risk of CRC with aspirin and other non-steroidal anti-inflammatory drugs (NSAID), which inhibit COX-2, thereby inhibiting PG production (Jones et al., 2003).

It has been reported that physical exercise decreased COX-2 expression in the colon mucosa of healthy untreated rats (Buehlmeyer et al., 2007) and DMH-treated rats (Demarzo et al., 2008). Exercise was found to inhibit one of the products of COX activities, PGE_2, in intestinal tumors and serum of ApcMin mice (Ju et al., 2008). In rat colon mucosa, exercise was found to reduce the expression of $iPLA_2$, which is one of the PLA_2 implicated in arachidonic acid release (Buehlmeyer et al., 2008). Exercise has also been found to reduce PGE_2 levels in rectal tissue among individuals with higher levels of self-reported exercise. On the other hand, in another study, exercise had no significant effect on PGE_2 levels in colon mucosa (Abrahamson et al., 2007).

The body of evidence is currently too limited to reach any final conclusions.

2.4.6 Effects on apoptosis, proliferation, gene expression

An alteration in the control of cellular proliferation and survival may be an important step in the development of colonic neoplasms. New cells are produced rapidly and continuously from stem cells at the base of the colonic crypt. Older cells undergo apoptosis (programmed cell death) and are sloughed into the colonic lumen. To maintain crypt organization and structure, cellular proliferation and apoptosis must be tightly controlled. Failure of these controls may lead to the formation of colonic neoplasms. It has been hypothesized that exercise-induced colon cancer risk reduction might be through alterations to colon crypt cell architecture and proliferation. It has been reported that a 12-month moderate-to-vigorous intensity exercise program (60 minutes per day, 6 days per week) increased colon crypt height and decreased proliferation in men (McTiernan et al., 2006) and changed the expression of Bcl-2 and Bax protein in colonic crypts (Campbell et al., 2007).

2.4.7 Effects on oxidative status

There is growing support for the concept that reactive oxygen species (ROS), which are already implicated in a range of diseases, may be important progenitors in the pathogenesis of colon cancer. Namely, an excess of intracellular ROS results in an environment that modulates gene expression, damages cellular molecules, including DNA, which ultimately leads to mutations. In order to counteract these deleterious actions of increased levels of ROS, cells possess an antioxidant defence system, which plays a central role in protecting cells from oxidative injury. It is belived that exercise may help to prevent colon cancer due to an improvement in the cell's antioxidant defence system. It has already been demonstrated that exercise improves the antioxidant defence system in various tissues. Exercise stimulates various signaling pathways in cells, such as MAPK and NFκB, which results in increased expression of important enzymes associated with cell defence (MnSOD and GPx) and adaptation to exercise (eNOS and iNOS). Many of the biological effects of antioxidants appear to be related to their ability not only to scavenge deleterious free radicals but also to modulate cell-signalling pathways. The modulation of signalling pathways by antioxidants could thus help to prevent cancer by preserving normal cell cycle regulation, inhibiting proliferation and inducing apoptosis, inhibiting tumor invasion and angiogenesis, suppressing inflammation and stimulating detoxification enzyme activity (Kramer & Goodyear, 2007; Scheele et al., 2009; Valko et al., 2007). Exercise has been found to decrease the expression of inducible nitric oxide synthase (iNOS), as well as TNF-α, in the colon of AOM-treated mice (Aoi et al., 2010).

3. Dietary fat and CRC

In contrast to physical activity, the association between fat intake and CRC is less conclusive. In the past, dietary fat has received considerable attention as a possible risk factor in the etiology of CRC but subsequent analysis of case control studies has indicated that the positive association was at least in part due to increased energy intake (Johnson & Lund, 2007).

While epidemiological studies have produced contradictory results (Johnson & Lund, 2007), experimental studies under isocaloric conditions have provided unequivocal evidence that a diet high in saturated fatty acids (SFA), such as lard or beef tallow, and n-6 polyunsaturated fatty acid (PUFA), such as corn or sunflower oil, increases the risk of developing CRC (Dai et al., 2002; Reddy, 2000). It was recently shown that long-term consumption of a high-fat, low-calcium and vitamin D diet induces colon neoplasia in mice, without any other treatment (Erdelyi et al., 2009). Interestingly, a recent expert review on nutrition and cancer published by the World Cancer Research Fund (American Institute for Cancer Research, 2007) found suggestive evidence that food rich in animal fat (rich in SFA) is associated with an increased risk of CRC. This means that epidemiological studies are mainly supportive but are limited in quantity, quality or consistency.

In contrast, diets high in olive oil or n-9 monounsaturated fatty acid (MUFA) have shown a protective or no effect on colon carcinogenesis in animal models, while diets with fish oil or n-3 PUFA have been shown to reduce colon tumorigenesis in both initiation and post-initiation phases (reviewed in Perše, 2010). Epidemiological reports investigating the effect of n-3 PUFA on CRC are scarce. However, some studies have shown that an n-3 PUFA-rich diet suppressed the risk of colon cancer in humans. The preventive or inhibitory effect of n-3 PUFA on experimental colon carcinogenesis has been widely evaluated (Biondo et al., 2008). All these results suggest that the composition of ingested dietary fatty acids is a more critical risk factor than the total amount of fat. This is further supported by their different mode of action, which is described in the following section.

However, at the same time, it is worth emphasizing that studies on animal models have shown that the promoting effects of SFA and n-6 PUFA on CRC can be modified by various dietary factors. A relatively small fraction of n-3 PUFA (25%) in total dietary fat or supplemental calcium or antioxidants, such as vitamin D (Pence & Buddingh, 1988), vitamin A (Delage et al., 2004), as well as green tea, vitamin B6 (Ju et al., 2003) and poliphenolic extract of red wine (Femia et al., 2005), have shown an appreciable beneficial effect in lowering the risk of CRC in animal models on a high fat diet. The influence of different amounts of calcium, antioxidants and other beneficial compounds in combination with dietary lipids may therefore be complex and difficult to elucidate, particularly in epidemiological investigations. Because many dietary, as well as environmental or lifestyle factors such as physical activity, can modify the promoting effects of dietary fat on CRC, results obtained from animal models under standardized conditions may represent an important contribution to understanding the mechanisms of dietary fat involvement in colorectal carcinogenesis (Hoffman-Goetz, 2003).

3.1 Mechanisms of dietary fat modulation

Dietary fats are an important energy reserve in an organism. However, this is not their only function. Linoleic acid (n-6 PUFA) and linolenic acid (n-3 PUFA) are considered essential, since they can not be synthesized by mammals and must therefore be obtained from diet.

Lipids and fatty acids obtained from dietary fats are metabolized and incorporated into the phospholipids of the cell membranes of many cell types and serve as precursors for many biologically active molecules, as well as being important for cell signaling (Jones et al., 2003). It is generally accepted that the balance of n-6 to n-3 PUFA in the diet is of importance to human health and disease, including CRC. An alteration in fatty acid composition in the cell as a result of altered dietary fat consumption may lead to changes in all these functions, which are briefly outlined below.

3.1.1 Effects on the concentration of secondary bile acids

Experimental and epidemiological studies have shown that diets high in beef tallow, lard or corn oil increase the concentration of colonic luminal (fecal) secondary bile acids, i.e. deoxycholic acid (DOC) and lithocholic acid, whereas high dietary fish oil has no such enhancing effect. It has been found and confirmed that these secondary bile acids induce cell proliferation and act as promoters in colon carcinogenesis. Recent experiments have provided new insight into their effects on colonic epithelial cells. The results indicate that secondary bile acid DOC may act as a carcinogen, not merely a promoter (explained in detail in Bernstein et al., 2011).

3.1.2 Effects on energy balance

Energy balance has become an important concept in exploring the etiology of a number of chronic diseases, including cancer, because of its close association with weight gain and overweight - conditions known to increase the risk of many chronic diseases.

The amount of energy that is required depends in part on the composition of the food. In this regard, it is worth noting that dietary fats are more readily converted to body fat and require less energy for transformation than carbohydrates. A high fat diet therefore contributes indirectly to CRC due to increased body mass index.

3.1.3 Effects on immune function

One of the most thoroughly evaluated associations between nutrition and the immune system is that related to dietary fat. Although total fat intake has been found to increase the risk of various types of cancer, it is the type of fat that has a more important effect on the immune response and, consequently, on cancer development. PUFA have been shown to modulate cytokine production, lymphocyte proliferation, expression of surface molecules, phagocytosis, apoptosis and natural killer cell activity (the last two are closely related to cancer development). An increase in n-3 PUFA helps control the production of pro-inflammatory eicosanoids, as well as cytokine production (Valdes-Ramos & Benitez-Arciniega, 2007).

3.1.4 Effects on arachidonic acid metabolism

It has been suggested that dietary n-3 PUFA has an anti-carcinogenic role in reduction of n-6 PUFA-derived eicosanoid biosynthesis and direct inhibition of COX-2.

Dietary n-6 PUFA incorporates into the membrane phospholipids as arachidonic acid (AA), while dietary n-3 PUFA does so as eicosapentaenoic acid (EPA). AA and EPA compete for prostaglandin and leukotriene synthesis. Pro-inflammatory eicosanoids of AA metabolism are released from membrane phospholipids in response to inflammatory activation. EPA is released to compete with AA for enzymatic metabolism, inducing the production of less inflammatory and chemotactic derivatives. Eicosanoids produced from EPA are much less potent (up to 100-fold) than the analogues produced from AA and even have anti-thrombotic and anti-inflammatory properties. The relative amounts of n-6 and n-3 PUFA provided by the diet, and so present in blood and tissues, may thus be of importance in the development of inflammatory diseases and cancers. The production of inflammatory eicosanoids is increased in response to many inflammatory stimuli (Simopoulos, 2002a). When the production of these substances is excessive, it may lead to chronic inflammation and an increased risk of cancer, since inflammation has been linked to the promotion phase of carcinogenesis (Federico et al., 2007). The increased n-6/n-3 ratio in Western diets probably contributes to reduced levels of EPA in phospholipids and, consequently, to an increased incidence of cardiovascular disease and inflammatory disorders (Simopoulos, 2002b).

Another indication of the importance of diet and n-6 PUFA in the induction and progression of CRC may be the upregulation in fatty acid binding protein (FABP)-5 during tumorigenesis, with concomitant inhibition of $\Delta 6$ desaturase activity, which are important steps in the production of AA (explained in Jones et al., 2003). Most AA in the human body derives from dietary linoleic acid (essential n-6 PUFA), which comes from vegetable oils and animal fats.

Animal studies have demonstrated that a high fat diet significantly increases the expression of PLA_2, COX-2 and PGE_2 in colon mucosa and tumors of carcinogen treated rats (Rao et al., 1996; Rao et al., 2001).

3.1.5 Effects on cell proliferation and apoptosis

The expression of Polo-like kinase-3 (PLK-3) results in cell cycle arrest or induces apoptosis. It is significantly suppressed in tumor tissue of the colon but has been found to be unchanged in colon mucosa isolated from rats on different diets. Suppression of PLK-3 was lower in tumors from rats fed n-3 PUFA than those fed n-6 PUFA (Dai et al., 2002).

Dietary corn oil and beef tallow increased BrdU incorporation and decreased apoptosis of the colon mucosa. Long-term (44 wks) high intake of corn oil and beef tallow enhanced cell proliferation through Wnt signaling and modulated the distribution of proliferating cells (Fujise et al., 2007).

High corn oil consumption decreased apoptosis and increased cell proliferation in colon of AOM treated rats (Wu et al., 2004). On the other hand, studies have indicated that n-3 PUFA has an inhibitory effect at least in part due to increased apoptosis in colonic mucosa (Hong et al., 2000; Wu et al., 2004).

3.1.6 Effects on cell signaling pathways

Studies have suggested that different types of fat may be implicated in different cell signaling pathways, rather than at the level of mutations. n-3 PUFA may interfere with Ras activation by decreasing its membrane localization and may thereby potentiate the effects of anti-Ras therapies. EPA and/or docosahexaenoic acid (DHA; another n-3 PUFA) have also been reported to prevent Akt phosphorylation or activation. n-3 PUFA incorporation into rafts or caveolae may alter the distribution or function of raft-associated signaling proteins – reduced epithelial growth factor receptor (EGFR) levels in the rafts, decreased levels of H-ras and eNOS in colonic caveolae. Alterations in raft lipid composition by PUFA have also been shown to displace signaling proteins from rafts in immune cells. n-3 PUFA decreases NFκB activity or expression in cancer cells, as well as monocytes, macrophages and T cells (Biondo et al., 2008). Peroxisome proliferators and retinoic acid–activated receptors (PPAR and RAR, RXR) are key transcription factors regulating gene expression in response to nutrient-activated signals. A high-fat diet containing various sources of fat, such as commonly consumed in Western countries (the majority SFA), induced PPARγ and RARβ expression, concomitant with an increase in levels of COX-2 and β-catenin in colon mucosa of DMH treated rats (Delage et al., 2004). Various fatty acids have different effects on the Wnt signaling pathway (Kim & Milner, 2007). Long-term (44 wks) high intake of corn oil and beef tallow enhanced Wnt signaling. Dietary corn oil and beef tallow increased the expression of cytosolic β-catenin and cyclin D1. Expressions of Wnt2 and Wnt3 in rats fed with beef tallow and Wnt5a in rats fed with corn oil increased, with or without AOM-treatment (Fujise et al., 2007).

3.1.7 Effects on oxidative status

It has been demonstrated that dietary fatty acids affect the lipid content of tissue and the lipid peroxidation process, due to the ratio of polyunsaturated versus saturated fatty acid. A substantial increase in the PUFA content may overcome the protective action of the antioxidant system and increase susceptibility to lipid peroxidation (Avula & Fernandes, 1999). We have recently demonstrated that long-term consumption of an high-fat mixed-lipid (HFML) diet together with physical inactivity significantly increased the production of lipid peroxides in the skeletal muscle (Perse et al., 2009), suggesting that an HFML diet is an important contributor to the development of chronic diseases, including CRC. There is growing support for the concept that an excess of intracellular ROS, results in an environment that modulates gene expression, damages cellular molecules, including DNA, which ultimately leads to mutations (Valko et al., 2006). On the other hand, fish oil has been found to reduce oxidative DNA damage (Bancroft et al., 2003; Wu et al., 2004).

The large intestine is constantly exposed to ROS originating from endogenous and exogenous sources, due to oxidized food debris, toxins and high levels of iron. It has been demonstrated that dietary fatty acids affect the lipid content of tissue and result in differential susceptibility to peroxidation (Kuratko & Pence, 1991; Kuratko & Becker, 1998; Kuratko & Constante, 1998; Wu et al., 2004). It was recently shown that a high-fat, low-calcium and vitamin D diet induces oxidative stress in the colon (Erdelyi et al., 2009).

3.1.8 Beneficial role of n-3 PUFA before or during chemotherapy

Based on considerable evidence showing different beneficial effects of n-3 PUFA, it has been suggested that n-3 PUFA may improve the outcome of patients undergoing abdominal cancer surgery (Valdes-Ramos & Benitez-Arciniega, 2007). Since n-3 PUFA enrichment can affect the physical properties of cell membranes, altering membrane fluidity and increasing the permeability of tumor cells, it has been proposed that n-3 PUFA consumption may modify the influx and efflux of drugs into or out of tumor cells. However, elucidation of mechanisms is essential for ensuring both the optimal efficacy of a drug and for identifying the target level at which to modify the diet or supplement with n-3 PUFA, in order to optimize the benefits to the patient (Biondo et.al, 2008).

4. Conclusion

Evidence that physical activity affects the risk of colon cancer has been provided by numerous epidemiological and experimental studies and reviewed extensively. Although strong evidence exists that regular physical activity is associated with decreased risk of colon cancer, little is known about the type, intensity, frequency and duration of physical activity that is most benefical. Evidence is consistent that both occupational and leisure-time physical activity can affect the risk of colon cancer. Based on the current level of knowledge, it is believed that 30-60 min/day of regular moderate to vigorous intensity physical activity is sufficient to decrease the risk of colon cancer in the general population.

The relation between dietary fat and CRC is less conclusive. Experimental studies suggest that the composition of ingested dietary fatty acids is a more critical risk factor than the total amount of fat. This is further supported by their different modes of action. It has been proposed that the increased n-6/n-3 ratio in Western diets probably contributes to an increased incidence of cardiovascular disease and inflammatory disorders, as well as at least in part CRC. There is increasing body of evidence that the consumption of n-3 PUFA can impact on immune functions, as well as alter gene expression and transcription factor activity in normal and cancer cells. It has also been found to reduce CRC risk and is suggested to have a beneficial role before or during chemotherapy, and even improve drug uptake.

5. Acknowledgement

This work was in part supported by ARRS (Slovenian Research Agency, Program P3-054).

6. References

Abrahamson, P.E., King, I.B., Ulrich, C.M., Rudolph, R.E., Irwin, M.L., Yasui, Y., Surawicz, C., Lampe, J.W., Lampe, P.D., Morgan, A., Sorensen, B.E., Ayub, K., Potter, J.D., & McTiernan, A. (2007) No Effect of Exercise on Colon Mucosal Prostaglandin Concentrations: a 12-Month Randomized Controlled Trial. *Cancer Epidemiol Biomarkers Prev*, Vol.16, No.11, pp. 2351-2356,

Aoi, W., Naito, Y., Takagi, T., Kokura, S., Mizushima, K., Takanami, Y., Kawai, Y., Tanimura, Y., Hung, L.P., Koyama, R., Ichikawa, H., & Yoshikawa, T. (2010) Regular Exercise Reduces Colon Tumorigenesis Associated With Suppression of INOS. *Biochem Biophys Res Commun*, Vol.399, No.1, pp. 14-19,

Avula, C.P. & Fernandes, G. (1999) Modulation of Antioxidant Enzymes and Apoptosis in Mice by Dietary Lipids and Treadmill Exercise. *J Clin Immunol*, Vol.19, No.1, pp. 35-44,

Bancroft, L.K., Lupton, J.R., Davidson, L.A., Taddeo, S.S., Murphy, M.E., Carroll, R.J., & Chapkin, R.S. (2003) Dietary Fish Oil Reduces Oxidative DNA Damage in Rat Colonocytes. *Free Radic Biol Med*, Vol.35, No.2, pp. 149-159,

Basterfield, L., Reul, J.M., & Mathers, J.C. (2005) Impact of Physical Activity on Intestinal Cancer Development in Mice. *J Nutr*, Vol.135, No.12 Suppl, pp. 3002S-3008S,

Biondo, P.D., Brindley, D.N., Sawyer, M.B., & Field, C.J. (2008) The Potential for Treatment With Dietary Long-Chain Polyunsaturated N-3 Fatty Acids During Chemotherapy. *J Nutr Biochem*, Vol.19, No.12, pp. 787-796,

Buehlmeyer, K., Doering, F., Daniel, H., Kindermann, B., Schulz, T., & Michna, H. (2008) Alteration of Gene Expression in Rat Colon Mucosa After Exercise. *Ann Anat*, Vol.190, No.1, pp. 71-80,

Buehlmeyer, K., Doering, F., Daniel, H., Schulz, T., & Michna, H. (2007) Exercise Associated Genes in Rat Colon Mucosa: Upregulation of Ornithin Decarboxylase-1. *Int J Sports Med*, Vol.28, No.5, pp. 361-367,

Campbell, K.L., McTiernan, A., Li, S.S., Sorensen, B.E., Yasui, Y., Lampe, J.W., King, I.B., Ulrich, C.M., Rudolph, R.E., Irwin, M.L., Surawicz, C., Ayub, K., Potter, J.D., & Lampe, P.D. (2007) Effect of a 12-Month Exercise Intervention on the Apoptotic Regulating Proteins Bax and Bcl-2 in Colon Crypts: a Randomized Controlled Trial. *Cancer Epidemiol Biomarkers Prev*, Vol.16, No.9, pp. 1767-1774,

Colbert, L.H., Davis, J.M., Essig, D.A., Ghaffar, A., & Mayer, E.P. (2000) Exercise and Tumor Development in a Mouse Predisposed to Multiple Intestinal Adenomas. *Med Sci Sports Exerc*, Vol.32, No.10, pp. 1704-1708,

Colbert, L.H., Mai, V., Perkins, S.N., Berrigan, D., Lavigne, J.A., Wimbrow, H.H., Alvord, W.G., Haines, D.C., Srinivas, P., & Hursting, S.D. (2003) Exercise and Intestinal Polyp Development in APCMin Mice. *Med Sci Sports Exerc*, Vol.35, No.10, pp. 1662-1669,

Colbert, L.H., Mai, V., Tooze, J.A., Perkins, S.N., Berrigan, D., & Hursting, S.D. (2006) Negative Energy Balance Induced by Voluntary Wheel Running Inhibits Polyp Development in APCMin Mice. *Carcinogenesis*, Vol.27, No.10, pp. 2103-2107,

Coups, E.J., Hay, J., & Ford, J.S. (2008) Awareness of the Role of Physical Activity in Colon Cancer Prevention. *Patient Educ Couns*, Vol.72, No.2, pp. 246-251,

Dai, W., Liu, T., Wang, Q., Rao, C.V., & Reddy, B.S. (2002) Down-Regulation of PLK3 Gene Expression by Types and Amount of Dietary Fat in Rat Colon Tumors. *Int J Oncol*, Vol.20, No.1, pp. 121-126,

Delage, B., Groubet, R., Pallet, V., Bairras, C., Higueret, P., & Cassand, P. (2004) Vitamin A Prevents High Fat Diet-Induced ACF Development and Modifies the Pattern of Expression of Peroxisome Proliferator and Retinoic Acid Receptor M-RNA. *Nutr Cancer*, Vol.48, No.1, pp. 28-36,

Demarzo, M.M. & Garcia, S.B. (2004) Exhaustive Physical Exercise Increases the Number of Colonic Preneoplastic Lesions in Untrained Rats Treated With a Chemical Carcinogen. *Cancer Lett*, Vol.216, No.1, pp. 31-34,

Demarzo, M.M., Martins, L.V., Fernandes, C.R., Herrero, F.A., Perez, S.E., Turatti, A., & Garcia, S.B. (2008) Exercise Reduces Inflammation and Cell Proliferation in Rat Colon Carcinogenesis. *Med Sci Sports Exerc*, Vol.40, No.4, pp. 618-621,

Erdelyi, I., Levenkova, N., Lin, E.Y., Pinto, J.T., Lipkin, M., Quimby, F.W., & Holt, P.R. (2009) Western-Style Diets Induce Oxidative Stress and Dysregulate Immune Responses in the Colon in a Mouse Model of Sporadic Colon Cancer. *J Nutr*, Vol.139, No.11, pp. 2072-2078,

Federico, A., Morgillo, F., Tuccillo, C., Ciardiello, F., & Loguercio, C. (2007) Chronic Inflammation and Oxidative Stress in Human Carcinogenesis. *Int J Cancer*, Vol.121, No.11, pp. 2381-2386,

Femia, A.P., Caderni, G., Vignali, F., Salvadori, M., Giannini, A., Biggeri, A., Gee, J., Przybylska, K., Cheynier, V., & Dolara, P. (2005) Effect of Polyphenolic Extracts From Red Wine and 4-OH-Coumaric Acid on 1,2-Dimethylhydrazine-Induced Colon Carcinogenesis in Rats. *Eur J Nutr*, Vol.44, No.2, pp. 79-84,

Flood, D.M., Weiss, N.S., Cook, L.S., Emerson, J.C., Schwartz, S.M., & Potter, J.D. (2000) Colorectal Cancer Incidence in Asian Migrants to the United States and Their Descendants. *Cancer Causes Control*, Vol.11, No.5, pp. 403-411,

Friedenreich, C., Norat, T., Steindorf, K., Boutron-Ruault, M.C., Pischon, T., Mazuir, M., Clavel-Chapelon, F., Linseisen, J., Boeing, H., Bergman, M., Johnsen, N.F., Tjonneland, A., Overvad, K., Mendez, M., Quiros, J.R., Martinez, C., Dorronsoro, M., Navarro, C., Gurrea, A.B., Bingham, S., Khaw, K.T., Allen, N., Key, T., Trichopoulou, A., Trichopoulos, D., Orfanou, N., Krogh, V., Palli, D., Tumino, R., Panico, S., Vineis, P., Bueno-de-Mesquita, H.B., Peeters, P.H., Monninkhof, E., Berglund, G., Manjer, J., Ferrari, P., Slimani, N., Kaaks, R., & Riboli, E. (2006) Physical Activity and Risk of Colon and Rectal Cancers: the European Prospective Investigation into Cancer and Nutrition. *Cancer Epidemiol Biomarkers Prev*, Vol.15, No.12, pp. 2398-2407,

Friedenreich, C. & Orenstein, M.R. (2004) Review of Physical Activity and the IGF Family. *Journal of Physical Activity and Health*, Vol.1, No.4, pp. 291-320,

Friedenreich, C.M. & Orenstein, M.R. (2002) Physical Activity and Cancer Prevention: Etiologic Evidence and Biological Mechanisms. *J Nutr*, Vol.132, No.11 Suppl, pp. 3456S-3464S,

Fujise, T., Iwakiri, R., Kakimoto, T., Shiraishi, R., Sakata, Y., Wu, B., Tsunada, S., Ootani, A., & Fujimoto, K. (2007) Long-Term Feeding of Various Fat Diets Modulates Azoxymethane-Induced Colon Carcinogenesis Through Wnt/Beta-Catenin Signaling in Rats. *Am J Physiol Gastrointest Liver Physiol*, Vol.292, No.4, pp. G1150-G1156,

Fuku, N., Ochiai, M., Terada, S., Fujimoto, E., Nakagama, H., & Tabata, I. (2007) Effect of Running Training on DMH-Induced Aberrant Crypt Foci in Rat Colon. *Med Sci Sports Exerc*, Vol.39, No.1, pp. 70-74,

Giovannucci, E. (2001) Insulin, Insulin-Like Growth Factors and Colon Cancer: a Review of the Evidence. *J Nutr*, Vol.131, No.11 Suppl, pp. 3109S-3120S,

Hoffman-Goetz, L. (2003) Physical Activity and Cancer Prevention: Animal-Tumor Models. *Med Sci Sports Exerc*, Vol.35, No.11, pp. 1828-1833,

Hong, M.Y., Lupton, J.R., Morris, J.S., Wang, N., Carroll, R.J., Davidson, L.A., Elder, R.H., & Chapkin, R.S. (2000) Dietary Fish Oil Reduces O6-Methylguanine DNA Adduct Levels in Rat Colon in Part by Increasing Apoptosis During Tumor Initiation. *Cancer Epidemiol Biomarkers Prev*, Vol.9, No.8, pp. 819-826,

Howard, R.A., Freedman, D.M., Park, Y., Hollenbeck, A., Schatzkin, A., & Leitzmann, M.F. (2008) Physical Activity, Sedentary Behavior, and the Risk of Colon and Rectal Cancer in the NIH-AARP Diet and Health Study. *Cancer Causes Control*, Vol.19, No.9, pp. 939-953,

Jemal, A., Bray, F., Center, M.M., Ferlay, J., Ward, E., & Forman, D. (2011) Global Cancer Statistics. *CA Cancer J Clin*, Vol.61, No.2, pp. 69-90,

Johnson, B.L., Trentham-Dietz, A., Koltyn, K.F., & Colbert, L.H. (2009) Physical Activity and Function in Older, Long-Term Colorectal Cancer Survivors. *Cancer Causes Control*, Vol.20, No.5, pp. 775-784,

Johnson, I.T. & Lund, E.K. (2007) Review Article: Nutrition, Obesity and Colorectal Cancer. *Aliment Pharmacol Ther*, Vol.26, No.2, pp. 161-181,

Jones, R., Adel-Alvarez, L.A., Alvarez, O.R., Broaddus, R., & Das, S. (2003) Arachidonic Acid and Colorectal Carcinogenesis. *Mol Cell Biochem*, Vol.253, No.1-2, pp. 141-149,

Ju, J., Liu, Y., Hong, J., Huang, M.T., Conney, A.H., & Yang, C.S. (2003) Effects of Green Tea and High-Fat Diet on Arachidonic Acid Metabolism and Aberrant Crypt Foci Formation in an Azoxymethane-Induced Colon Carcinogenesis Mouse Model. *Nutr Cancer*, Vol.46, No.2, pp. 172-178,

Ju, J., Nolan, B., Cheh, M., Bose, M., Lin, Y., Wagner, G.C., & Yang, C.S. (2008) Voluntary Exercise Inhibits Intestinal Tumorigenesis in Apc(Min/+) Mice and Azoxymethane/Dextran Sulfate Sodium-Treated Mice. *BMC Cancer*, Vol.8, pp. 316-

Keighley, M.R., O'Morain, C., Giacosa, A., Ashorn, M., Burroughs, A., Crespi, M., Delvaux, M., Faivre, J., Hagenmuller, F., Lamy, V., Manger, F., Mills, H.T., Neumann, C., Nowak, A., Pehrsson, A., Smits, S., & Spencer, K. (2004) Public Awareness of Risk Factors and Screening for Colorectal Cancer in Europe. *Eur J Cancer Prev*, Vol.13, No.4, pp. 257-262,

Kim, Y.S. & Milner, J.A. (2007) Dietary Modulation of Colon Cancer Risk. *J Nutr*, Vol.137, No.11 Suppl, pp. 2576S-2579S,

Kramer, H.F. & Goodyear, L.J. (2007) Exercise, MAPK, and NF-KappaB Signaling in Skeletal Muscle. *J Appl Physiol*, Vol.103, No.1, pp. 388-395,

Kruk, J. & Aboul-Enein, H.Y. (2006) Physical Activity in the Prevention of Cancer. *Asian Pac J Cancer Prev*, Vol.7, No.1, pp. 11-21,

Kuratko, C. & Pence, B.C. (1991) Changes in Colonic Antioxidant Status in Rats During Long-Term Feeding of Different High Fat Diets. *J Nutr*, Vol.121, No.10, pp. 1562-1569,

Kuratko, C.N. & Becker, S.A. (1998) Dietary Lipids Alter Fatty Acid Composition and PGE2 Production in Colonic Lymphocytes. *Nutr Cancer*, Vol.31, No.1, pp. 56-61,

Kuratko, C.N. & Constante, B.J. (1998) Linoleic Acid and Tumor Necrosis Factor-Alpha Increase Manganese Superoxide Dismutase Activity in Intestinal Cells. *Cancer Lett*, Vol.130, No.1-2, pp. 191-196,

Larsson, S.C., Orsini, N., & Wolk, A. (2005) Diabetes Mellitus and Risk of Colorectal Cancer: a Meta-Analysis. *J Natl Cancer Inst*, Vol.97, No.22, pp. 1679-1687,

Larsson, S.C., Rutegard, J., Bergkvist, L., & Wolk, A. (2006) Physical Activity, Obesity, and Risk of Colon and Rectal Cancer in a Cohort of Swedish Men. *Eur J Cancer*, Vol.42, No.15, pp. 2590-2597,

Lee, I.M. (2003) Physical Activity and Cancer Prevention-Data From Epidemiologic Studies. *Med Sci Sports Exerc*, Vol.35, No.11, pp. 1823-1827,

Lee, K.J., Inoue, M., Otani, T., Iwasaki, M., Sasazuki, S., & Tsugane, S. (2007) Physical Activity and Risk of Colorectal Cancer in Japanese Men and Women: the Japan Public Health Center-Based Prospective Study. *Cancer Causes Control*, Vol.18, No.2, pp. 199-209,

Lunz, W., Peluzio, M.C., Dias, C.M., Moreira, A.P., & Natali, A.J. (2008) Long-Term Aerobic Swimming Training by Rats Reduces the Number of Aberrant Crypt Foci in 1,2-Dimethylhydrazine-Induced Colon Cancer. *Braz J Med Biol Res*, Vol.41, No.11, pp. 1000-1004,

Mai, P.L., Sullivan-Halley, J., Ursin, G., Stram, D.O., Deapen, D., Villaluna, D., Horn-Ross, P.L., Clarke, C.A., Reynolds, P., Ross, R.K., West, D.W., Anton-Culver, H., Ziogas, A., & Bernstein, L. (2007) Physical Activity and Colon Cancer Risk Among Women in the California Teachers Study. *Cancer Epidemiol Biomarkers Prev*, Vol.16, No.3, pp. 517-525,

Mathur, N. & Pedersen, B.K. (2008) Exercise As a Mean to Control Low-Grade Systemic Inflammation. *Mediators Inflamm*, Vol.2008, pp. 109502-

Matsumoto, M., Inoue, R., Tsukahara, T., Ushida, K., Chiji, H., Matsubara, N., & Hara, H. (2008) Voluntary Running Exercise Alters Microbiota Composition and Increases N-Butyrate Concentration in the Rat Cecum. *Biosci Biotechnol Biochem*, Vol.72, No.2, pp. 572-576,

McTiernan, A., Yasui, Y., Sorensen, B., Irwin, M.L., Morgan, A., Rudolph, R.E., Surawicz, C., Lampe, J.W., Ayub, K., Potter, J.D., & Lampe, P.D. (2006) Effect of a 12-Month Exercise Intervention on Patterns of Cellular Proliferation in Colonic Crypts: a Randomized Controlled Trial. *Cancer Epidemiol Biomarkers Prev*, Vol.15, No.9, pp. 1588-1597,

Mehl, K.A., Davis, J.M., Clements, J.M., Berger, F.G., Pena, M.M., & Carson, J.A. (2005) Decreased Intestinal Polyp Multiplicity Is Related to Exercise Mode and Gender in ApcMin/+ Mice. *J Appl Physiol*, Vol.98, No.6, pp. 2219-2225,

Murthy, N.S., Mukherjee, S., Ray, G., & Ray, A. (2009) Dietary Factors and Cancer Chemoprevention: an Overview of Obesity-Related Malignancies. *J Postgrad Med*, Vol.55, No.1, pp. 45-54,

Nielsen, S. & Pedersen, B.K. (2008) Skeletal Muscle As an Immunogenic Organ. *Curr Opin Pharmacol*, Vol.8, No.3, pp. 346-351,

Nilsen, T.I., Romundstad, P.R., Petersen, H., Gunnell, D., & Vatten, L.J. (2008) Recreational Physical Activity and Cancer Risk in Subsites of the Colon (the Nord-Trondelag Health Study). *Cancer Epidemiol Biomarkers Prev*, Vol.17, No.1, pp. 183-188,

Orlando, F.A., Tan, D., Baltodano, J.D., Khoury, T., Gibbs, J.F., Hassid, V.J., Ahmed, B.H., & Alrawi, S.J. (2008) Aberrant Crypt Foci As Precursors in Colorectal Cancer Progression. *J Surg Oncol*, Vol.98, No.3, pp. 207-213,

Pedersen, B.K. & Hoffman-Goetz, L. (2000) Exercise and the Immune System: Regulation, Integration, and Adaptation. *Physiol Rev*, Vol.80, No.3, pp. 1055-1081,

Pence, B.C. & Buddingh, F. (1988) Inhibition of Dietary Fat-Promoted Colon Carcinogenesis in Rats by Supplemental Calcium or Vitamin D3. *Carcinogenesis*, Vol.9, No.1, pp. 187-190,

Perse, M. & Cerar, A. (2011) Morphological and Molecular Alterations in 1,2 Dimethylhydrazine and Azoxymethane Induced Colon Carcinogenesis in Rats. *J Biomed Biotechnol*, Vol.2011, pp. 473964-

Perse, M., Injac, R., Strukelj, B., & Cerar, A. (2009) Effects of High-Fat Mixed-Lipid Diet and Exercise on the Antioxidant System in Skeletal and Cardiac Muscles of Rats With Colon Carcinoma. *Pharmacol Rep*, Vol.61, No.5, pp. 909-916,

Perse, M. (2010) *Effects of Physical Activity and High-fat-mixed-Lipid Diet on the Development of Chemically Induced Colorectal Tumors in Wistar Rat*, University of Ljubljana: Ljubljana

Petersen, A.M. & Pedersen, B.K. (2005) The Anti-Inflammatory Effect of Exercise. *J Appl Physiol*, Vol.98, No.4, pp. 1154-1162,

Petersen, A.M. & Pedersen, B.K. (2006) The Role of IL-6 in Mediating the Anti-Inflammatory Effects of Exercise. *J Physiol Pharmacol*, Vol.57 Suppl 10, pp. 43-51,

Pisani, P. (2008) Hyper-Insulinaemia and Cancer, Meta-Analyses of Epidemiological Studies. *Arch Physiol Biochem*, Vol.114, No.1, pp. 63-70,

Rao, C.V., Hirose, Y., Indranie, C., & Reddy, B.S. (2001) Modulation of Experimental Colon Tumorigenesis by Types and Amounts of Dietary Fatty Acids. *Cancer Res*, Vol.61, No.5, pp. 1927-1933,

Rao, C.V., Simi, B., Wynn, T.T., Garr, K., & Reddy, B.S. (1996) Modulating Effect of Amount and Types of Dietary Fat on Colonic Mucosal Phospholipase A2, Phosphatidylinositol-Specific Phospholipase C Activities, and Cyclooxygenase Metabolite Formation During Different Stages of Colon Tumor Promotion in Male F344 Rats. *Cancer Res*, Vol.56, No.3, pp. 532-537,

Reddy, B.S. (2000) The Fourth DeWitt S. Goodman Lecture. Novel Approaches to the Prevention of Colon Cancer by Nutritional Manipulation and Chemoprevention. *Cancer Epidemiol Biomarkers Prev*, Vol.9, No.3, pp. 239-247,

Samad, A.K., Taylor, R.S., Marshall, T., & Chapman, M.A. (2005) A Meta-Analysis of the Association of Physical Activity With Reduced Risk of Colorectal Cancer. *Colorectal Dis*, Vol.7, No.3, pp. 204-213,

Sandhu, M.S., Dunger, D.B., & Giovannucci, E.L. (2002) Insulin, Insulin-Like Growth Factor-I (IGF-I), IGF Binding Proteins, Their Biologic Interactions, and Colorectal Cancer. *J Natl Cancer Inst*, Vol.94, No.13, pp. 972-980,

Scheele, C., Nielsen, S., & Pedersen, B.K. (2009) ROS and Myokines Promote Muscle Adaptation to Exercise. *Trends Endocrinol Metab*, Vol.20, No.3, pp. 95-99,

Simopoulos, A.P. (2002a) Omega-3 Fatty Acids in Inflammation and Autoimmune Diseases. *J Am Coll Nutr*, Vol.21, No.6, pp. 495-505,

Simopoulos, A.P. (2002b) The Importance of the Ratio of Omega-6/Omega-3 Essential Fatty Acids. *Biomed Pharmacother*, Vol.56, No.8, pp. 365-379,

Slattery, M.L. & Potter, J.D. (2002) Physical Activity and Colon Cancer: Confounding or Interaction? *Med Sci Sports Exerc*, Vol.34, No.6, pp. 913-919,

Souglakos, J. (2007) Genetic Alterations in Sporadic and Hereditary Colorectal Cancer: Implementations for Screening and Follow-Up. *Dig Dis*, Vol.25, No.1, pp. 9-19,

Steinberg, G.R. (2007) Inflammation in Obesity Is the Common Link Between Defects in Fatty Acid Metabolism and Insulin Resistance. *Cell Cycle*, Vol.6, No.8, pp. 888-894,

Tammariello, A.E. & Milner, J.A. (2010) Mouse Models for Unraveling the Importance of Diet in Colon Cancer Prevention. *J Nutr Biochem*, Vol.21, No.2, pp. 77-88,

Thorling, E.B., Jacobsen, N.O., & Overvad, K. (1994) The Effect of Treadmill Exercise on Azoxymethane-Induced Intestinal Neoplasia in the Male Fischer Rat on Two Different High-Fat Diets. *Nutr Cancer*, Vol.22, No.1, pp. 31-41,

Thune, I. & Furberg, A.S. (2001) Physical Activity and Cancer Risk: Dose-Response and Cancer, All Sites and Site-Specific. *Med Sci Sports Exerc*, Vol.33, No.6 Suppl, pp. S530-S550,

Valdes-Ramos, R. & Benitez-Arciniega, A.D. (2007) Nutrition and Immunity in Cancer. *Br J Nutr*, Vol.98 Suppl 1, pp. S127-S132,

Valko, M., Leibfritz, D., Moncol, J., Cronin, M.T., Mazur, M., & Telser, J. (2007) Free Radicals and Antioxidants in Normal Physiological Functions and Human Disease. *Int J Biochem Cell Biol*, Vol.39, No.1, pp. 44-84,

Valko, M., Rhodes, C.J., Moncol, J., Izakovic, M., & Mazur, M. (2006) Free Radicals, Metals and Antioxidants in Oxidative Stress-Induced Cancer. *Chem Biol Interact*, Vol.160, No.1, pp. 1-40,

Wolin, K.Y., Yan, Y., Colditz, G.A., & Lee, I.M. (2009) Physical Activity and Colon Cancer Prevention: a Meta-Analysis. *Br J Cancer*, Vol.100, No.4, pp. 611-616,

World Cancer Research Fund/American Institute for Cancer Research. (2007) *Food, nutrition, physical activity, and prevention of cancer: a global perspective.* Washington, DC: American Institute of Cancer Research,

Wu, B., Iwakiri, R., Ootani, A., Tsunada, S., Fujise, T., Sakata, Y., Sakata, H., Toda, S., & Fujimoto, K. (2004) Dietary Corn Oil Promotes Colon Cancer by Inhibiting Mitochondria-Dependent Apoptosis in Azoxymethane-Treated Rats. *Exp Biol Med (Maywood)*, Vol.229, No.10, pp. 1017-1025,

7

Polyunsaturated Fatty Acids, Ulcerative Colitis and Cancer Prevention

Karina Vieira de Barros[1], Ana Paula Cassulino[1] and
Vera Lucia Flor Silveira[1,2]
[1]*Department of Physiology, Federal University of São Paulo, São Paulo, SP,*
[2]*Department of Biological Sciences, Federal University of São Paulo, Diadema, SP,*
Brazil

1. Introduction

Fatty acids (FA) – lipid constituents – are carboxylic acids that can be represented by the form RCO2H. Most often, the group R is a long carbon chain, unbranched and with an even number of carbon atoms and may be saturated or contain one (monounsaturated) or more double bonds (polyunsaturated) (Calder et al. 2002). Fatty acids are often referred to by their common names, but they are correctly identified by a systematic nomenclature. This nomenclature indicates first the number of carbon atoms in the hydrocarbon chain, followed by the number of double bonds, and the position of the first double bond from the terminal methyl group, which is indicated by n-9, n-7, n-6 or n -3 (Figure 1). There are two main families of polyunsaturated FA (PUFA), n-6 (or w-6) and of n-3 (or w-3) (Curi et al. 2002).

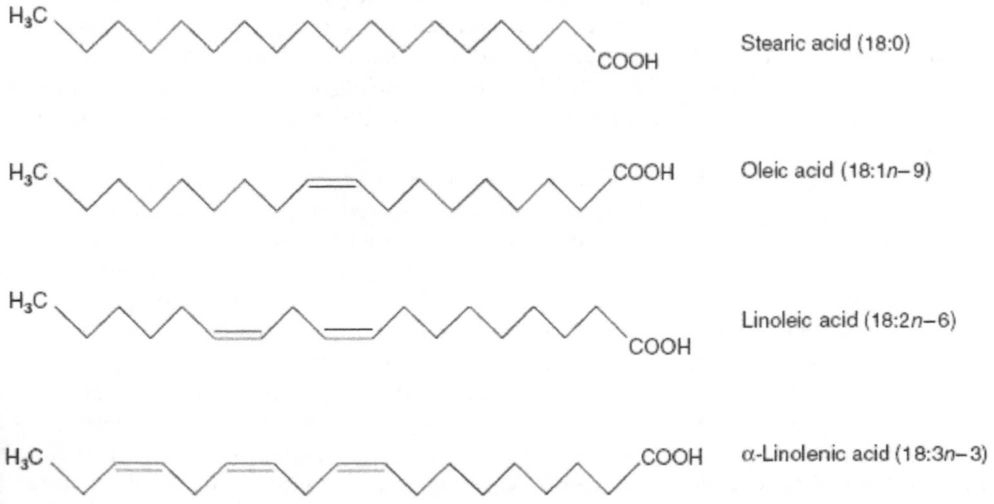

Fig. 1. Structure of some fatty acids (Sala-Vila et al. 2008).

Triacylglycerols (TAG), formed by three FA esterified to glycerol, are the main form of fat present in the human diet. TAG of animal origin are rich in saturated fatty acids and are characterised by being solid at ambient temperature (fats), while those of vegetable origin are rich in unsaturated fatty acids and liquid at room temperature (oils). TAG act as reserve lipids found in the form of oily microdroplets, emulsified in the cytosol (Lanning 1993). In addition to TAG, other lipids are present in small amounts in the diet, such as phospholipids, cholesterol, cholesterol esters and traces of free FA. Phospholipids are the major lipid components of the cell membrane, acting as structural elements, precursors of second messengers, and affecting the activity of some enzymes, such as phospholipase A2 and protein kinase C. Thus lipids, besides being a source of energy (immediate or reserve), act as key components of our body, both in terms of structure (cellular constituents) and function (Burr & Burr 1929, 1930).

Mammals synthesise saturated fatty acids from non-lipid precursors and unsaturated n-9 series and n-7; normally the diet provides adequate amounts of these fatty acids. However, the cell membrane also needs unsaturated FA of n-3 and n-6 families to maintain their structure, fluidity and function measures. As mammals lack the enzyme delta-12 desaturase and delta-15 (found in most plants), which insert double bonds at positions 3 and 6, they do not synthesise n-3 or n-6 PUFA. As such, these FA have to be consumed in the diet and are therefore called essential fatty acids (Semplecine & Valle 1994, Burr & Burr 1929).

The PUFA most commonly consumed are linoleic acid (LA, 18:2 n-6) and α-linolenic acid (ALA, 18:3 n-3). These two FA can be converted to other unsaturated derivatives. Linoleic acid can be converted to γ-Lilolênico (18:3 n-6), Dihomo-γ-linolenic (20:3 n-6) and arachidonic acid (AA, 20:4 n-6) sequentially. Similarly, the α-linolenic acid (18:3 n-3) is converted into eicosapentaenoic acid (EPA, 20:5 n-3) and Docosapentaenoico acid (DHA, 22:5 n-3) (Calder 2003) (Figure 2). The main dietary sources of acids LA and ALA are oils which are rich in polyunsaturated fats. The PUFA of n-6 series are derived from plants found, for example, in soybean, sunflower and evening primrose oils. The PUFA of n-3 series are predominantly found in fish oils and marine mammals, and deep cold water fish, such as mackerel, sardines, trout, salmon and tuna (Connor 1996). This occurs because many marine plants, especially phytoplankton algae, also synthesize EPA and DHA from-linolenic acid-α. This synthesis of long-chain PUFA n-3 by marine algae, and their transfer through the food chain to fish, explains their abundance in some fish oils and marine mammals (Semplecine & Valle 1994).

Up until 1929, the FAs were viewed exclusively as efficient energy storage. Between 1929 and 1930, George and Mildred Burr published articles reporting the essentiality of PUFA. The authors found that the administration of diets completely devoid of fat in rats caused severe changes in relation to growth and the physiological functions of various organs, which were attributed to the lack of long-chain PUFA. Similar changes were observed in newborns undergoing a diet based on skimmed milk and then reversed by the administration of whole milk. These findings led to a systematic study being carried out by Hensen et al. In 1958, it was found that the administration of skimmed milk to infants was associated with diarrhoea and skin abnormalities, among other things. The supplementation of milk with linoleic acid reversed all symptoms. These observations therefore characterise the effects of PUFA deficiency in humans (Hensen et al. 1958, Holman et al. 1998). With the development of parenteral nutrition, which initially did not contain essential fatty acids, it became evident that a deficiency of n-type PUFA-6 caused the death of patients. This led the

FDA (Food and Drug Administration), in 1982, approving the supplementation of parenteral nutrition with PUFA n-6 (Holman et al. 1998).

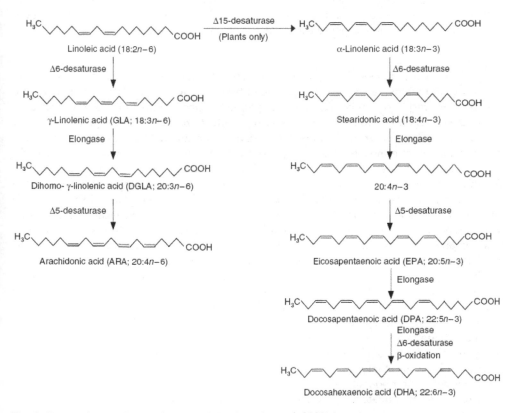

Fig. 2. Biosynthesis of some fatty acids (Sala-Vila et al. 2008)

2. Inflammation and PUFA

The relationship between inflammatory response and PUFA enriched diets has been investigated in recent years. Several studies show that PUFA can modify immunological and inflammatory reactions, and that it can be used as a complementary therapy in chronic diseases (Kinsella et al. 1990, Serhan et al. 2004).

Inflammation is a body's response to tissue injury, which can be triggered by mechanical stimuli, chemical or microbial invasion, as well as hypersensitivity reactions. This response includes complex processes that involve the immune system cells and biological mediators (Rankin et al. 2004). The acute phase response is characterised by increased blood flow and vascular permeability, increased accumulation of fluid, leukocytes and inflammatory mediators; meanwhile the chronic phase is characterised by the development of specific cellular and humoral immune responses against pathogens present at the site of injury (Saadi et al. 2002). Inflammation is characterised by redness, swelling, heat and pain. These signs occur primarily due to: vasodilatation, which allows increased blood flow to the affected area; increased vascular permeability, which facilitates the diffusion of molecules such as antibodies; cytokines and other plasma proteins to the site of injury and cellular infiltration, which occur through chemotaxis and diapedesis and the direct movement of inflammatory cells through the vessel wall towards the site of inflammation. In addition, during the inflammatory response catabolic and metabolic changes may occur, as well as biosynthetic activation in various organs and enzyme systems and cells of the immune system.

The inflammatory response begins the process of immune elimination of invading pathogens and toxins for the repair of damaged tissue (Rang & Dale 1995). The nonspecific inflammatory response can be seen, for example, in the phagocytosis of bacteria or leftover tissue, the secretion of proteolytic enzymes, the production of reactive oxygen species and the secretion of molecular modulators. It can also be immune-mediated, where there is the participation of lymphocytes and antigen-presenting cells. This second type is closely associated with the onset and maintenance of chronic inflammation (Pompei et al. 1999).

The inflammatory process is controlled by cellular and molecular components. Among the cellular components are neutrophils, monocytes, lymphocytes, macrophages fixed, dendritic cells, mast cells and eosinophils. These cells accumulate in inflamed tissues and interact with the endothelial cells of the microcirculation. Different adhesion molecules participate in these interactions, including selectins, integrins and intercellular adhesion molecules (ICAM) (Rang & Dale 1995). Neutrophils constitute 60% of circulating leukocytes and act as the first line of cellular defence, and they may participate in both reactions as a nonspecific defence and as specific antigen reactions (Curi et al. 1997). Monocytes represent approximately 3-6% of circulating leukocytes in human blood, and they migrate to different tissues where they differentiate into macrophages in response to different stimuli. These cells participate in a variety of functions related to the host's defence, the most well known being the phagocytosis of microorganisms and cell debris, and cytotoxic activity against microorganisms, virus-infected cells and tumour cells (Curi et al. 2002).

The molecular components of inflammation include vasoactive substances (kinins, histamine), proinflammatory cytokines (such as Tumour Necrose Factor (TNF), Interleukin (IL)-1 and IL-6), anti-inflammatory cytokines (such as IL-4, IL-10 and IL-13), chemokines, acute phase proteins, bioactive lipids (such as eicosanoids derived from AA), Platelet Activating Factor, diacylglycerol, ceramides, cAMP, and inositol triphosphate, amongst others.

3. Inflammatory bowel disease and carcinogenesis

Inflammatory bowel diseases (IBDs) are chronic disorders of the gastrointestinal (GI), which generally refer to two conditions, namely ulcerative colitis and Crohn's disease (Galvez et al. 2006). IBDs are characterised by chronic diarrhoea, malabsorption, mucosal barrier dysfunction and inflammatory intestinal process, being incurable clinically (Benedetti & Plum 1996). Ulcerative colitis encompasses a spectrum of diffuse inflammation and the continuous surface of the colon, which begins in the rectum and may extend to the proximal level. Crohn's disease is characterised by transmural inflammation affecting any asymmetric portion of the GI tract, from the mouth to the anus (Benedetti & Plum 1996).

IBDs cause nutritional deficiencies, such as calorie and protein malnutrition, and deficiencies in vitamins, minerals and trace elements. This underscores the importance of nutritional therapy in their treatment (Ferguson et al. 2007, Pizato et al. 2005, Razack et al. 2007). Malnutrition is common in these patients, and interventions through adequate nutritional therapy so as to restore the nutritional status have been associated with an improved recovery process involving the improvement of the immune system during periods of the exacerbation of the disease (Razack et al. 2007). Several characteristics contribute to the malnutrition observed in patients: 1) there is a decrease in the oral intake of nutrients associated with abdominal pain and anorexia; 2) the mucosal inflammation associated with diarrhoea leads to a loss of protein, minerals, blood, electrolytes and trace elements. In addition, multiple resections or bacterial overgrowth in the colon can cause adverse effects, such as the poor nutritional absorption of micronutrients: 3) drug therapies can lead to malnutrition. For example, sulfasalazine reduces the absorption of folic acid, and corticosteroids reduce calcium absorption and adversely affect the protein metabolism (Wild et al. 2007).

Although much progress has been made in understanding IBD, its aetiology is not fully elucidated. However, it is believed that there is involvement of immune factors, both genetic and environmental (Laroux et al. 2001, Cheon et al. 2006, Sainathan et al. 2008). Some studies have suggested that IBDs represent an inappropriate and exaggerated response of the intestinal mucosal immune system to normal intestinal microflora – in genetically susceptible individuals – which can be attributed in part to an imbalance between effector T cells (T eff) cells and T regulatory cells (T reg). (Sanchez-Muñoz et al. 2008, Ma et al. 2007). Effector T cells are helper T lymphocytes (lymph CD4 +) and cytolytic T lymphocytes (lymph CD8 +) that are activated during the adaptive or acquired immune response. The helper T cells secrete cytokines, whose function is to stimulate the proliferation and differentiation of T cells, as well as other cells including B lymphocytes, macrophages and other leukocytes (Sanchez-Muñoz et al. 2008, Sainathan et al. 2008). Cytolytic T lymphocytes destroy cells that produce antigens, such as cells infected by viruses or other intracellular microbes. Since regulatory T cells are cells capable of blocking the activation and effector function of T lymphocytes (Abbas & Lichtman 2005), some studies indicate that the suppressive action of these cells is linked to the secretion of immunosuppressive cytokines, such as IL-10 and Transforming Growth Factor Beta (TGF-β). TGF-β inhibits the proliferation of T and B cells, whereas IL-10 inhibits macrophage activation and is the main antagonist of Macrophage Activating Factor and Interferon Gamma (IFN-γ) (Sanchez-Muñoz et al. 2008).

The innate immune response in IBDs also plays an important role. This response is the first line of defence of the immune system, attended by phagocytic cells, natural killer cells, blood proteins, and including fractions of complements and other mediators of inflammation such as cytokines (Abbas & Lichtman 2005). Cytokines are polypeptides – produced mainly by immune cells – that facilitate communication between cells, stimulate the proliferation of antigen-specific effector cells, and mediate systemic inflammation and local roads in the endocrine, paracrine and autocrine (Muños-Sanchez et al. 2008). Dendritic cells and activated macrophages secrete various cytokines that regulate the inflammatory response. Once secreted, these cytokines promote the differentiation of T cells, activating the adaptive immune response (Abbas & Lichtman 2005). The T-helper cells or CD4 + T cells can differentiate into subpopulations of effector T cells that produce different sets of cytokines and, therefore, play different effector functions. The most well-defined sub-populations of effector T cells are T helper cells type 1 (Th1) and type 2 (Th2) (Abbas &

Lichtman 2005, Fuss et al. 2004). IFN-γ is associated with Th1 cells, while IL-4 and IL-5 are associated with Th2 cells. Today it is clear that individual cells can express various mixtures of cytokines, and that there may be many sub-populations with heterogeneous patterns of cytokine production. However, chronic immune reactions are often dominated by either Th1 or Th2 populations (Kampen et al. 2005). These sub-populations show differences in the expression of several cytokine receptors, and these differences may reflect the activation state of the cell, determine their effectors' functions, and participate in the development and expansion of their sub-populations (Abbas & Lichtman 2005). IBDs can cause an imbalance between regulatory T cells and T effector cells Th1/ Th2. The lack of appropriate regulation of T cells and the overproduction of effector T cells are related to the development and exacerbation of IBDs (Muños-Sanchez et al. 2008, Zhang et al. 2005).

Patients with IBDs, particularly ulcerative colitis, are at risk of developing cancer that is 10 times higher than that of the general population, indicating that chronic intestinal inflammation is an important risk factor for developing colon cancer (Gommeaux et al. 2007). Some studies have shown that the risk of developing cancer increases exponentially with the duration of the illness, and the extent and intensity of inflammation in the intestinal mucosa (Burstein & Fearon 2008).

The process of carcinogenesis seems to involve a sequence of events, where the chronically inflamed and hyperplastic epithelium progresses to initially flat foci of dysplasia, adenoma and finally to adenocarcinoma. Uncontrolled inflammation is associated with oxidative stress and oxidative cell damage. During cell proliferation, oxidative DNA lesions induce mutations that are commonly observed in oncogenesis and tumour suppressor genes, such as p53 (Gommeaux et al. 2007, Seril et al. 2003). It is likely that the cells of the colonic mucosa, persistently subjected to oxidizing agents, suffer progressive oxidative damage in their DNA, which can cause mutations in tumour suppressor genes (p53), oncogenes (k-ras) and genes that encode the repair of proteins (MSH2 and MLH1) (Gommeaux et al. 2007). The initiation of carcinogenesis is caused by an irreversible alteration of the DNA through the reaction of this molecule with carcinogenic substances. Thus, mechanisms of carcinogen detoxification, DNA repair, and the elimination of cells that have modified DNA (apoptosis, for example), are important for protection against cancer initiation (Brown et al. 1994). For initiation to occur requires not only the modification of DNA, but also its replication and cell proliferation, so that the original mutation can be fixed. Most human cancers originate from epithelial cells (carcinoma), as these are exposed to carcinogens (in the air or in food) and they are rapidly proliferating (Bartsch et al. 1996). In general, electrophilic substances are carcinogens or are metabolised to carcinogens substancesduring the process of detoxification. Such substances are attracted to molecules with high electron densities – such as DNA bases – which end up calling and leading to the formation of adducts (Bartsch et al., 2006).

The basis of the DNA which is more susceptible to this type of attack is guanine, but the adducts thereby formed have been reported in other bases. Being formed in DNA by specific chemical mechanisms, such adducts may lead to mutations in proto-oncogenesis or tumour suppressor genes, and they start the process of carcinogenesis (Lehman et al. 1994, Kinzler et al. 1996).

It is well established that inflammation facilitates the progression of normal cells to malignant cells, the production of pro-inflammatory cytokines such as TNF, IL-1, IL-6, IL-23 and reactive oxygen species (ROS) and nitrogen (Bartsch et al. 2006, Roessner et. al. 2008).

ROS – which are the cellular consequences of oxidative stress – may cause DNA oxidation, resulting in damage to all four bases and in the deoxy-ribose-molecule triggering the appearance of genetic mutations and initiating colorectal carcinogenesis (Chapkin et al. 2007).

With the large number of cytokines and growth factors released during inflammation, the immune cells and nonimmune cells may influence the process of carcinogenesis (Fantini et al. 2008). These mediators activate NF-kB, inducible nitric oxide synthase, and cyclooxygenase-2-related signalling pathways, which are associated with the delay or suppression of the apoptosis of intestinal epithelial cells and the modulation of angiogenesis (Chapkin et al. 2007, Fantini et al. 2008). Apoptosis – programmed cell death – is the mechanism by which the intestine eliminates cells with irreparable DNA damage, and the inhibition of this response is a characteristic of colon cancer (Bancroft et al. 2003).

The integrity of DNA is vital for cell division, and oxidative changes may interfere with transcription, translation and DNA replication, and may also increase mutations, senescence and cell death (Miranda et al. 2008).

4. Inflammatory bowel disease and dietary fatty acids

Epidemiological studies have been conducted in an attempt to correlate nutritional factors with chronic diseases and carcinogenesis on set. In this context, we can observe in recent years a drastic alteration in dietetic habits, mainly in lipids' composition and contents (Wild et al. 2007), leading to an association with the type and amount of fatty acid intake by diet, and the development of diseases (Figler et al. 2007). Asian countries that have changed from a traditional diet (i.e. high in fish and cruciferous vegetables) to a Western diet lifestyle (i.e. high in red meat and saturated fat), such as Singaporean Chinese (who have had a historically low risk for colorectal cancer), have doubled this risk in the past three decades, after dietetic modification (Stern et al. 2009).

Linoleic acid intake, in western countries, increased considerably in the 20th century, followed by vegetable oil and margarine introduction, which resulted in a significant rise in the n-6:n-3 PUFA ratio in the diet (Calder 2008). The incidence of IBDs is higher in western populations and has increased in developing countries which have adopted industrialised urban lifestyles associated with changes in dietetic habits, including an increased fast food intake with high lipids content (Wild et al. 2007).

PUFA n-6 and n-3 are incorporated in cell membrane phospholipids and can influence immunological and inflammatory responses by modifying fluidity, the antioxidant defence system and the inflammatory mediators (Calder 2008, Kinsella et al. 1990, Simopoulos 2003).

N-3 PUFA, EPA and DHA competitively inhibit AA oxygenation by cyclooxigenase, decreasing the synthesis of eicosanoids from series 2 and 4 from AA, with a concomitant increase in prostaglandin (PG), tromboxanes (TX) from 3 series and leukotrienes from 5 series (Yaqoob & Calder 1995). On the other hand, an excessive amount of n-6 PUFA, in diet poor in n-3 PUFA, can contribute to PGE_2, TXA2 and LTB_4 overproduction – potent inflammatory mediators. Eicosanoids produced from EPA (n-3 PUFA) are, in general, less active in inflammatory process than derived AA eicosanoids (Calder 1996, 1998, Kikuchi et al. 1998).

The inflammatory response is designed to remove the inciting stimulus and resolve tissue damage. However, excessive inflammatory response can cause local tissue damage and remodelling, which may lead to a significant and chronic injury. Therefore, acute inflammation in healthy individuals is self-limited and has an active termination program (Seki et al. 2009). In the past, it was believed that this termination program was a passive mechanism but, nowadays, it is known that the process of the resolution of inflammation is an active and well controlled event. In part, this is due to the formation of newly endogenous mediators that act as local autacoids stimulating proresolving mechanisms (Serhan 2007, Gilroy et al. 2004). These proresolving mediators are derived from essential fatty acids, and include lipoxins (LX) from AA and resolvines (Rv) and protectins from EPA and DHA (Gilroy et al. 2004), that are biosynthesised in inflammatory exudates during spontaneous resolution (Figure 3).

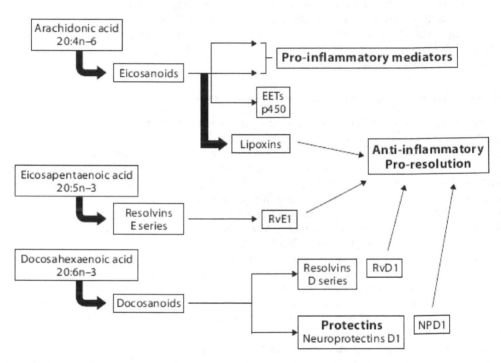

Fig. 3. News inflammatory mediators (Galli & Calder 2009)

The process of the resolution of inflammation has become a topic of interest because of expanding views of their action, particularly in chronic disorders where unresolved inflammation is a key factor leading to colon carcinogenesis. These newly identified LXs and Rvs have proven to be potent regulators of both leukocyte and cytokine production, thereby regulating the events of interest in inflammation and resolution. In light of the existing knowledge of the interconnected pathways of pro-inflammatory mediators (leukotrienes, chemokines (IL8, SDF-1α, MIP-1α, MCP-1,2 etc), and cytokines (IL3, IL6, IL12, IL-1β, GM-CSF, B94, TNF-α etc)), the anti-inflammatory properties of pro-resolving mediators in preventing the chronic inflammation which leads to carcinogenesis requires further study. Clinical trials have demonstrated the beneficial effects of fish oil supplementation – rich in EPA and DHA – in chronic and acute inflammatory conditions (Innis et al. 2006, Simopoulos et al. 2002, Harbige 1998, MacLean 2005). Fish oil supplementation seems to increase apoptosis on top of colonic crypts, where tumours and polyps are usually developed (Paulsen et al. 1997; Courtney et al. 2006, Hong et al. 2005). Bégin et al. (1991) showed that under some specific conditions, long chain PUFA – mainly GLA, AA, EPA, and DHA – are the most effective for inducing tumour cell death. However, this effect depends upon the type of cancer cells tested and the concentration of the fatty acid used.

The role of n-3 and n-6 PUFA on cancer development has been extensively investigated in epidemiological and experimental studies. The contrasting role of these fatty acids in carcinogenesis – n-3 as protectors and n-6 as promoters – remains as an intriguing question in the fields of nutritional and cancer research (Eder et al. 2008).

In rats with colitis induced by Dextran Sulphate Sodium (DSS), our group showed that a normal fat PUFA rich diet, with a balance on the n-6:n-3 ratio, can increase IL-10 cytokine – an immunoregulatory cytokine that influences the immunological system – both on the innate and cell-mediated response, reduce disease activity and the loss of weight, improve the histological score and protect against DNA damage (Barros et al., 2010). IL-10 is considered an immunoregulatory cytokine which exerts effects in both the innate immune response and in the adaptive immune response. IL-10 Knochout animals, for example, develop colitis spontaneously, and 30 to 60% of these animals show invasive carcinoma of the colon between 3 and 6 months of age (Hegazi et al. 2006, McCafferty et al. 2000). These animals have two important characteristics: 1) an increased intestinal permeability in an early age, and before the onset of the disease; 2) the development of colitis, dependent on the microbiological presence in the intestinal lumen. These characteristics suggest that the colitis observed in these animals can develop as a consequence of the high intestinal permeability that increases in the luminal agent's mucosal immune system (Arrieta et al. 2008). Some studies have demonstrated the role of IL-10 on gastrointestinal mucosal homeostasis maintenance. The mechanism by which this cytokine regulates mucosal inflammation is probably multifactorial; however, it is associated with reduced antigen presentation (Hegazi et al. 2006, McCafferty et al. 2000), an increased release of IFN-☐ and IL-12 – a cytokine that inhibits the differentiation of T lymphocytes into Th1 lymphocytes (Rennick & Fort 2000). There is strong evidence that IL-10 promotes the differentiation and the increase of the activity of the regulatory T cells (Hegazi et al. 2006). *In vitro* studies have demonstrated that the administration of IL-10 reduces the release of pro-inflammatory cytokines in lamina propria mononuclear cells amongst patients with Crohn's Disease. In addition, high doses of IL-10 administered intraperitoneally into mice with colitis, induced by Trinitrobenzenesulphonic acid (TNBS), are able to restore the tolerance of the lamina propria mononuclear cells (Duchmann et al. 1996).

Considering the abundance of fatty acids in cells and its susceptibility to oxidation, PUFA are – for the oxidants – more likely targets than DNA (Shimizu et al., 2001, Wagner et al., 1994). It is estimated that approximately 60 molecules of linoleic acid and 200 of arachidonic acid are consumed by oxidants that react with the lipid bilayer. Autocatalytic oxidation triggers a cascade that generates numerous genotoxic substances, and such damage to lipids has important implications for the integrity of DNA (Wagner et al., 1994). The peroxidation of membrane lipids initiates autocatalytic breaks with the consequent formation of cytotoxic and genotoxic metabolites, such as malondialdehyde and hidroxinomenal. The degradation of these products can interfere with intracellular signalling cascades, involving replication and cell death (Eder et al. 2008).

The dietary lipids that are related to the pro-oxidative attack of the colonic epithelial cells may be an important contributor to carcinogenesis (Nowak et al. 2007, Udilova et al. 2003). So far, there is still no specific treatment for IBDs and the best strategy to regulate the exacerbated inflammatory response is to interfere with the multiple phases of the inflammatory cascade with anti-inflammatory and immunosuppressive drugs. These drugs, however, have serious side-effects that limit their use (Stein et al., 2000). Dietary treatment may be an alternative to drug therapy (Camuesco et al., 2005, Nowak et al., 2007).

Although the high intake of PUFA has been related to colorectal cancer, several studies show that, besides the genotoxic effects of lipid peroxidation, epigenetic factors may also be responsible for an increased cancer risk after excessive PUFA intake (Nystrom et al. 2009). Using a model of DSS colitis and a high fat diet (20%), in our laboratory, we did not observe an exacerbation of experimental ulcerative colitis in relation to the diet control group (5%). Besides, the great balance in the n-6:n-3 PUFA ratio (2:1) caused beneficial effects on both pro- and anti-inflammatory cytokine balance and protected the DNA against damage (Barros et al. 2010).

Sasasuki et al. (2010) in an epidemiological study where it was inquired as to whether the intake of n-3 and n-6 PUFA are related to a decreased risk of colorectal cancer development. They found that, in a population with high fish consumption and a wide range of n-3 PUFA intakes, the PUFAs originating with marine consumption may be inversely related to the risk of cancer in proximal sites of the large bowel. On the other hand, Dahm et al. (2010), in a case-control study nested within seven prospective UK cohort studies, comprising 579 cases of the incidence of colorectal cancer and 1996 matched controls, did not find any association between total dietary fat, saturated, monounsaturated and PUFA intakes, and colorectal cancer risk.

5. Polymorphisms

Conclusive evidence between colorectal cancer and PUFA in epidemiological studies may be related to genetic influence. The relationship between genes and the environment has been recognised as central to knowledge of disease and health. During the last two decades, advances in molecular biology have demonstrated that genetic factors determine disease susceptibility, while environmental factors determine whether or not genetically susceptible individuals will be affected (Simopoulos et al. 2008, Paolini-Giacobini et al. 2003). In this context, nutritional aspects are beginning to be considered as one of the most important environmental factors (Simopoulos et al. 2008). Several studies have shown the mechanisms by which genes may influence the metabolism of nutrients, as well as the mechanisms by which nutrients can influence gene expression (Simopoulos et al. 2008, Paolini-Giacobini et al. 2003, Calder 2007). With advances in science, and emphasis on the study of nutrigenomics and nutrigenetics, it has been shown that certain nutrients can influence the inflammatory response, accelerating or regressing the development of many diseases (Heller et al. 2002, Weiss et al. 2002, Mayer et al. 2003, Paolini-Giacobini et al. 2003, Simopoulos et al. 2008).

Stern et al. (2009), from the Singapore Chinese Health Study, through analyses taking into account variants in genes that are relevant for the proposed PUFAs mechanism of action – hypothesised that the genes which play key roles in the pathways that repair PUFA-induced damage might modify the effect of these FA on colorectal cancer. This study also showed that diets high in marine n–3 PUFA were positively associated with colorectal cancer risk

(Stern et. al. 2009). However, using a subset of this prospective cohort, Stern et al. (2009) reported that the marine n–3 PUFA association with rectal cancer is confined to those who carry the PARP codon 762 Ala allele. The PARP protein plays an important role in maintaining genomic stability, apoptosis, and in regulating transcription.

In this regard, some studies have shown that genetic variability in the FADS1-FADS-2 gene cluster, and the encoding delta-5 (D5D) and delta-6 (D6D) desaturases, have been associated with plasma long-chain PUFA and lipid levels in adults (Bokor et al. 2010). Desaturases and elongases catalyse the conversion of PUFAs in humans. The D5D and D6D desaturases are known to be the key enzyme of this pathway. Both desaturases are expressed in a majority of human tissue, with the highest levels in liver, but also with major amounts in the brain, the heart and the lungs. The hypothesis that they play a key role in inflammatory diseases is strengthened by functional studies in mice, where selective D5D and D6D inhibitors showed an anti-inflammatory response.

Several single nucleotide polymorphisms (SNP) in FADS genes were reported in humans, and some showed association between FADS SNPs and fatty acids in serum or plasma phospholipids, and erythrocyte membrane and adipose tissue (Schaeffer et al. 2006, Malerba et al. 2008, Rzehak et al. 2009), demonstrating that these concentrations are influenced not only by diet, but also to a large extent by genetic variants common in the world population (Koletzko et al. 2011).

6. References

Abbas AK, Lichtman AH, Pillai S. Celular and Molecular Immunology, Elsevier, 6th edition, 2007.

Arrieta MC, Madsen K, Doyle J, Meddings J. Reducing small intestinal permeability attenuates colitis in the IL-10 gene deficient mouse. Gut. 58:41-8, 2008.

Barros KV, Xavier RA, Abreu GG, Martinez CA, Ribero ML Gambero A, Carvalho PO, Nascimento CM, Silveira VL. Soybean and fish oil mixture protects against DNA damage and decrease colonic inflammation in rats with dextran sulfate sodium (DSS). Lipids Health Dis. 68:8-14, 2010.

Barstch H. DNA adducts in human carcinogenesis: etiological relevance and structure activity relationship. Mutat. Res. 340: 67-79, 1996.

Bartsch H and Nair J. Chronic inflammation and oxidative stress in the genesis and perpetuation of cancer: role of lipid peroxidation, DNA damage and repair. Arch Surg. 391:499-510, 2006.

Bégin ME, Ells G, Das UN, Horrobin DF. Differential killing of human carcinoma cells supplemented with n-3 and n-6 polyunsaturated fatty acids. J. Natl.Cancer Inst., 77(5):1053-1062, 1986.

Benedett JC & Plum F. Doença inflamatória intestinal. In: Cecil: Tratado de medicina interna, 20° ed, V1, Guanabara Koogan, 1996.

Bokor S, Dumont J, Spinneker A, Gonzalez-Gross M, et al., Single nucleotide polymorphisms in the FADS gene cluster are associated with delta-5 and delta-6 desaturase activities estimated by serum fatty acid ratios. J Lipid Res. 51(8):2325-33, 2010.

Brown K et al. Distribution and reactivity of inhaled 14C-labeled toluene diisocyanate (TDI) in rats.Arch toxicol. 16 (suppl);68:434-43, 1994.

Burr GO, Burr MM. A new deficiency disease produced by the rigid exclusion of fat from the diet. Nutr Rev. 31:248–9, 1973.

Burstein E and Fearon ER. Colitis and cancer: a tale of inflammatory cells and theirs cytokines. J Clin Invest. 118:464-467, 2008.

Calder PC. Effects of fatty acids and dietary lipids on cell of the immune system. Proc. Nutr Soc. 55:127-150, 1996.

Calder PC. Long-chain n-3 fatty acids and inflammation: potential application in surgical and trauma patients. Braz J Med Biol Res. 36: 433-446, 2003.

Calder PC. Immunoregulatory and anti-inflammatory effects of n-3 polyunsaturated fatty acids. Brazilian Journal of Medical and Biological Research. 31:67-490, 1998.

Calder PC. Immunomodulation by omega-3 fatty acids. Prostaglandins Leukot Essent Fatty Acids. 77:327-35, 2007.

Calder PC. Polyunsaturated fatty acids, inflammatory processes and inflammatory bowel disease. Mol Nutr Food Res. 52:885-897, 2008.

Camuesco D, Comalada M, Concha A, Nieto A, Sierra S, Xaus J, Zarzuelo A, Gálvez J. Intestinal anti-inflammatory activity of combined quercitrin and dietary olive oil supplemented with fish oil, rich in EPA and DHA (n-3) polyunsaturated fatty acids, in rats with DSS-induced colitis. Clin Nutr. 25:466-76, 2006.

Chapkin RS, Davidson LA, Weeks BR, Lupton JR, McMurray DN. Immunomodulatory effects of (n-3) fatty acids: Putative link to inflammation and colon cancer. J Nutr. 137:200S-204S, 2007.

Cheon JH, Kim JS, Kim JM, Kim N, Jung HC, Song S. Plant sterol guggulsterone inhibits nuclear factor-kb sinaling in intestinal epithelial cells by blocking IkB kinase and ameliorates acute murine colitis. Inflamm Bowel Dis. 12:1152-1161, 2006.

Connor WE. Omega-3 essential fatty acids in infant neurological development. PUFA Information. 1 (1):1-6, 1996.

Courtney ED, Matthews S, Finlayson C et al. Eicosapentaenoic acid (EPA) reduces crypt cell proliferation and increases apoptosis In normal colonic mucosa in subjects with a history of colorectal adenomas. J Colorectal Dis. 22:765-76, 2007.

Curi TP, Melo MP, Azevedo RB et al. Glutamine utilization by rat neutrophils: presence of phosphate-dependent glutaminase. Am. J. Physiol, 273:C1124-9, 1997.

Curi R, Pompeia C, Miyasaka CK, Procopio J. Entendendo a gordura – os ácidos graxos. Manole, 1ed., 2002.

Dahm CC, Keogh RH, Lentjes MAH, et al. Intake of dietary fats and colorectal cancer risk: Prospective findings from the UK Dietary Cohort Consortium. Cancer Epidemiology 34:562–567, 2010.

Duchmann R, Schimitt E, Knolle P et al. Tolerance towards resident intestinal flora in mice is abrogated in experimental colitis and restored by treatment with interleukin-10 or antibodies to interleukin-12. Eur J Immuno. 26:934-938, 1996.

Eder E, Wacker M, Wanek P. Lipid peroxidation-related 1, N2-propanodeoxyguanosine-DNA adducts induced by endogenously formed 4-hydroxy-2-nonenal in organs of female rats fed diets supplemented with sunflower, rapeseed, olive or coconut oil. Mutat Res. 654:101-107, 2008.

Fantini MC, Palloni F. Cytokines: from gut inflammation to colorectal cancer. Curr Drug Targets. 29:375-80, 2008.

Ferguson LR, Peterman I, Hubner C, Philpott M, Shellin AN. Uncoupling gene-diet interactions in inflammatory bowel disease (IBD). Genes Nutr. 2:71-73, 2007.

Figler M, Gasztonyi B, Cseh J et al. Association of n-3 and n-6 long-chain polyunsaturated fatty acids in plasma lipid classes with inflammatory bowel diseases. British Journal of Nutrition. 97:1154-1161, 2007.

Fuss IJ, Heller F, Boirivant M, Leon F, Yoshida M et al. Nonclassical CD1 d-restricted NK T cells that produce IL-13 characterize an atypical Th2 response in ulcerative colitis. J Clin Invest. 113:1490-1497, 2004.

Galvez J, Gracioso JS, Camuesco D et al. Intestinal anti-inflammatory activity of a lyophilized infusion of Turnera ulmifolia in TNBS rat colits. Fitoterapia. 77:515-20, 2006.

Galli C & Calder PC. Effects of fat and fatty acid intake on inflammatory and immune responses: A critical review. Ann Nutr Metab 55:123–139, 2009.

Gilroy DW, Newson J, Sawmynaden P, Willoughby DA, and Croxtall JD. A novel role for phospholipase A2 isoforms in the checkpoint control of acute inflammation. FASEB J. 18:489–498, 2004.

Gommeaux J, Cano C, Garcia S, Gironella M, Petri S et al. Colitis and colitis-associated cancer are exacerbated in mice deficient for tumour protein 53-induced nuclear protein 1. Molecular and cellular biology. 27:2215-228, 2007.

Hang HP, Dale MM. Farmacologia. 3 ed. Guanabara Koogan, 1995.

Harbidgel LS. Dietary w-6 e w-3 fatty acids in immunity and autoimmune disease. Proc Nutr Soc. 57:555-62,1998.

Hegazi RAF, Saad RS , Mady H et al., Dietary fatty acids modulate chronic colitis, colitis-associated colon neoplasia and COX-2 expression in IL-10 Knockout mice. Nutrition. 22:275-282, 2006.

Heller AR, Fischer S, Rossel T et al., Impact of n-3 fatty acid supplemented parenteral nutrition on haemostasis patters after major abdominal surgery. Brit J Nutr. 87:S95 - S101; 2002.

Hensen AE, Haggard ME, et al. Essential fatty acids in infant nutrition. J Nutr, 66: 565-76, 1958.

Holman RT. The slow discovery of the importance of n-3 essential fatty acids in human health. J. Nutr. 128:427S-433S, 1998.

Hong MY, Bancroft LK, Turner ND et al., Fish oil decreases oxidative stress DNA damage by enhancing apoptosis in rat colon. Nutr Cancer. 52:166-175, 2005.

Innis SM. Essential fatty acids in growth and development. Prog. Lip. Res., 30:39-108, 1991.

Innis SM, Pinsk V, Jacobson K. Dietary lipids and intestinal inflammatory disease. J Pediatr. 149:S89-S96, 2006.

Kampen CV, Gauldie J, Collins SM. Proinflammatry proprieties of IL-4 in the intestinal microenvironment. Am J Physiol Gastrointest Liver Physiol. 288:G111-G117, 2005.

Kinsella JE, Lokesh B, Brougton KS, Whelan J. Dietary polyunsaturated fatty acids and eicosanoids potencial effects on the modulation of inflammatory and immune cells: an overview. Nutrition. 5:24-44, 1990.

Kinzler KW, Vogelstein B. Life (and death) in a malignant tumour. Nature 4;379(6560):19-20, 1996.

KIkuchi S, Sakomoto T, Ishikawa C, Yazawa K, Torii S. Modulation of eosinophil chemotatic activities to leukotriene B4 by n-3 polyunsaturated fatty acids. Prost, LK and Essential Fatty Acids. 58 (3):243-248, 1998.

Koletzko B, Lattka E, Zeilinger S, Lllig T, Steer C. Genetic variants of the fatty acid desaturase gene cluster predict amounts of red blood cell docosahexaenoic and other polyunsaturated fatty acids in pregnant women: findings from the Avon Longitudinal Study of Parents and Children. Am J Clin Nutr. 93(1):211-9, 2011.

Laroux FS, Pavlick KP, Wolf RE, Grisham MB. Dysregulation of intestinal mucosal immunity: implications in inflammatory bowel disease. News Physiol Sci. 16:272-277, 2001.

Lehman TA and Harris CC. Mutational spectra of protooncogenes and tumour suppressor genes: clues in predicting cancer aetiology. IARC Sci. 125:399-412, 1994.

Lehninger AL, Nelson DL, Cox MM. Princíples of Biochemistry, 4th edition, New York, NY: W.H. Freeman and Company, 2005.

Ma X, Torbenson M, Hamad ARA, Soloski MJ, Li Z. High-fat diet modulates non-CD1d-restricted natural killer T cells and regulatory T cells in mouse colon and exacerbates experimental colitis. Clinical and Experimental Immunology. 151:130-138, 2007.

MacLean C, Mojica WA, Newberry SJ et al., Systematic review of the effects of n-3 fatty acids in inflammatory bowel disease. Am J Clin Nutr. 82:611-9, 2005.

McCafferty DM, Sihota E, Muscara M, Wallace JL, Sharkey KA, Kubes P. Spontaneously developing chronic colitis in IL-10/iNOS double-deficient mice. Am J Physiol Gastrointest Liver Physiol. 279:G90-G99, 2000.

Malerba G, Schaeffer L, Xumerle L, et al. SNPs of the FADS gene cluster are associated with polyunsaturated fatty acids in a cohort of patients with cardiovascular disease. Lipids, 2008.

Mayer K, Gokorsc S, Fegbeutel C, Hattar K et al. Parenteral nutrition with fish oil modulates cytokine response in patients with sepsis. Am J Resp Crit Care Med. 167:1321-1328, 2003.

McCafferty DM, Sihota E, Muscara M, Wallace JL, Sharkey KA, Kubes P. Spontaneously developing chronic colitis in IL-10/iNOS double-deficient mice. Am J Physiol Gastrointest Liver Physiol. 279:G90-G99, 2000.

Miranda DC, Arçari DP, Pedrazolli Jr, Carvalho PO, Cerutti SM, Bastos DHM, Ribeiro ML. Protective effects of mate tea (Ilex paraguariensis) on H2O2-induced DNA damage and DNA repais in mice. Mutagenesis. 23:261-5, 2008.

Nowak J, W, Weylandt KH, Habbel P, Wang J, Dignass A, Glickman J, Kang J. Colitis-associated colon tumorigenesis is suppressed in transgenic mice rich in endogenous n-3 fatty acids. Carcinogenesis. 28:1991-1995, 2007.

Nystrom M & Mutanen M. Diet and epigenetics in colon cancer. World J Gastroenterol, 15:257-63, 2009.

Paoloni-Giacobino A, Grimble R, and Pichard C. Genomic interactions with disease and nutrition. Clin Nutr. 22:507-514, 2003.

Paulsen JE, Elvsaas IK, Steffensen IL, Alexander J. A fish oil derived concentrate enriched in eicosapentaenoic and docosahexaenoic acid as ethyl ester suppresses the formation and growth of intestinal polyps in the min mouse. Carcinogenesis 18:1905-10, 1997.

Pizato N, Bonatto S, Yamazaki RK, Aikawa J, et al., Ratio of n-6 to n-3 fatty acids in the diet affects tumour growth and cachexia in Walker 256 tumour-bearing rats. Nutrition and cancer. 53:194-201, 2005.

Pompéia C, Lopes LR, Miyasaka CK, Procópio J, Sannomiya P. Effect of fatty acids on leukocyte function. Med. Res. 33 (11): 1255-68, 1999.

Razack R, Seidner DL. Nutrition in inflammatory bowel disease. Curr Opin Gastroenterol. 23:400-405, 2007.

Rankin Ja. Biological mediators of acute inflammation. AACN Clin Issues. 15(1): 3-17, 2004.

Rennick DM, Fort MM. Lessons from genetically engineered animal models. XII. IL-10-deficient (IL-10(-/-) mice and intestinal inflammation. Am J Physiol Gastrointest Liver Physiol. 278:829-33, 2000.

Ribeiro ML, Priolli DG, Miranda DC, Arçari DP, Pedrazzoli J, Martinez CAR. Analysis of oxidative DNA damage in patients with colorectal cancer. Clinical Colorectal Cancer. 267-272, 2008.

Roessner A, Kuester D, Malfertheiner P, Schneider-Stock. Oxidative stress in ulcerative colitis-associated carcinogenesis. Pathology - Research and Practices. 204:511-524, 2008.

Rzehak P, Heinrich J, Klopp N, et al., Evidence for an association between genetic variants of the fatty acid desaturase 1 fatty acid desaturase 2 (FADS1 FADS2) gene cluster and the fatty acid composition of erythrocyte membranes. Br J Nutr. 101:20-6, 2009.

Saadi S, Wrenshall LE, Platt JL. Regional manifestations and control of the immune system. FASEB J. 16(8):849-56. 2002.

Sainathan SK, Hanna EM, Gong Q et al., Granulocyte macrophage colony-stimulating factor ameliorates DSS-induced experimental colitis. Inflamm Bowel Dis. 14:88-98, 2008.

Sala-Vila A, Miles E.A, Calder PC. Fatty acid composition abnormalities in atopic disease: evidence explored and role in the disease process examined. Clinical and Experimental Allergy, 38:1432–1450, 2008.

Sanchez-Muñoz F, Dominguez-Lopes A, Yamamoto-Furusho JK. Role of cytokines in inflammatory bowel disease. World J Gastroenterol. 21:4280-4288, 2008.

Sasazuki S, Inoue M, Iwasaki M, et al., Intake of n-3 and n-6 polyunsaturated fatty acids and development of colorectal cancer by subsite: Japan Public Health Center–based prospective study. Int. J. Cancer. 000: 000–000, 2010.

Schaeffer L, Gohlke H, Muller M, et al., Common genetic variants of the FADS1 FADS2 gene cluster and their reconstructed haplotypes are associated with the fatty acid composition in phospholipids. Human Molecular Genetics. 15 (11):1745-1756, 2006.

Seki H, Tani Y, Arita M. Omega-3 PUFA derived anti-inflammatory lipid mediator resolving E1. Prostaglandins Other Lipid Mediat. 89(3-4):126-30, 2009.

Semplecine A and Valle R. Fish oils and their possible role in the treatment of cardiovascular diseases., Pharmac Ther. 61: 385-387, 1994.

Serhan, C.N. A search for endogenous mechanisms of anti-inflammation uncovers novel chemical mediators: missing links to resolution. Histochem Cell Biol. 122:305-321, 2004.

Serhan CN. Resolution phases of inflammation: novel endogenous anti-inflammatory and pro-resolving lipid mediators and pathways. Annu. Rev. Immunol. 25:101–137, 2007.

Serhan CN, Arita M, Hong S, Gotlinger K. Resolvins, docosatrienes, and neuroprotectins, novel omega-3-derived mediators, and their endogenous aspirin-triggered epimers. Lipids. 39:1125–32, 2004.

Seril DN, Liao J, Yang GY, Yang CS. Oxidative stress and ulcerative colitis-associated carcinogenesis: studies in humans and animal models. Carcinogenesis. 24:353-62, 2003.

Shimizu T, Igarashi J, Ohtuka Y, Oguchi S, Kaneko K, Yamashiro Y. Effects of n-3 polyunsaturated fatty acids and vitamin E on colonic mucosal leukotriene generation, lipid peroxidation, and microcirculation in rats with experimental colitis. Digestion. 63:49-54, 2001.

Simopoulos AP. Importance of the ratio of omega-6/omega-3 essential fatty acids: evolutionary aspects. World Rev Nutr Diet. 92:1-22, 2003.

Simopoulos AP. Omega-3 fatty acids in inflammation and autoimmune diseases. J Am Coll Nutr. 21:495-505, 2002.

Simopoulos AP. The importance of the omega-6/omega-3 fatty acid ratio in cardiovascular disease and other chronic diseases. ExpBiolMed(Maywood). 233:674–88, 2008.

Stein RB, Hanauer SB. Comparative tolerability of treatments for inflammatory bowel disease. Drug Saf. 23:429-48, 2000.

Stern MC, Butler LM, Corral R, et al., Polyunsaturated Fatty Acids, DNA Repair Single Nucleotide Polymorphisms and Colorectal Cancer in the Singapore Chinese Health Study. J Nutrigenet Nutrigenomics. 2:273–279, 2009.

Udilova N, Jurck D, Marian B et al., Induction of peroxidation in biomembranes by dietary oil components. Food and chemical toxicology. 41:1481- 1489, 2003.

Wagner BA; Buettner GR and Burns. Free radical-mediated lipid peroxidation in cells: oxidizability is a function of cell lipid bis-allylic hydrogen content. Biochemistry. 33:4449, 1994.

Weiss G, Meyer F, Mathies B, Pross M, et al., Immunomodulation by perioperative administration of n-3 fatty acids. Brit J Nutr. 87:S89-S94, 2002.

Wild GE, Drozdowski L et al., Nutritional modulation of the inflammatory response in inflammatory bowel disease – from the molecular to the integrative to the clinical. World J Gastroenterol. 13:1-7, 2007.

YaqooB P & Calder PC. Effects of dietary lipid manipulation upon inflammatory mediator production murine macrophages. Cellular Immunology. 163: 120-128, 1996.

Zhang P, Smith R, Chapkin RS, McMurray DN. Dietary (n-3) polyunsaturated fatty acids modulates murine Th1/Th2 balance toward the pole by supression of Th1 development. J Nutr. 135:1745-1751, 2005.

8

Dietary Anthocyanins: Impact on Colorectal Cancer and Mechanisms of Action

Federica Tramer[1], Spela Moze[2], Ayokunle O. Ademosun[3],
Sabina Passamonti[1] and Jovana Cvorovic[4]
[1]University of Trieste,
[2]University of Ljubljana,
[3]Federal University of Technology, Ondo State,
[4]University of Trieste,
[1,4]Italy
[2]Slovenia
[3]Nigeria

1. Introduction

Colorectal cancer is the third most common malignancy in males and the second most common in females, with significant variations in the worldwide distribution, and remains among four leading causes of cancer deaths overall, shows global cancer statistics. The highest incident rates are found in economically developed countries, whereas the lowest rates are noted in Africa and South-Central (Jemal et al., 2011). However, striking increase in colorectal cancer incident trends is observed in areas historically at low risk, such as Spain and some Eastern European (the Czech Republic and Slovakia) and Eastern Asian countries (Japan). On the other hand, generally high incident rates over the past several decades are going down in the Unites States (Center et al., 2009). These recent "perturbations" in colorectal cancer trends probably result from a combination of risk factors, including obesity, sedentary lifestyle, increased prevalence of smoking, excessive alcohol consumption and "westernization" in dietary habits - a diet rich in red and processed meat and low intake of fruits and vegetables (Center et al., 2009; Chao et al., 2005; Jemal et al., 2011). Decreasing incident and mortality rates are mainly associated with colorectal cancer screening and improved treatment.

Prognosis of these patients depends on the stage of the cancer at diagnosis. As the AJCC (American Joint Committee on Cancer) stage increases from stage I to stage IV, the 5-year overall survival rates decrease dramatically, reaching 90% if the disease is detected early when still localized, though just 39% of colorectal cancers are found at this stage. Almost 25% of patients have a metastatic disease at diagnosis, with a 5-year survival of less than 10% (Goldberg et al., 2007). The primary treatment for colorectal cancer is surgical resection. More than two-thirds of patients undergo radical surgery, but 30-50% of patients who present with stage II or III tumors ultimately experience disease recurrence and distant metastases (Rodriguez-Moranta et al., 2006). Although a broader base of treatment options for metastatic colorectal cancer (mCRC) has evolved in recent years, 50 - 70% of mCRC patients still cannot be subjected to radical resection of metastases and are candidates for palliative therapy only (Fornaro et al., 2010).

The drugs commonly used to treat mCRC are fluoropyrimidines (fluorouracil and capecitabine), irinotecan – a semisynthetic derivative of the natural alkaloid camptothecin, and oxaliplatin – a diaminocyclohexane platinum compound. More recently, two monoclonal antibodies have been approved for the treatment of advanced stages of colorectal cancer. Bevacizumab, a humanized monoclonal antibody against vascular endothelial growth factor (VEGF), is broadly used in combination with fluoropyrimidine-based chemotherapy. Cetuximab, a chimeric monoclonal antibody against the epidermal growth factor receptor (EGFR), is used as monotherapy or together with irinotecan in irinotecan-resistant patients (Hess et al., 2010; Tol and Punt, 2010; Van Cutsem et al., 2009). These chemotherapy agents have significantly improved the prognoses and median overall survival. However, chemotherapy drug resistance occurs in nearly all patients and remains the most frequent cause of treatment failure (Candeil et al., 2004; Dallas et al., 2009), calling for finding novel agents capable of killing drug-resistant colorectal cancer cells.

2. Dietary compounds and cancer

2.1 Cancer prevention by diet

The possibility that fruit and vegetables might help to reduce the risk for various types of cancer raised great interest already in the 1970s. The first studies conducted to assess differences in cancer rates and diet between countries suggested that various dietary factors might have important effects on cancer risk (Armstrong and Doll, 1975; Bjelke, 1975).

In 1992, an epidemiological research with 156 studies on connection between the consumption of fruit and vegetables and cancer concluded that persons with a low fruit and vegetable intake face up to twice the risk of developing cancer compared to those with a high intake (Block et al., 1992). Several years later, a joint report by the World Cancer Research Fund together with the American Institute of Cancer Research found 'convincing' evidence that a high fruit and vegetable intake would reduce cancer of the colon and rectum (AIRC, 1997).

Unfortunately, 10 years later, an updated report released by the same organization and based on large prospective studies instead on case-control studies, downgraded these previous conclusions. The evidence that high intakes of fruit and/or vegetables decrease the risk for cancers of the mouth and pharynx, esophagus, stomach, colorectum and lung were judged 'probable' or 'limited- suggestive', so researchers did not confirm the earlier results (AIRC, 2007).

In a randomized dietary intervention trial, called The Polyp Prevention Trial, it was examined the effectiveness of a low-fat, high-fiber, high-fruit, and high-vegetable diet on adenoma recurrence. This study was the first to examine the association between flavonoid intake and colorectal adenoma recurrence. It was found that total flavonoid intake was not associated with colorectal adenoma recurrence, but they also detected during the trial a reduced risk of advanced adenoma recurrence with greater flavonol consumption (Bobe et al., 2008).

The European Prospective Investigation into Cancer and Nutrition in 2009 suggested that a high consumption of fruit and vegetables is associated with a reduced risk of CRC, especially of colon cancer but differs according to smoking status. An inverse association for never and former smokers and a statistically non significant positive association for current smokers was observed (van Duijnhoven et al., 2009).

Key, on the other hand, by summarizing data recorded from large prospective studies or pooled analyses, recommended a diet which contains moderate amounts of fruit and vegetables in order to prevent deficiencies of any nutrients. Nevertheless, the available data suggest that, at least in relatively well-nourished populations, general increases in fruit and vegetable intake would not have much effect on cancer rates (Key, 2011).

Due, at least in part, to their anti-oxidant and anti-inflammatory activities, epidemiologic studies suggest that the consumption of anthocyanins lowers the risk of cardiovascular disease, diabetes, arthritis and cancer (Prior and Wu, 2006). Their activities are associated to their action at different molecular level: direct ability to scavenge reactive oxygen species (Wang and Jiao, 2000) or to induce phase II antioxidant and detoxifying enzymes (Shih et al., 2005; Shih et al., 2007).

2.2 Dietary compounds and tumor progression

Cancer cells differ from normal cells due to the following properties: unlimited replication potential, the absence of apoptosis, the absence of telomere shortening, angiogenesis and metastasis. Dietary compounds have been shown to affect molecular events involved in the initiation, promotion and progression of cancer, thereby inhibiting carcinogenesis. Furthermore, their inhibitory activity may ultimately suppress the final steps of carcinogenesis as well, namely angiogenesis and metastasis. The relationship between the frequency of consumption of vegetables and fruit and cancer risk is linked to a class of phytochemicals which flavonoids belong to.

The unlimited replication potential of cancer cells is a result of the inactivation of tumour suppressor genes. For instance, mutated p21 gene products are no longer able to bind to cyclin, thus cyclin-dependent kinase remains active and cell division becomes uncontrolled. Targeting these protein kinases using natural products has been seen as a promising approach in solving the cancer menace (Omura et al., 1995; Yasuzawa et al., 1986). Although research on protein kinases is still at an early stage, there is enough evidence that dietary compounds have useful potency and specificity against protein kinases of medicinal importance.

Resveratol has been shown by numerous reports to inhibit cell proliferation through the inhibition of cell-cycle progression at different stages (Aggarwal and Shishodia, 2006; Liang et al., 2003; Takagaki et al., 2005). Down-regulation of the cyclin D1/Cdk4 complex by resveratrol has been reported in colon cancer cell lines (Wolter et al., 2001) as well as resveratrol-induced G2 arrest through the inhibition of Cdk7 and Cdc2 kinases in colon carcinoma HT-29cells (Liang et al., 2003). Furthermore, an anthocyanin-rich extract caused cell cycle arrest and increased expression of the p27kip1 and p21WAF1/Cip1 genes and a 60% cancer cell growth inhibition (Malik et al., 2003).

Abnormalities in the ubiquitin-proteasome system have been implicated in many protein degradation disorders, including several types of cancer. This has made the proteasome an important target for anti-cancer drug discovery. Proteasome inhibitors can be categorized as synthetic and natural, where natural molecules are often more specific and potent than synthetic ones (D'Alessandro et al., 2009). Chen and colleagues showed that dietary flavonoids apigenin and quercetin inhibit proteasome, and this inhibition may contribute to their cancer-preventative effects (Chen et al., 2005). Furthermore, Kazi and colleagues also showed that the tumor cell apoptosis-inducing ability of genistein (a soy flavonoid) is associated with its inhibition of proteosome activity (Kazi et al., 2003).

Apoptosis is triggered when normal cells are worn out. In cancer cells, the telomerase activity allows them to evade apoptosis by stabilizing and elongating telomeres through synthesis of de novo telomeric DNA (Naasani et al., 2003). Telomerase activity has been identified in most human tumors (Kim et al., 1994). A high telomerase activity has been linked to the degree of malignancy and likelihood of tumor progression (Fujiwara et al., 2000; Hiyama et al., 1995). Tea catechins, especially the degradation products of epigallocatechin gallate, epicatechin, quercetin, naringin and naringinin, have been found to inhibit telomerase activity (Naasani et al., 1998).

Angiogenesis, one of the hallmarks of cancer, vital to tumor growth and metastasis, is characterized by growth of new capillaries from preexisting vessels (Folkman, 1995). Cancer cells release vascular epithelial growth factor (VEGF), an angiogenic cytokine which stimulates blood vessel growth. Inhibition of VEGF has therefore become a primary target for anti-angiogenic strategies, and inhibitors directed against either VEGF or its receptor VEGFR-2, have been demonstrated to prevent vascularization and growth of a large number of experimental tumor types (Labrecque et al., 2005; Underiner et al., 2004). Ellagic acid (naturally occurring phenolic constituent in fruits and nuts) has been shown to inhibit VEGF-induced migration of endothelial cells (Labrecque et al., 2005). Green tea catechins inhibit vascular endothelial growth factor receptor phosphorylation (Lamy et al., 2002), and resveratol also inhibits vascular endothelial growth factor (VEGF)-induced angiogenic effects in the human umbilical vein endothelial cells through the abrogation of VEGF-mediated tyrosine phosphorylation of vascular endothelial (VE)-cadherin and its complex partner, b-catenin (Aggarwal and Shishodia, 2006; Lin et al., 2003). In addition, the flavonoid luteolin also inhibited both VEGF-induced survival and proliferation of the human umbilical vein endothelial cells (Bagchi et al., 2004). *In vitro* studies have shown that anthocyanin-rich berry extract formula exhibited a potent inhibitory effect on H_2O_2-induced VEGF expression. Anthocyanins suppress angiogenesis through the inhibition of H_2O_2- and tumor necrosis factor alpha (TNF-a)-induced VEGF expression, as well as through the inhibition of VEGF and VEGF receptor expression (Bagchi et al., 2004).

Metastasis occurs when cancer cells invade blood and lymphatic vessels and are transported to other cells and tissues in the body. Cancer cells produce proteinase enzymes that allow them to invade blood and lymphatic vessels. The matrix metalloproteinases (MMP) are a group of proteolytic enzymes that degrade the extracellular matrix (ECM) components (Nabeshima et al., 2002). MMP-2 and MMP-9 are two important MMPs in cell invasion as cancerous tissues and tumor cells have shown increased levels and activities of both MMP-2 and MMP-9 (Bernardo and Fridman, 2003).

Proanthocyanidins and flavonoids from cranberry and other *Vaccinium* berries have been shown to inhibit the expression of MMPs involved in remodeling the extracellular matrix (Pupa et al., 2002). Curcumin inhibits MMP-2, which is implicated in the formation of loose and primitive looking meshwork formed by aggressive cancers such as melanoma and prostate cancers (Aggarwal and Shishodia, 2006). Resveratrol has been found to cause a dose-dependent inhibition of PMA (Phorbol Myristate Aacetate)-induced increases in MMP-9 expression and activity and also the suppression of MMP-9 mRNA expression. Furthermore, Rose and colleagues found that phytochemicals from broccoli and rorripa have anti-invasive and anti-metalloproteinase activities (Rose et al., 2005). Purified ursolic acid and hydroxycinnamate esters from cranberry fruit strongly inhibited expression of MMP-2 and MMP-9 activities at micromolar concentrations in fibrosarcoma cells (Cha et al., 1996). Anthocyanins from mulberry fruits and highbush blueberry (*V. angustifolium*) inhibited MMP-2 and MMP-9 activities (Huang et al., 2008; Matchett et al., 2005; Matchett et al., 2006). Delphinidin can inhibit invasion of human fibrosarcoma cells through down-regulation of MMP-2 and MMP-9, expression (Nagase et al., 1998). More recently, it has been demonstrated that black rice anthocyanins, cyanidin 3-glucoside and peonidin 3-glucoside, significantly reduce the expression of MMP-9 in diverse types of cancer cells (Chen et al., 2006). Furthermore, it was also demonstrated that the activities of MMP-2 and -9 were dose-dependently suppressed by anthocyanin treatment on HT-29 human colon cancer cells (Yun et al., 2010) and in HCT-116 human colon cancer cells through the activation of 38-MAPK and suppression of the PI3K/Akt pathway (Shin et al., 2011).

2.3 Flavonoids

Bioactive compounds that impart protective properties to plants against various pathological conditions are grouped under the name of phytochemicals. Active components of dietary phytochemicals which have been identified to protect against cancer include curcumin, resveratrol, diallyl sulfide, S-allyl cysteine, allicin, lycopene, capsaicin, diosgenin, 6-gingerol, ellagic acid, ursolic acid, silymarin, anethol, eugenol, isoeugenol, dithiolthiones, isothiocyanates, indole-3-carbinol, protease inhibitors, saponins, phytosterols, inositol hexaphosphate, Vitamin C, D-limonene, lutein, folic acid, beta carotene, selenium, Vitamin E, flavonoids, and dietary fiber (Aggarwal and Shishodia, 2006).

Flavonoids represent one of the largest groups of secondary metabolites whose name refers to a class of more than 6500 molecules based upon a 15-carbon skeleton (Harborne and Williams, 2000; Ververidis et al., 2007). They are divided into six major classes: flavanols, flavonones, flavones, isoflavones, flavonols and anthocyanins. Flavonoids are not synthesized in animal cells, thus their detection in animal tissues is indicative of plant ingestion (Mennen et al., 2008). Dietary flavonoids play an important role in cancer prevention and inhibition influencing various cellular processes, such as reactive oxygen species production and cell signal transduction pathways related to cellular proliferation, apoptosis, and angiogenesis (Yao et al., 2011).

Flavonoids compounds are the most studied anticarcinogens among phytochemicals. Anthocyanins, a particular class of this group of molecules, are the most abundant flavonoid constituents of fruits and vegetables (Wang and Stoner, 2008).

2.3.1 Anthocyanins: Chemistry

Anthocyanins (Greek anthos = flower and kyanos = blue) are water-soluble pigments in fruits and vegetables, responsible for red, blue and purple colors. In plant cells, they are present in vacuoles in the form of various sized granules. Their basic anthocyanidin aglycone structures consist of an aromatic ring A bonded to a heterocyclic ring C that contains oxygen, which is also bound by carbon-carbon bond to a third aromatic ring B (Figure 1). Anthocyanins normally occur in nature in glycoside forms. The sugar moiety is mainly attached to the C ring (in the 3-position) or to the A ring (in the 5, 7-position). Glucose, galactose, arabinose, rhamnose and xylose are the most common sugars bonded to the anthocyanidins. These glycosylated forms are known as anthocyanins. More than 500 different anthocyanins have been found, among which the most common is cyanidin

3-glucoside. The most common anthocyanidins (anthocyanins aglycones) found in nature are pelargonidin, peonidin, cyanidin, malvidin, petunidin and delphinidin (Figure 1) (Castañeda-Ovando et al., 2009; Manach et al., 2004; Szajdek and Borowska, 2008).

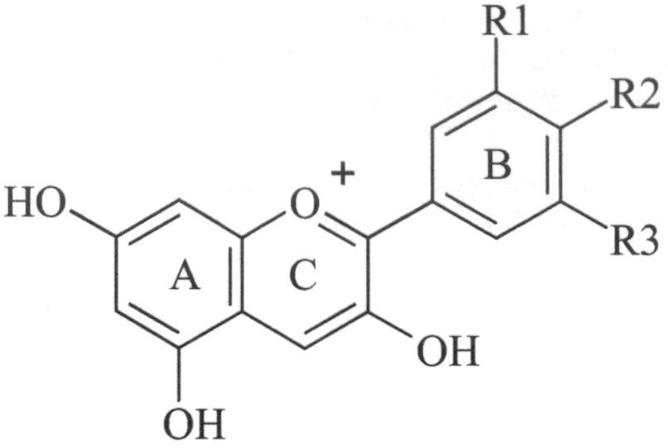

Anthocyanidin	R1	R2	R3
Pelargonidin	H	OH	H
Cyanidin	OH	OH	H
Delphinidin	OH	OH	OH
Peonidin	OCH$_3$	OH	H
Petunidin	OCH$_3$	OH	OH
Malvidin	OCH$_3$	OH	OCH$_3$

Fig. 1. Chemical structures of anthocyanidins (Prior and Wu, 2006).

2.3.2 Fate of anthocyanins in the gastro-intestinal tract

The lack of the knowledge of anthocyanin metabolism in the gastrointestinal tract has been studied by many authors (Aura, 2005; Hassimotto et al., 2008; He et al., 2009; McGhie and Walton, 2007; Vitaglione et al., 2007). The fate of anthocyanins in the gastrointestinal tract is summarized in Table 1.

Part of gastrointestinal tact	Anthocyanin fate
Mouth	Deglycosylation?
	(McGhie and Walton, 2007; Selma et al., 2009)
Stomach	Chemical stability
	(Hassimotto et al., 2008; McDougall et al., 2005) Absorption
	(Felgines et al., 2008; Passamonti et al., 2003b)
Small intestine	Deglycosylation, degradation, absorption
Large intestine	Deglycosylation, degradation (Talavera et al., 2004)

Table 1. Fate of anthocyanins through the gastrointestinal pathway

There are no data of the effect of saliva on anthocyanins but some publications suggest that flavonoid glycosides are hydrolyzed to corresponding aglycons (McGhie and Walton, 2007; Selma et al., 2009).

In the stomach, anthocyanins remain intact due to the low pH that shifts the molecules toward the most stabile flavylium cation. Anthocyanins absorption takes place in the stomach through active transport (including transport carriers such as bilitranslocase (Passamonti et al., 2003b) and sodium dependent glucose transporter (Felgines et al., 2008)) and continues in the small intestine (Talavera et al., 2004).

At the intestine neutral pH anthocyanins exist in equilibrium of four molecular forms (flavylium cation, quinoidal base, carbinol pseudobase and chalcone pseudobase) thus they can be easily exposed to degradation (McDougall et al., 2005). First studies showed degradation of anthocyanins from tart cherries to phenolic acids (Seeram et al., 2001). Later, their degradation was demonstrated by two steps. The first step is deglycosylation of anthocyanins to anthocyanidin aglycon while the second step is degradation of the formed aglycon to phenolic acid and aldehyde (Ávila et al., 2009; Fleschhut et al., 2006).

Deglycosylation is the cleavage of the glycosyl moiety from anthocyanins structure to form anthocyanidin aglycons.

These reactions could take place due to intestinal microflora (Aura et al., 2005b; Ávila et al., 2009; Fleschhut et al., 2006), under intestinal conditions at pH 7 (Fleschhut et al., 2006), or spontaneously in the presence of intestinal epithelial cells (Hassimotto et al., 2008; Kay et al., 2009).

Degradation of anthocyanidin aglycon, achieved spontaneously or by microflora (Ávila et al., 2009; Fleschhut et al., 2006; Forester and Waterhouse, 2008), represents the breakdown of its heterocycle and cleavage of the C-ring to form phenolic acid and aldehyde (Keppler and Humpf, 2005). Spontaneous degradation is a consequence of the neutral pH because anthocyanidin aglycones are observed in chalcone form which is rather unstable and can be easily degraded (Fleschhut et al., 2006; Keppler and Humpf, 2005). Data showed that major degradation products of anthocyanidin aglycons degraded to corresponding phenolic acids (Table 2), as well to some other less present products still unidentified (Ávila et al., 2009; Fleschhut et al., 2006; Forester and Waterhouse, 2008). Further phenolic acids can be transformed to the benzoic acids in the presence of intestinal bacteria by cleavage of the hydroxyl group in the 4-position (Aura et al., 2005a; Selma et al., 2009).

Anthocyanidin aglycon	Corresponding phenolic acid
Cyanidin	Protocatechuic acid
Delphinidin	Gallic acid
Pelargonidin	4-hydroxybenzoic acid
Malvidin	Syringic acid
Peonidin	Vanilic acid
Petunidin	3-O-methylgallic acid

Table 2. Degradation products of anthocyanidin aglycons

The fastest degraded were anthocyanidin aglycons, much faster than anthocyanin monoglycosides (Keppler and Humpf, 2005). As well anthocyanin degradation by intestinal microflora was much faster than spontaneous one (Forester and Waterhouse, 2008).

Anthocyanins that are not absorbed or degraded in the gastrointestinal tract can be excreted as intact forms. Unchanged anthocyanins were detected in human fecal samples 24 hours after blood orange juice consumption (Vitaglione et al., 2007), as well as in fecal samples collected from rats previously fattened by chokeberries, bilberries and grapes (He et al., 2005).

3. Citotoxicity/apoptosis of anthocyanins on colon cancer cells

As mentioned above, naturally occurring dietary substances, in particular, flavonoids, have gained increased attention as agents interfering with processes involved in cancer development and progression. Among them, anthocyanins might be of particular interest since their daily intake is remarkably high compared to other flavonoids - it is estimated to vary between 180 and 215 mg (Hou, 2003) whereas the intake of other flavonoids reaches only 20-25 mg/day. Numerous recent studies indicate that anthocyanins are able to inhibit the growth of embryonic fibroblasts and of different cancer cells derived from malignant human tissues, suggesting their possible role as chemopreventive agents. This brings in focus their possible importance for public health as dietary components with preventive impact on cancer as well as effective, cheap and safe anticancer supplements.

3.1 Cytotoxicity in colon and other cancer cell lines

There are few reports on the inhibitory effects of anthocyanins on colon cancer cell growth. Extracts of grapes, bilberries and chokeberries rich in anthocyanins have been shown to inhibit the growth of human malignant HT-29 colon cancer cells but did not affect the growth of non-malignant colon-derived cells (Zhao et al., 2004). Similar effect was observed in highly and low tumorigenic colon cancer cell lines, LoVo/Adr and LoVo. While delphinidin and cyanidin were cytotoxic and induced apoptosis in the former, they failed to demonstrate a similar effect in the latter (Cvorovic et al., 2010). Anthocyanins from tart cherries significantly reduced proliferation of human colon cancer cells HT29 and HCT-116 as well (Kang et al., 2003; Marko et al., 2004). An anthocyanins extract from Vaccinium uliginosum suppressed the growth of human colorectal cancer cells DLD-1 and COLO205 in a dose-dependent manner through the induction of apoptosis. It was hypothesized that the anticancer efficacy might be attributed to its high percentage of malvidin (Zu et al., 2010). On the other hand, the antiproliferative and the anti-cancer potential of several berry extracts containing different profiles of phenolic compounds (anthocyanins, flavonols, and ellagitannins) was studied in human colon cancer HT-29 cells. All the berry extracts studied decreased the proliferation and the number of HT-29 cells in the G0/G1 phase of the cell cycle. This correlated with their anthocyanin concentration supporting the fact that the inhibitory effect of berry extracts is based on the concentration rather than the composition of anthocyanins (Coates et al., 2007; Johnson et al., 2011; Wu et al., 2007).

Numerous studies reported antiproliferative activity of anthocyanins in human cancer cells derived from malignant tissues of various origins such as breast, lung, uterus, stomach, central nervous system, vulva, prostate (Lazze et al., 2004; Meiers et al., 2001; Olsson et al., 2004; Seeram et al., 2004; Zhang et al., 2005). Anthocyanins were potent and selective in inhibiting human promyelocytic leukemia cell proliferation as well (Feng et al., 2007; Hou et al., 2003; Katsube et al., 2003).

Animal studies have also reported anticarcinogenic properties of anthocyanins. In induced rat colon cancer cell models they significantly decreased total tumors as well as aberrant crypts (Hagiwara et al., 2001; Hagiwara et al., 2002; Harris et al., 2001; Lala et al., 2006; Magnusson et al., 2003). Cai and colleagues demonstrated that Red grape pomace extract (oenocyanin) interferes with adenoma development in the Apc[Min] mouse by affecting tumor burden more prominently than tumor number. Oenocyanin efficacy was accompanied by the decreased adenoma cell proliferation and down-regulation of expression of the PI3 pathway component Akt, which supports cell proliferation (Cai et al., 2010). It was also demonstrated in the same animal model that anthocyanin-rich tart cherry extract added to the drinking water was associated with fewer and smaller tumors in the cecum, but none of the tested treatments influenced the number of tumors in the small intestine or the number or burden of tumors in the colon. It was supposed, therefore, that lack of effect of anthocyanins on colonic tumor development may be a consequence of their metabolism by intestinal bacteria or their spontaneous degradation in the cecal and colonic environment (Bobe et al., 2006; Kang et al., 2003). Moreover, it was shown in ApcMin mice that dietary consumption of anthocyanins in the form of either a mixture (Mirtoselect) or as a pure compound (cyanidin-3-glucoside) interferes with small intestinal adenoma development in a dose-dependent fashion. Authors remarked the presence of measurable levels of anthocyanins in the target organ and in the urine, and in concentrations near or below the detection limit in the systemic circulation. Unfortunately, the dietary dose, at which either agent was significantly efficacious when extrapolated by dose/ surface area comparison, suggested that equivalent for humans can be found in 740 g bilberries, that is a hefty dose. In terms of absolute dose of agent, cyanidin-3-glucoside was less efficacious than the Mirtoselect mixture. Furthermore, authors suggested that different results obtained, in comparison with other studies (Kang et al., 2003) were possibly due in part to the higher dose of anthocyanins employed but also due to the different way of administration since anthocyanins tend to be unstable in aqueous solution at neutral pH (Cooke et al., 2006). Recently, bilberry [(BB),Vaccinium myrtillus], lingonberry (LB, Vaccinium vitis-idaea), and cloudberry (CB, Rubus chamaemorus), rich in anthocyanins, proanthocyanidins and ellagic acid respectively, proved to be chemopreventive as demonstrated by a significant reduction in the number of intestinal tumors in Min/1 mice. Concerning their different chemical composition, authors suggested that the effects seen, may rather be a result of a mixture of compounds acting in synergy than an effect of a single active substance. Moreover, since the cellular levels of b-catenin are increased at all stages of colon carcinogenesis, it was demonstrated that two of these berries, LB and CB, markedly inhibited the growth of the adenomas and accumulation of nuclear b-catenin and cyclin D1. Unfortunately, also in this study, the amount of berries in the diets was high and could not be easily reached in a human diet (Misikangas et al., 2007).

Concerning other tumor models, the incidence, multiplicity and final mass of mammary tumors were significantly reduced in rats that would receive grape juice containing 15 different anthocyanins (Singletary et al., 2003). Cyanidin-3-glucoside reduced the size of lung cancer xenografts and significantly inhibited metastasis in nude mice (Ding et al., 2006). Lyophilized black raspberries prevented the development of NMBA (N-nitrosomethylbenzylamine)-induced esophageal tumors (Stoner et al., 2007), just like anthocyanin-containing pomegranate extract delayed the onset and reduced the incidence of DMBA (7,12-dimethylbenzanthracene)-induced skin tumors in CD-1 mice.

Epidemiological studies in humans are, however, still scarce and contradictory. Biopsies of tumor and normal-appearing tissues in colon cancer patients consuming black raspberry powder daily during several weeks, showed reduced proliferation and increased apoptosis in cancerous but not in normal tissue. Antiangiogenic effect was also observed in these patients (Wang et al., 2007). A phase I pilot study in colorectal cancer patients demonstrated that treatment with black raspberries caused positive modulation of biomarkers of tumor development, including cell proliferation, apoptosis, angiogenesis and Wnt pathway in both colorectal adenocarcinomas and adjacent normal tissues (Wang et al., 2007). In a clinical pilot study twenty-five colorectal cancer patients, scheduled to undergo resection of primary tumor or liver metastases, received different amount of mirtocyan. This is a standardized anthocyanin mixture extracted from bilberries administered daily for 7 days before surgery. In the immunohistochemical observations of colorectal tumors from all patients who had received mirtocyan, in comparison with the preintervention biopsy, the proliferation index, reflected by Ki-67 staining, was significantly decreased by 7%. The apoptotic index in colorectal cancer samples from all patients increased from 3.6% to 5.3% of epithelial cells. However, in the absence of a zero dose control group, authors couldn't determine if this increase could, at least, to some extent, be the consequence of inherent procedural differences in measurements. Nevertheless, the pharmacodynamic changes observed seemed to be more prominent in patients at a dose of anthocyanins, which elicited target tissue levels below the detection limit, than at higher one, which furnished detectable anthocyanin levels in colorectal tissue (Thomasset et al., 2009).

However, an Italian study aimed at investigating the relationship between anthocyanidins intake and risk for oral or pharyngeal cancer did not show any significant association (Rossi et al., 2007). There was no protective effect demonstrated on the development of prostate cancer either (Bosetti et al., 2006). Optimal tumor inhibition occurs when the berry anthocyanins are added to the diet before, during and after treatment with carcinogens, suggesting that consumption of berries throughout life may maximize their chemopreventive effectiveness in humans. The fact that berry diets show a variable effect on tumorigenesis suggests that the inhibitory components of berry extract are not completely absorbed and/or that molecules housed in berry extracts do not affect certain critical signaling pathways of carcinogenesis (Stoner, 2009). Although further proves are needed, these studies open a possibility for anthocyanins to be considered for use in cancer treatment in combination with other therapeutic methods.

3.2 How anthocyanins work – The mechanisms

Antimutagenic and anticarcinogenic activity of anthocyanins is generally ascribed to their antioxidant properties conveyed by their phenolic structure. The double bonds in the ring and the hydroxyl side chains confers them potent free-radical scavenging activities (the positively charged oxygen atom in their molecule makes them more generous hydrogen-donating antioxidants compared to other flavonoids), but also enables their metal chelation and protein binding properties (Kong et al., 2003). Apart from acting as direct free-radical scavengers, anthocyanins have been demonstrated to affect the activity of phase II enzymes well-known for their detoxifying and antioxidant properties and therefore important in cancer prevention. *In vivo* studies showed that the diet supplemented with freeze-dried blueberries or black raspberries, both rich in anthocyanins, led to increased glutathione S-transferase (GST) activity in rats (Boateng et al., 2007; Reen et al., 2006). On the other hand, intake of an anthocyanin-rich mixed berry juice reduced oxidative DNA damage in peripheral-blood mononuclear cells and significantly increased total glutathione (GSH) level and GSH status in whole blood in male healthy non-smoking probands (Weisel et al., 2006). All this speaks in favor of a multi-level antioxidant activity of anthocyanins.

However, numerous recent studies, on the anthocyanins role in tumor growth inhibition, point at their prooxidant properties. It has been shown that the apoptotic effect of anthocyanins in malignant cells could be result of their ability to induce ROS accumulation in these cells. Moreover, the apoptotic activity was directly correlated to the number of hydroxyl groups at the B-ring (Hou et al., 2003). Interestingly, ROS generation was observed in leukemia cells treated with cyanidin-3-rutinoside, but not in normal human peripheral-blood mononuclear cells. Parallel with the accumulation of ROS, Feng and colleagues demonstrated the increase of peroxides, but not superoxides in these cells, suggesting the reaction with the glutathione antioxidant system as one of the possible mechanisms for this prooxidant activity, together with ROS-dependent activation of p38 and JNK (Feng et al., 2007). Similarly, both delphinidin and cyanidin, showed prooxidant activity and induced apoptotic changes and cytotoxic effect in metastatic colorectal drug-resistant cells (LoVo/ADR), but not in cells originating from primary tumor site, Caco-2 (Cvorovic et al., 2010). This "inconsistent" behavior of the anthocyanidins might be influenced by cellular energy metabolism changes associated with neoplastic transformation (Warburg, 1956b). Indeed, the rate of lactate production is significantly higher in highly tumorigenic LoVo/ADR than in low tumorigenic LoVo cells (Fanciulli et al., 2000), and, presumably, in CaCo-2 as well. And even a slight decrease of pH might favor protonation of anthocyanidins, a mechanism causing loss of their free-radical scavenging activity (Borkowski et al., 2005). However, it is not clear if anthocyanidins directly promote oxidative stress in LoVo/ADR cells. One of the possible mechanisms proposed in this study is the interference with the glutathione antioxidant system. Delphinidin and cyanidin inhibited glutathione reductase (GR) activity in LoVo/ADR cells and significantly depleted their intracellular glutathione levels, while failing to induce any similar effect in CaCo-2 cells. These studies give evidence that anthocyanins preferentially kill cancer cells with high malignant characteristics and resistant to conventional treatment regimens, which could set the basis for the development of new sensitizing agents in the treatment of metastatic disease.

4. Biochemical features accompanying cytotoxicity/apoptosis

4.1 Membrane transport of anthocyanins

All the metabolic actions exerted by anthocyanins imply their cellular bioavailability. Previous *in vivo* studies have reported that anthocyanins are absorbed in the stomach and small intestine (Passamonti et al., 2003a; Talavera et al., 2003; Talavera et al., 2004). Felgines and colleagues administered an oral dose of a radiolabelled cyanidin 3-O-glucoside, demonstrating that the major site of absorption in mice is the intestine with a minimal accumulation of the radioactivity in tissues out of the gastrointestinal tract (Felgines et al., 2010).

Intestinal barrier is impermeable to most flavonoid glucosides because, based on their molecular structure, anthocyanins and their aglycones cannot cross the cell membrane passively (Dreiseitel et al., 2009). Among the influx carriers, the hexose transporters SGLT1 and GLUT 5 are expressed on apical membrane of the intestinal epithelium. Different groups suggested that anthocyanins, based on their glycosides moiety, could be transported by glucose carrier SGLT1. However, the involvement of this protein it is not completely understood (Milane et al., 2007; Talavera et al., 2004; Wolffram et al., 2002).

Recently, it was also demonstrated that GLUT2, another glucose transporter, is expressed not only at the basolateral but also at apical membranes of intestinal cells. Faria and colleagues showed that kinetic parameters of ^{3}H-2-deoxy-D-glucose-uptake of GLUT2 are changed after acute treatment with anthocyanins, supporting a favorable use of anthocyanins in diabetic population. Interestingly they also observed an increased GLUT2 expression (not for SGLT1 or GLUT5) after a chronic exposure to anthocyanins speculating that this behavior could increase their own bioavailability (Faria et al., 2009).

Bilitranslocase (BTL) is an organic anions transporter specific for bilirubin, initially found in the membranes of hepatic sinusoidal cells, but present also at the gastric mucosa and in renal tubules (Baldini et al., 1986; Elias et al., 1990; Sottocasa et al., 1989). Some of its substrates are nicotinic acid, bromosulfophthalein, cibacron blue and some flavonoids (Passamonti et al., 2009; Passamonti et al., 2002). Among flavonoids family, 17 anthocyanins showed competitive inhibitory behavior to specific transport assay with delphinidin as the most active molecule (Passamonti et al., 2002). It was also demonstrated that the BTL is directly involved in the vasoactivity of flavonoids: vasorelaxation induced by both, cyanidin 3-glucoside and bilberry anthocyanins, was significantly decreased in aorta rings pre-treated with anti-BTL antibodies (Ziberna et al., 2011). Recent studies have revealed that bilitranslocase is also expressed at the intestinal epithelial level, in particular, at the apical domain. Caco-2 cells express BTL as well and the uptake of BSP into these cells is strongly inhibited by anti-bilitranslocase antibodies (Passamonti et al., 2009).

The results reported should be further implemented to clarify the involvement of the influx membrane transporters.

More data are available on flavonoids efflux transporters. Major interest on these proteins is linked to their involvement in cancer resistance. These proteins belong to the class of the ABC transporters (ATP-binding cassette), and their role in cancer cells is to prevent the accumulation of anticancer drugs. Some ABC transporters are MRP1 (multidrug resistance-associated protein 1, ABCC1) (Cole et al., 1992), MRP2 (ABCC2) and MRP3 (ABCC3) (Borst et al., 1999) as well as BCRP/MXR1 (ABCG2) (Doyle et al., 1998; Miyake et al., 1999) and Breast Cancer Resistance Protein BCRP (ABCG2) however, P-glycoprotein (ABCB1) is overexpressed to the highest level and plays the major role. It was shown that flavonoids interact with these transporters but their effects are often contradictory depending on the type of cancer cells (Di Pietro et al., 2002). Moreover, a different behavior depending on the molecular structure was also demonstrated. Dreiseitel and colleagues showed that, depending on the sugar moiety, some flavonoids can act as BCRP stimulators while others act as inhibitors (Dreiseitel et al., 2009; Morris and Zhang, 2006).

However, the significance of these flavonoid–efflux transporter interactions has not been unequivocally demonstrated since it is impossible to exclude the involvement of other drugs transporters and of intracellular metabolizing enzymes that modify the substrate disposition (Morris and Zhang, 2006).

4.2 Oxidative stress and apoptosis

Reactive oxygen species (ROS) and reactive nitrogen species (RONS) are a collective term that broadly describes O_2-derived free radicals such as superoxide anions ($O2^{\bullet-}$), hydroxyl radicals ($HO\bullet$), peroxyl ($RO_2\bullet$) and alkoxyl radicals ($RO\bullet$), nitrogen monoxide ($NO\bullet$), peroxynitrite ($ONOO^-$), nitrogen dioxide ($NO_2\bullet$) as well as O_2-derived non-radical species such as hydrogen peroxide (H_2O_2) (Halliwell and Cross, 1994). Both reactive species are important mediators in the normal regulation of different physiological processes such as cellular proliferation or activation. On the other hand, the imbalance of cellular redox homeostasis is described at the base of many chronic diseases and is also involved in cancer development (Acharya et al., 2010).

Specific ROS such as H_2O_2 or superoxide have been implicated as crucial mediators of apoptotic cell death (Casado et al., 2002; Circu and Aw, 2010; Madeo et al., 1999). ROS tend to enhance survival or promote cell death by activating different factors such as members of the mitogen-activated protein kinases (MAPKs), phosphatidylinositol-3-kinase (PI3K)/Akt pathway, phospholipase C-g1 (PLCg1) signaling, protein kinase C, p53 signaling, ataxia-telangiectasia-mutated (ATM) kinase, nuclear factor-kappaB (NF-kB) signaling, and Jak/Stat pathway. ROS modulate the apoptotic signaling pathway through the cellular redox status by activating key protein kinases (Chan et al., 2010; Noguchi et al., 2005). Pro-oxidants such as H_2O_2 or other stressors, could induce apoptosis (or programmed cell death) by activating the intrinsic or "mitochondrial" apoptosis pathway that results in the damage of this sub-cellular compartment and the pro-apoptotic factors release (Circu and Aw, 2010; Mates et al., 2008). ROS involved in apoptosis derive both from environmental pro-oxidants or from intracellular respiratory dysfunction since mitochondria are the main site of intracellular source of ROS production. It was reported that oxidative stress plays an important role in the molecular mechanism of colorectal cancer (Keshavarzian et al., 1992) Flavones in HT-29 colon cancer cells increase the uptake of pyruvate or lactate into mitochondria, which is followed by an increase in O_2^- production that finally leads to apoptosis (Wenzel et al., 2005).

The prooxidant activity of anthocyanins through the increase of intracellular ROS production has been clearly explained in several studies (Feng et al., 2007; Hou et al., 2005).

4.3 GSH role in apoptosis

Intracellular glutathione (GSH) is a major buffer of cellular redox status due to its active SH-group that has reducing nucleophilic properties (Meister, 1983; Meister, 1991; Meister and Anderson, 1983). It acts as reducing agent, antioxidant and free-radical scavenger against ROS generated during oxidative metabolism and/or oxidative stress (Donati et al., 1990; Hall, 1999a; Hall, 1999b; Sies, 1999) and is also involved in the metabolism of xenobiotics and some cellular molecules (Wu et al., 2004). Free glutathione is present mainly in its reduced form maintained by the action of glutathione reductase (GR), but chemical oxidation of GSH to GSSG can occur as a result of numerous enzyme-catalysed reactions that use GSH to reduce hydrogen peroxide or other peroxides to water or the corresponding alcohol (Diaz Vivancos et al., 2010). GSH is preferentially (85-90%) located in the cytosolic-nuclear compartments and only a small amount is present in mitochondria and endoplasmic reticulum (Hwang et al., 1992; Meredith and Reed, 1982). The free-radical and antioxidant action of GSH depends on its involvement in different enzymatic reactions as those catalyzed by glutathione peroxidases (GPxs) (Lei, 2002), glutathione-S-transferases (GSTs), formaldehyde dehydrogenase, maleylacetoacetate isomerase, and glyoxalase I (Arrigo, 1999; Dickinson and Forman, 2002; Dickinson et al., 2002; Hayes and McLellan, 1999). Cancer cells present elevated GSH levels that generally increase antioxidant capacity and resistance to oxidative stress and regulate different mechanisms linked to carcinogenesis, sensitivity against cytotoxic drugs, ionizing radiation, and some cytokines, DNA synthesis, and cell proliferation (Estrela et al., 2006). There are yet a few reports on the possible role of flavonoids, as well as other phytochemicals, in modulating the glutathione antioxidant system activity, including regulation of GSH intracellular levels through targeting its synthesis (Ramos and Aller, 2008), induction of MRP-1 mediated GSH efflux (Kachadourian and Day, 2006), or inhibition of glutathione peroxidase enzyme activity (Trachootham et al., 2006). Upon grape seed extract treatment, HT29 colon cancer cells showed increased ROS production (that might result in oxidative stress in cells) and a decreased level of intracellular reduced glutathione (Kaur et al., 2011). In addition, after delphinidin and cyanidin treatment in primary (Caco-2) and metastatic (LoVo and LoVo/ADR) colorectal cancer cell lines, no significant changes in the total GSH levels were observed in Caco-2 and LoVo cells, while both were shown to deplete intracellular glutathione levels in LoVo/ADR cells. GSSG content was not measurable in Caco-2 and LoVo cells, suggesting a normal cellular GSH/GSSG ratio (30:1–300:1) (Cvorovic et al., 2010). Cells undergoing apoptosis appear to rapidly and selectively release GSH into the extracellular space (Ghibelli et al., 1995; Ghibelli et al., 1998; Hammond et al., 2007). Hammond and colleagues demonstrated that apoptotic GSH export is directly linked to MRPs. Indeed basal and apoptotic GSH releases were decreased after RNAi reduction of MRP1 expression in Jurkat cells, indicating that MRP1 is a major player in both processes (Hammond et al., 2007). MRP1-channelled GSH export from cells can be also increased by different xenobiotics, including arsenite, verapamil (VRP), and some naturally-occurring flavonoids (Leslie et al., 2003; Loe et al., 2000).

GSTs are known as a family of Phase II detoxification enzymes that catalyze the conjugation of GSH (S-glutathionylation) with different compounds as xenobiotics and drugs or their metabolites, to form mercapturates (Hayes et al., 2005).

It has been recently shown that anthocyanin fractions from selected cultivars of Georgia-Grown Blueberries at 50-150 íg/mL do induce apoptosis in HT-29 colon cancer cells but these same concentrations decrease GST activities rather than induce it (Srivastava et al., 2007).

There are several studies, in normal cells and tissues, in which it was demonstrated that anthocyanins, probably involving some protein kinases, modulate the activity of some GSH-dependent enzymes, thus ameliorating the antioxidant response (Hou et al., 2010; Suda et al., 2008; Veigas et al., 2008).

GSSG formed intracellularly is continuously reduced to GSH by the activity of GR. If oxidative stress or other factors limit the GR activity (e.g., glucose-6-phosphate dehydrogenase deficiency may limit NADPH supply), GSSG will accumulate (Deneke and Fanburg, 1989). In this respect, Cvorovic and colleagues showed that delphinidin and cyanidin did inhibit GR activity in LoVo/ADR cells but not in Caco2 and Lovo cells (Cvorovic et al., 2010). This has two important consequences: (i) the thiol redox status of the cell will shift, activating oxidant response transcriptional elements; and (ii) GSSG may be preferentially secreted out of the cell. (i) The protein sequences of many transcription factors contain cys residues, mainly localized in the DNA-binding domain that, when oxidized, cause a different modulation of gene expression (Arrigo, 1999). (ii) GSSG may be reduced back to GSH, but when GSSG is present in excess, it is also eliminated from the cell by export into the extracellular space. Strong evidence that this export step is mediated by MRP2 was provided by studies of GSSG transport with canalicular membrane-enriched vesicles derived from normal and EHBR (Eisai hyperbilirubinuric rats) rats (Ballatori et al., 2009).

4.4 Intracellular pH and apoptosis

Despite the genetic variability, two phenotypes common to all tumor cells are cellular alkalinization and a shift to glycolytic metabolism. In the first decade of the 20th century, Otto Warburg found that cancer cells, even in the presence of oxygen disposition and a higher request of ATP for fast growing cells, prefer to metabolize glucose via glycolysis instead of oxidative phosphorylation (Warburg, 1956a). The oxygen levels within a tumor vary both spatially and temporally. The elevated glycolytic pathway of cancer cells appears to be a response to hypoxia due to the growth of the tumor surpassing the available vascular supplied oxygen (Mathupala et al., 2001) and seems to be controlled directly by the antiapoptotic protein Akt that generates apoptotic resistance *in vitro* (Elstrom et al., 2004). Then, the decreased dependence on aerobic respiration becomes a selective advantage for survival and proliferation escaping from the apoptotic event. Cell metabolism is shifted toward the increased expression of glycolytic enzymes, glucose transporters, and inhibitors of mitochondrial metabolism that result in a transitional intracellular acidification (Hsu and Sabatini, 2008) and increased glucose uptake is observed coincident with the transition from colon adenomas to invasive cancer (Yasuda et al., 2001). Nevertheless, evidence that intracellular acidification is associated with the progression of apoptosis, has been steadily accumulating (Barry et al., 1993; Gottlieb et al., 1996; Li and Eastman, 1995; Rebollo et al., 1995). An important role in the intracellular acidification could be due to alterations of membrane pHi-regulating mechanisms, including the Na^+/H^+ exchanger (NHE) that might favor accumulation of the protons produced by energetic metabolism. NHE is ubiquitously expressed transporter in the plasma membrane with a main function to extrude H^+ from the cytoplasm.

Multidrug resistant tumor cells exhibit an altered pH gradient across different cell compartments, which favors a reduced intracellular accumulation of antineoplastic drugs and a decreased therapeutic effect. In fact, the activity and expression of NHE are increased in doxorubicin-resistant (HT29-dx) human colon carcinoma cells in comparison with doxorubicin-sensitive HT29 cells (Miraglia et al., 2005). On the other hand, it was demonstrated that activation of the NHE-1 and the resulting cellular alkalinization play a key role in oncogenic transformation (Reshkin et al., 2000). Cyanidin (10 microM), but not its glycosides, could inhibit the neurotensin- and EGF-induced increased rate of extracellular acidification in HT-29 human colon adenocarcinoma cell line probably by inhibiting cellular metabolism, rather than directly altering Na+/H+ exchange (Briviba et al., 2001).

The effect of anthocyanins on metabolism involved in pH modulation of apoptosis is anyway a poor-trodden path.

5. Roadmap for further investigations

5.1 Role of flavonoids on DNA methylation

In humans, multistage carcinogenesis was previously considered a consequence of genetic alterations that cause activation of oncogenes and inactivation of tumor suppressor genes. In addition to genetic events, epigenetic events are another leading player in carcinogenesis (Link et al., 2010). Indeed, it is believed that majority of cancers result from changes that accumulate throughout the life due to the exposure to various endogenous factors and arguably diet and environment-mediated epigenetic perturbations play a crucial role in cancer progression in humans (Herceg, 2007). It was first recognized more than 25 years ago that in colorectal cancer cells, global DNA methylation patterns differed considerably from those in their normal counterparts (Venkatachalam et al., 2010).

The developmental biologist Conrad H. Waddington coined the term 'epigenetics' in 1942, trying to describe reversible heritable changes in gene expression that occur without alteration in DNA sequence sufficiently powerful to regulate the dynamics of gene expression (Waddington, 1951 as cited in (Hitchler and Domann, 2009).

One of the "epigenome" processes is DNA methylation, a covalent chemical modification resulting in addition of a methyl (CH3) group at the carbon 5 position of the cytosine ring in CpG dinucleotides (Kanai and Hirohashi, 2007). This process plays important roles in chromatin structure modulation, transcriptional regulation and genomic stability, and is essential for the development of mammals (Ducasse and Brown, 2006; Li, 2002). CpG dinucleotides are not uniformly distributed throughout the human genome, but are often enriched in the promoter regions of genes. Short CpG-rich regions are also called as "CpG islands", and these are present in more than 50% of human gene promoters and can lead to gene silencing and proliferation or to affect the metabolic processes associated with energy metabolism. (Link et al., 2010). This mechanism is an enzymatic process mediated by DNA methyltransferases (DNMT): DNMT1, also called a "maintenance methyltransferase", preserves existing methylation patterns following DNA replication; DNMT3a and DNMT3b, on the other hand, serve as *de novo* methyltransferases, which act independently of replication on both strands, altering the epigenetic information content (Yu et al., 2011).

Recent studies havedemonstrated that all three DNMTs are overexpressed in several tumor types, including tumors of the colon and rectum, bladder, and kidney. When DNMT1 and DNMT3b are knocked out in colon cancer cell lines, methylation of tumor suppressor genes such as p16 is almost entirely eliminated and the gene is re-expressed (Rhee et al., 2002), as well as it has been established that the inhibition of DNA methyltransferase activity can strongly inhibit the formation of tumors (Stresemann et al., 2006).

It is known that some nutrients like folic acid, B vitamins and SAM (S-adenosylmethionine) and anthocyanins are key components of the methyl-metabolism pathway (Vanzo et al., 2011). Their methyl-donating mechanism can rapidly alter gene expression by modulating the availability of methyl donors as well as DNMT activity (Ross, 2003). There is a growing interest in the role of polyphenols in prevention of DNA methylation. It was demonstrated that epigallocatechin-3-gallate (EGCG), a tea polyphenol, through its methylation exerted by catechol-O-methyltransferase (COMT), indirectly inhibited DNMT. Indeed, S-adenosyl-L-homocysteine (SAH), produced by COMT reaction is a potent inhibitor of DNMT (Fang et al., 2003). On the other hand, EGCG can directly inhibit DNMT through the hydrogen bonds formation with different residues in the catalytic pocket of the enzyme (Lee et al., 2005). Moreover, Fang et al. showed that reactivation of some methylation-silenced genes by EGCG was also demonstrated in human colon cancers and prostate cancer cells (Fang et al., 2003).

5.2 Apoptosis and ATP/ADP ratio

Oxygen consumption in cells is regulated by a respiratory control system which depends on ADP and Pi. When the amount of ATP is high, the amount of ADP is limited and therefore, use of oxygen declines. In other words, oxygen consumption increases as the need for ATP arises (Valle et al., 2010). ATP generation through oxygen conversion is not a fully efficient process because a percentage of the energy of the electrochemical gradient is lost and not coupled to ATP production (Matsuyama and Reed, 2000). This situation arises due to a phenomenon called 'proton leak' which causes protons to return to the mitochondrial matrix via alternative pathways that by-pass ATP synthase (Brand, 1990; Brown and Brand, 1991; Valle et al., 2010). Lynen suggested that the increased dependence of cancer cells on glycolysis stemmed not from their inability to reduce oxygen, but rather from their inability to synthesize ATP in response to the mitochondrial proton gradient (Lynen, 1951 as cited in (Samudio et al., 2009).

Although, some explanations for the 'proton leak' come from the biophysical properties of the inner membrane, much of the explanation comes from the activities of a family of mitochondrial proteins termed uncoupling proteins (UCPs) (Klingenberg, 1999; Valle et al., 2010). UCPs exploit the gap in pH concentration to transfer the proton through the inner membrane into the matrix where they are released. Consequently, the mitochondrial membrane potential decreases, reduction of O_2 via the respiratory chain is no longer linked to ATP synthesis and ATP/ADP exchange is not longer maintained (Vander Heiden et al., 1999). The influence of anthocyanins on ATP/ADP ratio and on UCPs role could be the aim of further studies.

5.3 Apoptosis and oxygen consumption

Cancer cells seem to show high glycolytic rates even when oxygen is sufficient for oxidative phosphorylation (OXPHOS). This condition leads to a survival benefit of the tumor providing protection from oxidative stress and resulting in apoptosis avoidance (Kondoh et al., 2007a; Kondoh et al., 2007b). The importance of glycolysis in the survival of cancer cells was demonstrated by Bonnet and colleagues. Their experimental approach aimed at inhibiting the anaerobic glycolisys by repressing the activity of pyruvate dehydrogenase kinase (PDK) with dichloroacetate (DCA). PDK acts as a negative modulator of pyruvate dehydrogenase, a gate-keeping mitochondrial enzyme which controls the glucose oxidative fate into the cell. DCA changes the metabolism of cancer cells from the cytoplasm-based glycolysis to the mitochondria- based glucose oxidation. This led to increased ROS production and decreased mitochondrial membrane potential, efflux of pro-apoptotic mediators from mitochondria, and induction of mitochondria-dependent apoptosis only in cancer cells (Bonnet et al., 2007). On the other hand, in the majority of mammalian cells, glycolysis is inhibited by the presence of oxygen, which allows the mitochondria to oxidize pyruvate to CO_2 and H_2O.

The transcription factor p53 regulates cellular energy metabolism and antioxidant defense mechanisms. Emerging evidence has shown that these two functions of p53 contribute greatly to p53's role in tumor suppression (Bensaad and Vousden, 2007; Matoba et al., 2006; Sablina et al., 2005). Loss of p53 results in decreased oxygen consumption and impaired mitochondrial respiration and promotes a switch to high glucose utilization in aerobic glycolysis in cells (Maddocks and Vousden).

It was shown that p53 regulates the OXPHOS dependence of cell by modulating the assembly of a key complex in the mitochondrial electron chain transport: cytochrome c oxidase (COX) (Ma et al., 2007; Matoba et al., 2006). It was demonstrated, in fact, that in HCT116 cells, p53 controls the expression of SCO 2 (Synthesis of Cytochrome c Oxidase 2). SCO2 is required for the assembly of mitochondrial DNA-encoded COX II subunit (MTCO2 gene) into the COX, so, p53 directly regulates mitochondrial oxygen consumption. p53 mutations in cancer cells induce a loss in SCO2, thereby resulting in a switch from an aerobic mitochondrial respiration to anaerobic glycolysis. p53 induces SCO2 expression to enhance mitochondrial respiration and induces TIGAR expression to slow glycolysis (Won et al., 2011).

The metabolic implications of anthocyanins through the oxidative use of glucose could be appreciated indirectly. In fact, it is known that anthocyanins induce p53 expression (Fimognari et al., 2005; Lo et al., 2007; Renis et al., 2008), but a direct involvement of this compounds on glucose metabolic use it is not yet demonstrated.

6. Conclusions

The different observations found in epidemiological studies in comparison to the *in vitro* ones are linked, partly to the relatively low flavonoid intake and complexity of metabolism in humans, and partly to the lack of adequate molecular biomarkers for monitoring the earliest stages of disease development in humans (Pierini et al., 2008). Moreover, the relevance of the *in vitro* studies to the *in vivo* situation needs to be confirmed in view of the high concentrations of polyphenols employed in the *in vitro* studies.

All the data recorded about the role of polyphenols and flavonoids has been obtained through the use of classical cell biology and biochemistry methods. Maybe nutrigenomics, that is the study of the effects of foods and food constituents on gene expression could deepen our understanding of these and other phytochemicals (Corthesy-Theulaz et al., 2005; Davis and Hord, 2005; Mariman, 2006).

7. References

Acharya, A., Das, I., Chandhok, D., and Saha, T. (2010): Redox regulation in cancer: a double-edged sword with therapeutic potential. *Oxid Med Cell Longev* 3, 23-34.

Aggarwal, B. B., and Shishodia, S. (2006): Molecular targets of dietary agents for prevention and therapy of cancer. *Biochem Pharmacol* 71, 1397-421.

AIRC (1997): World Cancer Research Fund/American Institute for Cancer Research. Food, Nutrition, Physical Activity and the Prevention of Cancer: A Global Perspective. , Washington, DC: AIRC, 1997.

AIRC (2007): World Cancer Research Fund / American Institute for Cancer Research.Food, Nutrition, Physical Activity, and the Prevention of Cancer: a Global Perspective, pp. 216–251, Washington DC: AICR, 2007.

Armstrong, B., and Doll, R. (1975): Environmental factors and cancer incidence and mortality in different countries, with special reference to dietary practices. *Int J Cancer* 15, 617-31.

Arrigo, A. P. (1999): Gene expression and the thiol redox state. *Free Radic Biol Med* 27, 936-44.

Aura, A. M. (2005): In vitro digestion models for dietary phenolic compounds: *Department of Chemical Technology*, Helsinki University of Technology (Finland), Espoo.

Aura, A. M., Martin-Lopez, P., O'Leary K, A., Williamson, G., Oksman-Caldentey, K. M., Poutanen, K., and Santos-Buelga, C. (2005a): In vitro metabolism of anthocyanins by human gut microflora. *Eur J Nutr* 44, 133-42.

Aura, A. M., Martin-Lopez, P., O'Leary, K. A., Williamson, G., Oksman-Caldentey, K. M., Poutanen, K., and Santos-Buelga, C. (2005b): In vitro metabolism of anthocyanins by human gut microflora. *Eur J Nutr* 44, 133-42.

Ávila, M., Hidalgo, M., Sánchez-Moreno, C., Pelaez, C., Requena, T., and de Pascual-Teresa, S. (2009): Bioconversion of anthocyanin glycosides by Bifidobacteria and Lactobacillus. *Food Research International* 42, 1453-1461.

Bagchi, D., Sen, C. K., Bagchi, M., and Atalay, M. (2004): Anti-angiogenic, antioxidant, and anti-carcinogenic properties of a novel anthocyanin-rich berry extract formula. *Biochemistry (Mosc)* 69, 75-80, 1 p preceding 75.

Baldini, G., Passamonti, S., Lunazzi, G. C., Tiribelli, C., and Sottocasa, G. L. (1986): Cellular localization of sulfobromophthalein transport activity in rat liver. *Biochim Biophys Acta* 856, 1-10.

Ballatori, N., Krance, S. M., Marchan, R., and Hammond, C. L. (2009): Plasma membrane glutathione transporters and their roles in cell physiology and pathophysiology. *Mol Aspects Med* 30, 13-28.

Barry, M. A., Reynolds, J. E., and Eastman, A. (1993): Etoposide-induced apoptosis in human HL-60 cells is associated with intracellular acidification. *Cancer Res* 53, 2349-57.

Bensaad, K., and Vousden, K. H. (2007): p53: new roles in metabolism. *Trends Cell Biol* 17, 286-91.

Bernardo, M. M., and Fridman, R. (2003): TIMP-2 (tissue inhibitor of metalloproteinase-2) regulates MMP-2 (matrix metalloproteinase-2) activity in the extracellular environment after pro-MMP-2 activation by MT1 (membrane type 1)-MMP. *Biochem J* 374, 739-45.

Bjelke, E. (1975): Dietary vitamin a and human lung cancer. *International Journal of Cancer* 15, 561-565.

Block, G., Patterson, B., and Subar, A. (1992): Fruit, vegetables, and cancer prevention: a review of the epidemiological evidence. *Nutr Cancer* 18, 1-29.

Boateng, J., Verghese, M., Shackelford, L., Walker, L. T., Khatiwada, J., Ogutu, S., Williams, D. S., Jones, J., Guyton, M., Asiamah, D., Henderson, F., Grant, L., DeBruce, M., Johnson, A., Washington, S., and Chawan, C. B. (2007): Selected fruits reduce azoxymethane (AOM)-induced aberrant crypt foci (ACF) in Fisher 344 male rats. *Food Chem Toxicol* 45, 725-32.

Bobe, G., Sansbury, L. B., Albert, P. S., Cross, A. J., Kahle, L., Ashby, J., Slattery, M. L., Caan, B., Paskett, E., Iber, F., Kikendall, J. W., Lance, P., Daston, C., Marshall, J. R., Schatzkin, A., and Lanza, E. (2008): Dietary flavonoids and colorectal adenoma recurrence in the Polyp Prevention Trial. *Cancer Epidemiol Biomarkers Prev* 17, 1344-53.

Bobe, G., Wang, B., Seeram, N. P., Nair, M. G., and Bourquin, L. D. (2006): Dietary anthocyanin-rich tart cherry extract inhibits intestinal tumorigenesis in APC(Min) mice fed suboptimal levels of sulindac. *J Agric Food Chem* 54, 9322-8.

Bonnet, S., Archer, S. L., Allalunis-Turner, J., Haromy, A., Beaulieu, C., Thompson, R., Lee, C. T., Lopaschuk, G. D., Puttagunta, L., Harry, G., Hashimoto, K., Porter, C. J., Andrade, M. A., Thebaud, B., and Michelakis, E. D. (2007): A mitochondria-K+ channel axis is suppressed in cancer and its normalization promotes apoptosis and inhibits cancer growth. *Cancer Cell* 11, 37-51.

Borkowski, T., Szymusiak, H., Gliszczynska-Rwiglo, A., Rietjens, I. M., and Tyrakowska, B. (2005): Radical scavenging capacity of wine anthocyanins is strongly pH-dependent. *J Agric Food Chem* 53, 5526-34.

Borst, P., Evers, R., Kool, M., and Wijnholds, J. (1999): The multidrug resistance protein family. *Biochim Biophys Acta* 1461, 347-57.

Bosetti, C., Bravi, F., Talamini, R., Parpinel, M., Gnagnarella, P., Negri, E., Montella, M., Lagiou, P., Franceschi, S., and La Vecchia, C. (2006): Flavonoids and prostate cancer risk: a study in Italy. *Nutr Cancer* 56, 123-7.

Brand, M. D. (1990): The proton leak across the mitochondrial inner membrane. *Biochim Biophys Acta* 1018, 128-33.

Briviba, K., Abrahamse, S. L., Pool-Zobel, B. L., and Rechkemmer, G. (2001): Neurotensin- and EGF-induced metabolic activation of colon carcinoma cells is diminished by dietary flavonoid cyanidin but not by its glycosides. *Nutr Cancer* 41, 172-9.

Brown, G. C., and Brand, M. D. (1991): On the nature of the mitochondrial proton leak. *Biochim Biophys Acta* 1059, 55-62.

Cai, H., Marczylo, T. H., Teller, N., Brown, K., Steward, W. P., Marko, D., and Gescher, A. J. (2010): Anthocyanin-rich red grape extract impedes adenoma development in the Apc(Min) mouse: pharmacodynamic changes and anthocyanin levels in the murine biophase. *Eur J Cancer* 46, 811-7.

Candeil, L., Gourdier, I., Peyron, D., Vezzio, N., Copois, V., Bibeau, F., Orsetti, B., Scheffer, G. L., Ychou, M., Khan, Q. A., Pommier, Y., Pau, B., Martineau, P., and Del Rio, M. (2004): ABCG2 overexpression in colon cancer cells resistant to SN38 and in irinotecan-treated metastases. *Int J Cancer* 109, 848-54.

Casado, F. J., Lostao, M. P., Aymerich, I., Larrayoz, I. M., Duflot, S., Rodriguez-Mulero, S., and Pastor-Anglada, M. (2002): Nucleoside transporters in absorptive epithelia. *J Physiol Biochem* 58, 207-16.

Castañeda-Ovando, A., Pacheco-Hernández, M. L., Páez-Hernández, M. E., Rodríguez, J. A., and Galán-Vidal, C. A. (2009): Chemical studies of anthocyanins: A review. *Food Chemistry* 113, 859-871.

Center, M. M., Jemal, A., and Ward, E. (2009): International trends in colorectal cancer incidence rates. *Cancer Epidemiol Biomarkers Prev* 18, 1688-94.

Cha, H. J., Bae, S. K., Lee, H. Y., Lee, O. H., Sato, H., Seiki, M., Park, B. C., and Kim, K. W. (1996): Anti-invasive activity of ursolic acid correlates with the reduced expression of matrix metalloproteinase-9 (MMP-9) in HT1080 human fibrosarcoma cells. *Cancer Res* 56, 2281-4.

Chan, H. L., Chou, H. C., Duran, M., Gruenewald, J., Waterfield, M. D., Ridley, A., and Timms, J. F. (2010): Major role of epidermal growth factor receptor and Src kinases in promoting oxidative stress-dependent loss of adhesion and apoptosis in epithelial cells. *J Biol Chem* 285, 4307-18.

Chao, A., Thun, M. J., Connell, C. J., McCullough, M. L., Jacobs, E. J., Flanders, W. D., Rodriguez, C., Sinha, R., and Calle, E. E. (2005): Meat consumption and risk of colorectal cancer. *JAMA* 293, 172-82.

Chen, D., Daniel, K. G., Chen, M. S., Kuhn, D. J., Landis-Piwowar, K. R., and Dou, Q. P. (2005): Dietary flavonoids as proteasome inhibitors and apoptosis inducers in human leukemia cells. *Biochem Pharmacol* 69, 1421-32.

Chen, P. N., Kuo, W. H., Chiang, C. L., Chiou, H. L., Hsieh, Y. S., and Chu, S. C. (2006): Black rice anthocyanins inhibit cancer cells invasion via repressions of MMPs and u-PA expression. *Chem Biol Interact* 163, 218-29.

Circu, M. L., and Aw, T. Y. (2010): Reactive oxygen species, cellular redox systems, and apoptosis. *Free Radic Biol Med* 48, 749-62.

Coates, E. M., Popa, G., Gill, C. I., McCann, M. J., McDougall, G. J., Stewart, D., and Rowland, I. (2007): Colon-available raspberry polyphenols exhibit anti-cancer effects on in vitro models of colon cancer. *J Carcinog* 6, 4.

Cole, S. P., Bhardwaj, G., Gerlach, J. H., Mackie, J. E., Grant, C. E., Almquist, K. C., Stewart, A. J., Kurz, E. U., Duncan, A. M., and Deeley, R. G. (1992): Overexpression of a transporter gene in a multidrug-resistant human lung cancer cell line. *Science* 258, 1650-4.

Cooke, D., Schwarz, M., Boocock, D., Winterhalter, P., Steward, W. P., Gescher, A. J., and Marczylo, T. H. (2006): Effect of cyanidin-3-glucoside and an anthocyanin mixture from bilberry on adenoma development in the ApcMin mouse model of intestinal carcinogenesis--relationship with tissue anthocyanin levels. *Int J Cancer* 119, 2213-20.

Corthesy-Theulaz, I., den Dunnen, J. T., Ferre, P., Geurts, J. M., Muller, M., van Belzen, N., and van Ommen, B. (2005): Nutrigenomics: the impact of biomics technology on nutrition research. *Ann Nutr Metab* 49, 355-65.

Cvorovic, J., Tramer, F., Granzotto, M., Candussio, L., Decorti, G., and Passamonti, S. (2010): Oxidative stress-based cytotoxicity of delphinidin and cyanidin in colon cancer cells. *Arch Biochem Biophys* 501, 151-7.

D'Alessandro, A., Pieroni, L., Ronci, M., D'Aguanno, S., Federici, G., and Urbani, A. (2009): Proteasome inhibitors therapeutic strategies for cancer. *Recent Pat Anticancer Drug Discov* 4, 73-82.

Dallas, N. A., Xia, L., Fan, F., Gray, M. J., Gaur, P., van Buren, G., 2nd, Samuel, S., Kim, M. P., Lim, S. J., and Ellis, L. M. (2009): Chemoresistant colorectal cancer cells, the cancer stem cell phenotype, and increased sensitivity to insulin-like growth factor-I receptor inhibition. *Cancer Res* 69, 1951-7.

Davis, C. D., and Hord, N. G. (2005): Nutritional "omics" technologies for elucidating the role(s) of bioactive food components in colon cancer prevention. *J Nutr* 135, 2694-7.

Deneke, S. M., and Fanburg, B. L. (1989): Regulation of cellular glutathione. *Am J Physiol* 257, L163-73.

Di Pietro, A., Conseil, G., Perez-Victoria, J. M., Dayan, G., Baubichon-Cortay, H., Trompier, D., Steinfels, E., Jault, J. M., de Wet, H., Maitrejean, M., Comte, G., Boumendjel, A., Mariotte, A. M., Dumontet, C., McIntosh, D. B., Goffeau, A., Castanys, S., Gamarro, F., and Barron, D. (2002): Modulation by flavonoids of cell multidrug resistance mediated by P-glycoprotein and related ABC transporters. *Cell Mol Life Sci* 59, 307-22.

Diaz Vivancos, P., Wolff, T., Markovic, J., Pallardo, F. V., and Foyer, C. H. (2010): A nuclear glutathione cycle within the cell cycle. *Biochem J* 431, 169-78.

Dickinson, D. A., and Forman, H. J. (2002): Cellular glutathione and thiols metabolism. *Biochem Pharmacol* 64, 1019-26.

Dickinson, D. A., Iles, K. E., Watanabe, N., Iwamoto, T., Zhang, H., Krzywanski, D. M., and Forman, H. J. (2002): 4-hydroxynonenal induces glutamate cysteine ligase through JNK in HBE1 cells. *Free Radic Biol Med* 33, 974.

Ding, M., Feng, R., Wang, S. Y., Bowman, L., Lu, Y., Qian, Y., Castranova, V., Jiang, B. H., and Shi, X. (2006): Cyanidin-3-glucoside, a natural product derived from blackberry, exhibits chemopreventive and chemotherapeutic activity. *J Biol Chem* 281, 17359-68.

Donati, Y. R., Slosman, D. O., and Polla, B. S. (1990): Oxidative injury and the heat shock response. *Biochem Pharmacol* 40, 2571-7.

Doyle, L. A., Yang, W., Abruzzo, L. V., Krogmann, T., Gao, Y., Rishi, A. K., and Ross, D. D. (1998): A multidrug resistance transporter from human MCF-7 breast cancer cells. *Proc Natl Acad Sci U S A* 95, 15665-70.

Dreiseitel, A., Oosterhuis, B., Vukman, K. V., Schreier, P., Oehme, A., Locher, S., Hajak, G., and Sand, P. G. (2009): Berry anthocyanins and anthocyanidins exhibit distinct affinities for the efflux transporters BCRP and MDR1. *Br J Pharmacol* 158, 1942-50.

Ducasse, M., and Brown, M. A. (2006): Epigenetic aberrations and cancer. *Mol Cancer* 5, 60.

Elias, M. M., Lunazzi, G. C., Passamonti, S., Gazzin, B., Miccio, M., Stanta, G., Sottocasa, G. L., and Tiribelli, C. (1990): Bilitranslocase localization and function in basolateral plasma membrane of renal proximal tubule in rat. *Am J Physiol* 259, F559-64.

Elstrom, R. L., Bauer, D. E., Buzzai, M., Karnauskas, R., Harris, M. H., Plas, D. R., Zhuang, H., Cinalli, R. M., Alavi, A., Rudin, C. M., and Thompson, C. B. (2004): Akt stimulates aerobic glycolysis in cancer cells. *Cancer Res* 64, 3892-9.

Estrela, J. M., Ortega, A., and Obrador, E. (2006): Glutathione in cancer biology and therapy. *Crit Rev Clin Lab Sci* 43, 143-81.

Fanciulli, M., Bruno, T., Giovannelli, A., Gentile, F. P., Di Padova, M., Rubiu, O., and Floridi, A. (2000): Energy metabolism of human LoVo colon carcinoma cells: correlation to drug resistance and influence of lonidamine. *Clin Cancer Res* 6, 1590-7.

Fang, M. Z., Wang, Y., Ai, N., Hou, Z., Sun, Y., Lu, H., Welsh, W., and Yang, C. S. (2003): Tea polyphenol (-)-epigallocatechin-3-gallate inhibits DNA methyltransferase and reactivates methylation-silenced genes in cancer cell lines. *Cancer Res* 63, 7563-70.

Faria, A., Pestana, D., Azevedo, J., Martel, F., de Freitas, V., Azevedo, I., Mateus, N., and Calhau, C. (2009): Absorption of anthocyanins through intestinal epithelial cells - Putative involvement of GLUT2. *Mol Nutr Food Res* 53, 1430-7.

Felgines, C., Krisa, S., Mauray, A., Besson, C., Lamaison, J. L., Scalbert, A., Merillon, J. M., and Texier, O. (2010): Radiolabelled cyanidin 3-O-glucoside is poorly absorbed in the mouse. *Br J Nutr* 103, 1738-45.

Felgines, C., Texier, O., Besson, C., Vitaglione, P., Lamaison, J. L., Fogliano, V., Scalbert, A., Vanella, L., and Galvano, F. (2008): Influence of glucose on cyanidin 3-glucoside absorption in rats. *Mol Nutr Food Res* 52, 959-64.

Feng, R., Ni, H. M., Wang, S. Y., Tourkova, I. L., Shurin, M. R., Harada, H., and Yin, X. M. (2007): Cyanidin-3-rutinoside, a natural polyphenol antioxidant, selectively kills leukemic cells by induction of oxidative stress. *J Biol Chem* 282, 13468-76.

Fimognari, C., Berti, F., Nusse, M., Cantelli-Fortii, G., and Hrelia, P. (2005): In vitro anticancer activity of cyanidin-3-O-beta-glucopyranoside: effects on transformed and non-transformed T lymphocytes. *Anticancer Res* 25, 2837-40.

Fleschhut, J., Kratzer, F., Rechkemmer, G., and Kulling, S. E. (2006): Stability and biotransformation of various dietary anthocyanins in vitro. *Eur J Nutr* 45, 7-18.

Folkman, J. (1995): Angiogenesis in cancer, vascular, rheumatoid and other disease. *Nat Med* 1, 27-31.

Forester, S. C., and Waterhouse, A. L. (2008): Identification of Cabernet Sauvignon anthocyanin gut microflora metabolites. *J Agric Food Chem* 56, 9299-304.

Fornaro, L., Masi, G., Loupakis, F., Vasile, E., and Falcone, A. (2010): Palliative treatment of unresectable metastatic colorectal cancer. *Expert Opin Pharmacother* 11, 63-77.

Fujiwara, M., Okayasu, I., Takemura, T., Tanaka, I., Masuda, R., Furuhata, Y., Noji, M., Oritsu, M., Kato, M., and Oshimura, M. (2000): Telomerase activity significantly correlates with chromosome alterations, cell differentiation, and proliferation in lung adenocarcinomas. *Mod Pathol* 13, 723-9.

Ghibelli, L., Coppola, S., Rotilio, G., Lafavia, E., Maresca, V., and Ciriolo, M. R. (1995): Non-oxidative loss of glutathione in apoptosis via GSH extrusion. *Biochem Biophys Res Commun* 216, 313-20.

Ghibelli, L., Fanelli, C., Rotilio, G., Lafavia, E., Coppola, S., Colussi, C., Civitareale, P., and Ciriolo, M. R. (1998): Rescue of cells from apoptosis by inhibition of active GSH extrusion. *FASEB J* 12, 479-86.

Goldberg, R. M., Rothenberg, M. L., Van Cutsem, E., Benson, A. B., 3rd, Blanke, C. D., Diasio, R. B., Grothey, A., Lenz, H. J., Meropol, N. J., Ramanathan, R. K., Becerra, C. H., Wickham, R., Armstrong, D., and Viele, C. (2007): The continuum of care: a paradigm for the management of metastatic colorectal cancer. *Oncologist* 12, 38-50.

Gottlieb, R. A., Nordberg, J., Skowronski, E., and Babior, B. M. (1996): Apoptosis induced in Jurkat cells by several agents is preceded by intracellular acidification. *Proc Natl Acad Sci U S A* 93, 654-8.

Hagiwara, A., Miyashita, K., Nakanishi, T., Sano, M., Tamano, S., Kadota, T., Koda, T., Nakamura, M., Imaida, K., Ito, N., and Shirai, T. (2001): Pronounced inhibition by a natural anthocyanin, purple corn color, of 2-amino-1-methyl-6-phenylimidazo[4,5-b]pyridine (PhIP)-associated colorectal carcinogenesis in male F344 rats pretreated with 1,2-dimethylhydrazine. *Cancer Lett* 171, 17-25.

Hagiwara, A., Yoshino, H., Ichihara, T., Kawabe, M., Tamano, S., Aoki, H., Koda, T., Nakamura, M., Imaida, K., Ito, N., and Shirai, T. (2002): Prevention by natural food anthocyanins, purple sweet potato color and red cabbage color, of 2-amino-1-methyl-6-phenylimidazo[4,5-b]pyridine (PhIP)-associated colorectal carcinogenesis in rats initiated with 1,2-dimethylhydrazine. *J Toxicol Sci* 27, 57-68.

Hall, A. G. (1999a): Glutathione and the regulation of cell death. *Adv Exp Med Biol* 457, 199-203.

Hall, A. G. (1999b): Review: The role of glutathione in the regulation of apoptosis. *Eur J Clin Invest* 29, 238-45.

Halliwell, B., and Cross, C. E. (1994): Oxygen-derived species: their relation to human disease and environmental stress. *Environ Health Perspect* 102 Suppl 10, 5-12.

Hammond, C. L., Marchan, R., Krance, S. M., and Ballatori, N. (2007): Glutathione export during apoptosis requires functional multidrug resistance-associated proteins. *J Biol Chem* 282, 14337-47.

Harborne, J. B., and Williams, C. A. (2000): Advances in flavonoid research since 1992. *Phytochemistry* 2000, 481-504.

Harris, G. K., Gupta, A., Nines, R. G., Kresty, L. A., Habib, S. G., Frankel, W. L., LaPerle, K., Gallaher, D. D., Schwartz, S. J., and Stoner, G. D. (2001): Effects of lyophilized black raspberries on azoxymethane-induced colon cancer and 8-hydroxy-2'-deoxyguanosine levels in the Fischer 344 rat. *Nutr Cancer* 40, 125-33.

Hassimotto, N. M. A., Genovese, M. I., and Lajolo, F. M. (2008): Absorption and metabolism of cyanidin-3-glucoside and cyanidin-3-rutinoside extracted from wild mulberry (Morus nigra L.) in rats. *Nutrition Research* 28, 198-207.

Hayes, J. D., Flanagan, J. U., and Jowsey, I. R. (2005): Glutathione transferases. *Annu Rev Pharmacol Toxicol* 45, 51-88.

Hayes, J. D., and McLellan, L. I. (1999): Glutathione and glutathione-dependent enzymes represent a co-ordinately regulated defence against oxidative stress. *Free Radic Res* 31, 273-300.

He, J., Magnuson, B. A., and Giusti, M. M. (2005): Analysis of anthocyanins in rat intestinal contents--impact of anthocyanin chemical structure on fecal excretion. *J Agric Food Chem* 53, 2859-66.

He, J., Wallace, T. C., Keatley, K. E., and Failla, M. L. G., M.M. (2009): Stability of black raspberry anthocyanins in the digestive tract lumen and transport efficiency into gastric and small intestinal tissues in the rat. *J Agric Food Chem.* 57, 3141-8.

Herceg, Z. (2007): Epigenetics and cancer: towards an evaluation of the impact of environmental and dietary factors. *Mutagenesis* 22, 91-103.

Hess, G. P., Wang, P. F., Quach, D., Barber, B., and Zhao, Z. (2010): Systemic Therapy for Metastatic Colorectal Cancer: Patterns of Chemotherapy and Biologic Therapy Use in US Medical Oncology Practice. *J Oncol Pract* 6, 301-7.

Hitchler, M. J., and Domann, F. E. (2009): Metabolic defects provide a spark for the epigenetic switch in cancer. *Free Radic Biol Med* 47, 115-27.

Hiyama, E., Hiyama, K., Yokoyama, T., Matsuura, Y., Piatyszek, M. A., and Shay, J. W. (1995): Correlating telomerase activity levels with human neuroblastoma outcomes. *Nat Med* 1, 249-55.

Hou, D. X. (2003): Potential mechanisms of cancer chemoprevention by anthocyanins. *Curr Mol Med* 3, 149-59.

Hou, D. X., Ose, T., Lin, S., Harazoro, K., Imamura, I., Kubo, M., Uto, T., Terahara, N., Yoshimoto, M., and Fujii, M. (2003): Anthocyanidins induce apoptosis in human promyelocytic leukemia cells: structure-activity relationship and mechanisms involved. *Int J Oncol* 23, 705-12.

Hou, D. X., Tong, X., Terahara, N., Luo, D., and Fujii, M. (2005): Delphinidin 3-sambubioside, a Hibiscus anthocyanin, induces apoptosis in human leukemia cells through reactive oxygen species-mediated mitochondrial pathway. *Arch Biochem Biophys* 440, 101-9.

Hou, Z., Qin, P., and Ren, G. (2010): Effect of anthocyanin-rich extract from black rice (Oryza sativa L. Japonica) on chronically alcohol-induced liver damage in rats. *J Agric Food Chem* 58, 3191-6.

Hsu, P. P., and Sabatini, D. M. (2008): Cancer cell metabolism: Warburg and beyond. *Cell* 134, 703-7.

Huang, H. P., Shih, Y. W., Chang, Y. C., Hung, C. N., and Wang, C. J. (2008): Chemoinhibitory effect of mulberry anthocyanins on melanoma metastasis involved in the Ras/PI3K pathway. *J Agric Food Chem* 56, 9286-93.

Hwang, C., Sinskey, A. J., and Lodish, H. F. (1992): Oxidized redox state of glutathione in the endoplasmic reticulum. *Science* 257, 1496-502.

Jemal, A., Bray, F., Center, M. M., Ferlay, J., Ward, E., and Forman, D. (2011): Global cancer statistics. *CA Cancer J Clin* 61, 69-90.

Johnson, J. L., Bomser, J. A., Scheerens, J. C., and Giusti, M. M. (2011): Effect of black raspberry (Rubus occidentalis L.) extract variation conditioned by cultivar, production site, and fruit maturity stage on colon cancer cell proliferation. *J Agric Food Chem* 59, 1638-45.

Kachadourian, R., and Day, B. J. (2006): Flavonoid-induced glutathione depletion: potential implications for cancer treatment. *Free Radic Biol Med* 41, 65-76.

Kanai, Y., and Hirohashi, S. (2007): Alterations of DNA methylation associated with abnormalities of DNA methyltransferases in human cancers during transition from a precancerous to a malignant state. *Carcinogenesis* 28, 2434-42.

Kang, S. Y., Seeram, N. P., Nair, M. G., and Bourquin, L. D. (2003): Tart cherry anthocyanins inhibit tumor development in Apc(Min) mice and reduce proliferation of human colon cancer cells. *Cancer Lett* 194, 13-9.

Katsube, N., Iwashita, K., Tsushida, T., Yamaki, K., and Kobori, M. (2003): Induction of apoptosis in cancer cells by Bilberry (Vaccinium myrtillus) and the anthocyanins. *J Agric Food Chem* 51, 68-75.

Kaur, M., Tyagi, A., Singh, R. P., Sclafani, R. A., Agarwal, R., and Agarwal, C. (2011): Grape seed extract upregulates p21 (Cip1) through redox-mediated activation of ERK1/2 and posttranscriptional regulation leading to cell cycle arrest in colon carcinoma HT29 cells. *Mol Carcinog* 50, 553-62.

Kay, C. D., Kroon, P. A., and Cassidy, A. (2009): The bioactivity of dietary anthocyanins is likely to be mediated by their degradation products. *Mol Nutr Food Res* 53 Suppl 1, S92-101.

Kazi, A., Urbizu, D. A., Kuhn, D. J., Acebo, A. L., Jackson, E. R., Greenfelder, G. P., Kumar, N. B., and Dou, Q. P. (2003): A natural musaceas plant extract inhibits proteasome activity and induces apoptosis selectively in human tumor and transformed, but not normal and non-transformed, cells. *Int J Mol Med* 12, 879-87.

Keppler, K., and Humpf, H. U. (2005): Metabolism of anthocyanins and their phenolic degradation products by the intestinal microflora. *Bioorg Med Chem* 13, 5195-205.

Keshavarzian, A., Zapeda, D., List, T., and Mobarhan, S. (1992): High levels of reactive oxygen metabolites in colon cancer tissue: analysis by chemiluminescence probe. *Nutr Cancer* 17, 243-9.

Key, T. J. (2011): Fruit and vegetables and cancer risk. *British Journal of Cancer* 104, 6-11.

Kim, N. W., Piatyszek, M. A., Prowse, K. R., Harley, C. B., West, M. D., Ho, P. L., Coviello, G. M., Wright, W. E., Weinrich, S. L., and Shay, J. W. (1994): Specific association of human telomerase activity with immortal cells and cancer. *Science* 266, 2011-5.

Klingenberg, M. (1999): Uncoupling protein--a useful energy dissipator. *J Bioenerg Biomembr* 31, 419-30.

Kondoh, H., Lleonart, M. E., Bernard, D., and Gil, J. (2007a): Protection from oxidative stress by enhanced glycolysis; a possible mechanism of cellular immortalization. *Histol Histopathol* 22, 85-90.

Kondoh, H., Lleonart, M. E., Nakashima, Y., Yokode, M., Tanaka, M., Bernard, D., Gil, J., and Beach, D. (2007b): A high glycolytic flux supports the proliferative potential of murine embryonic stem cells. *Antioxid Redox Signal* 9, 293-9.

Kong, J. M., Chia, L. S., Goh, N. K., Chia, T. F., and Brouillard, R. (2003): Analysis and biological activities of anthocyanins. *Phytochemistry* 64, 923-33.

Labrecque, L., Lamy, S., Chapus, A., Mihoubi, S., Durocher, Y., Cass, B., Bojanowski, M. W., Gingras, D., and Beliveau, R. (2005): Combined inhibition of PDGF and VEGF receptors by ellagic acid, a dietary-derived phenolic compound. *Carcinogenesis* 26, 821-6.

Lala, G., Malik, M., Zhao, C., He, J., Kwon, Y., Giusti, M. M., and Magnuson, B. A. (2006): Anthocyanin-rich extracts inhibit multiple biomarkers of colon cancer in rats. *Nutr Cancer* 54, 84-93.

Lamy, S., Gingras, D., and Beliveau, R. (2002): Green tea catechins inhibit vascular endothelial growth factor receptor phosphorylation. *Cancer Res* 62, 381-5.

Lazze, M. C., Savio, M., Pizzala, R., Cazzalini, O., Perucca, P., Scovassi, A. I., Stivala, L. A., and Bianchi, L. (2004): Anthocyanins induce cell cycle perturbations and apoptosis in different human cell lines. *Carcinogenesis* 25, 1427-33.

Lee, W. J., Shim, J. Y., and Zhu, B. T. (2005): Mechanisms for the inhibition of DNA methyltransferases by tea catechins and bioflavonoids. *Mol Pharmacol* 68, 1018-30.

Lei, X. G. (2002): In vivo antioxidant role of glutathione peroxidase: evidence from knockout mice. *Methods Enzymol* 347, 213-25.

Leslie, E. M., Deeley, R. G., and Cole, S. P. (2003): Bioflavonoid stimulation of glutathione transport by the 190-kDa multidrug resistance protein 1 (MRP1). *Drug Metab Dispos* 31, 11-5.

Li, E. (2002): Chromatin modification and epigenetic reprogramming in mammalian development. *Nat Rev Genet* 3, 662-73.

Li, J., and Eastman, A. (1995): Apoptosis in an interleukin-2-dependent cytotoxic T lymphocyte cell line is associated with intracellular acidification. Role of the Na(+)/H(+)-antiport. *J Biol Chem* 270, 3203-11.

Liang, Y. C., Tsai, S. H., Chen, L., Lin-Shiau, S. Y., and Lin, J. K. (2003): Resveratrol-induced G2 arrest through the inhibition of CDK7 and p34CDC2 kinases in colon carcinoma HT29 cells. *Biochem Pharmacol* 65, 1053-60.

Lin, M. T., Yen, M. L., Lin, C. Y., and Kuo, M. L. (2003): Inhibition of vascular endothelial growth factor-induced angiogenesis by resveratrol through interruption of Src-dependent vascular endothelial cadherin tyrosine phosphorylation. *Mol Pharmacol* 64, 1029-36.

Link, A., Balaguer, F., and Goel, A. (2010): Cancer chemoprevention by dietary polyphenols: promising role for epigenetics. *Biochem Pharmacol* 80, 1771-92.

Lo, C. W., Huang, H. P., Lin, H. M., Chien, C. T., and Wang, C. J. (2007): Effect of Hibiscus anthocyanins-rich extract induces apoptosis of proliferating smooth muscle cell via activation of P38 MAPK and p53 pathway. *Mol Nutr Food Res* 51, 1452-60.

Loe, D. W., Deeley, R. G., and Cole, S. P. (2000): Verapamil stimulates glutathione transport by the 190-kDa multidrug resistance protein 1 (MRP1). *J Pharmacol Exp Ther* 293, 530-8.

Ma, W., Sung, H. J., Park, J. Y., Matoba, S., and Hwang, P. M. (2007): A pivotal role for p53: balancing aerobic respiration and glycolysis. *J Bioenerg Biomembr* 39, 243-6.

Maddocks, O. D., and Vousden, K. H. Metabolic regulation by p53. *J Mol Med (Berl)* 89, 237-45.

Madeo, F., Frohlich, E., Ligr, M., Grey, M., Sigrist, S. J., Wolf, D. H., and Frohlich, K. U. (1999): Oxygen stress: a regulator of apoptosis in yeast. *J Cell Biol* 145, 757-67.

Magnusson, B. A., Lala, G., and Kwon, Y. J. (2003): Anthocyanin-rich extracts inhibit growth of human colon cancer cells and azoxymethane-induced colon aberrant crypts in rats: Implications for colon cancer Chemoprevention. *Cancer Epidemiol Biomark Prev* 12, 1323s-1324s.

Malik, M., Zhao, C., Schoene, N., Guisti, M. M., Moyer, M. P., and Magnuson, B. A. (2003): Anthocyanin-rich extract from Aronia meloncarpa E induces a cell cycle block in colon cancer but not normal colonic cells. *Nutr Cancer* 46, 186-96.

Manach, C., Scalbert, A., Morand, C., Remesy, C., and Jimenez, L. (2004): Polyphenols: food sources and bioavailability. *Am J Clin Nutr* 79, 727-47.

Mariman, E. C. (2006): Nutrigenomics and nutrigenetics: the 'omics' revolution in nutritional science. *Biotechnol Appl Biochem* 44, 119-28.

Marko, D., Puppel, N., Tjaden, Z., Jakobs, S., and Pahlke, G. (2004): The substitution pattern of anthocyanidins affects different cellular signaling cascades regulating cell proliferation. *Mol Nutr Food Res* 48, 318-25.

Matchett, M. D., MacKinnon, S. L., Sweeney, M. I., Gottschall-Pass, K. T., and Hurta, R. A. (2005): Blueberry flavonoids inhibit matrix metalloproteinase activity in DU145 human prostate cancer cells. *Biochem Cell Biol* 83, 637-43.

Matchett, M. D., MacKinnon, S. L., Sweeney, M. I., Gottschall-Pass, K. T., and Hurta, R. A. (2006): Inhibition of matrix metalloproteinase activity in DU145 human prostate cancer cells by flavonoids from lowbush blueberry (Vaccinium angustifolium): possible roles for protein kinase C and mitogen-activated protein-kinase-mediated events. *J Nutr Biochem* 17, 117-25.

Mates, J. M., Segura, J. A., Alonso, F. J., and Marquez, J. (2008): Intracellular redox status and oxidative stress: implications for cell proliferation, apoptosis, and carcinogenesis. *Arch Toxicol* 82, 273-99.

Mathupala, S. P., Rempel, A., and Pedersen, P. L. (2001): Glucose catabolism in cancer cells: identification and characterization of a marked activation response of the type II hexokinase gene to hypoxic conditions. *J Biol Chem* 276, 43407-12.

Matoba, S., Kang, J. G., Patino, W. D., Wragg, A., Boehm, M., Gavrilova, O., Hurley, P. J., Bunz, F., and Hwang, P. M. (2006): p53 regulates mitochondrial respiration. *Science* 312, 1650-3.

Matsuyama, S., and Reed, J. C. (2000): Mitochondria-dependent apoptosis and cellular pH regulation. *Cell Death Differ* 7, 1155-65.

McDougall, G. J., Fyffe, S., Dobson, P., and Stewart, D. (2005): Anthocyanins from red wine--their stability under simulated gastrointestinal digestion. *Phytochemistry* 66, 2540-8.

McGhie, T. K., and Walton, M. C. (2007): The bioavailability and absorption of anthocyanins: towards a better understanding. *Mol Nutr Food Res* 51, 702-13.

Meiers, S., Kemeny, M., Weyand, U., Gastpar, R., von Angerer, E., and Marko, D. (2001): The anthocyanidins cyanidin and delphinidin are potent inhibitors of the epidermal growth-factor receptor. *J Agric Food Chem* 49, 958-62.

Meister, A. (1983): Selective modification of glutathione metabolism. *Science* 220, 472-7.

Meister, A. (1991): Glutathione deficiency produced by inhibition of its synthesis, and its reversal; applications in research and therapy. *Pharmacol Ther* 51, 155-94.

Meister, A., and Anderson, M. E. (1983): Glutathione. *Annu Rev Biochem* 52, 711-60.

Mennen, L. I., Sapinho, D., Ito, H., Galan, P., Hercberg, S., and Scalbert, A. (2008): Urinary excretion of 13 dietary flavonoids and phenolic acids in free-living healthy subjects - variability and possible use as biomarkers of polyphenol intake. *Eur J Clin Nutr* 62, 519-25.

Meredith, M. J., and Reed, D. J. (1982): Status of the mitochondrial pool of glutathione in the isolated hepatocyte. *J Biol Chem* 257, 3747-53.

Milane, H. A., Al Ahmad, A., Naitchabane, M., Vandamme, T. F., Jung, L., and Ubeaud, G. (2007): Transport of quercetin di-sodium salt in the human intestinal epithelial Caco-2 cell monolayer 139. *Eur J Drug Metab Pharmacokinet* 32, 139-47.

Miraglia, E., Viarisio, D., Riganti, C., Costamagna, C., Ghigo, D., and Bosia, A. (2005): Na+/H+ exchanger activity is increased in doxorubicin-resistant human colon cancer cells and its modulation modifies the sensitivity of the cells to doxorubicin. *Int J Cancer* 115, 924-9.

Misikangas, M., Pajari, A. M., Paivarinta, E., Oikarinen, S. I., Rajakangas, J., Marttinen, M., Tanayama, H., Torronen, R., and Mutanen, M. (2007): Three Nordic berries inhibit intestinal tumorigenesis in multiple intestinal neoplasia/+ mice by modulating beta-catenin signaling in the tumor and transcription in the mucosa. *J Nutr* 137, 2285-90.

Miyake, K., Mickley, L., Litman, T., Zhan, Z., Robey, R., Cristensen, B., Brangi, M., Greenberger, L., Dean, M., Fojo, T., and Bates, S. E. (1999): Molecular cloning of cDNAs which are highly overexpressed in mitoxantrone-resistant cells: demonstration of homology to ABC transport genes. *Cancer Res* 59, 8-13.

Morris, M. E., and Zhang, S. (2006): Flavonoid-drug interactions: effects of flavonoids on ABC transporters. *Life Sci* 78, 2116-30.

Naasani, I., Oh-Hashi, F., Oh-Hara, T., Feng, W. Y., Johnston, J., Chan, K., and Tsuruo, T. (2003): Blocking telomerase by dietary polyphenols is a major mechanism for limiting the growth of human cancer cells in vitro and in vivo. *Cancer Res* 63, 824-30.

Naasani, I., Seimiya, H., and Tsuruo, T. (1998): Telomerase inhibition, telomere shortening, and senescence of cancer cells by tea catechins. *Biochem Biophys Res Commun* 249, 391-6.

Nabeshima, K., Inoue, T., Shimao, Y., and Sameshima, T. (2002): Matrix metalloproteinases in tumor invasion: role for cell migration. *Pathol Int* 52, 255-64.

Nagase, H., Sasaki, K., Kito, H., Haga, A., and Sato, T. (1998): Inhibitory effect of delphinidin from Solanum melongena on human fibrosarcoma HT-1080 invasiveness in vitro. *Planta Med* 64, 216-9.

Noguchi, T., Takeda, K., Matsuzawa, A., Saegusa, K., Nakano, H., Gohda, J., Inoue, J., and Ichijo, H. (2005): Recruitment of tumor necrosis factor receptor-associated factor family proteins to apoptosis signal-regulating kinase 1 signalosome is essential for oxidative stress-induced cell death. *J Biol Chem* 280, 37033-40.

Olsson, M. E., Gustavsson, K. E., Andersson, S., Nilsson, A., and Duan, R. D. (2004): Inhibition of cancer cell proliferation in vitro by fruit and berry extracts and correlations with antioxidant levels. *J Agric Food Chem* 52, 7264-71.

Omura, S., Sasaki, Y., Iwai, Y., and Takeshima, H. (1995): Staurosporine, a potentially important gift from a microorganism. *J Antibiot (Tokyo)* 48, 535-48.

Passamonti, S., Terdoslavich, M., Franca, R., Vanzo, A., Tramer, F., Braidot, E., Petrussa, E., and Vianello, A. (2009): Bioavailability of flavonoids: a review of their membrane transport and the function of bilitranslocase in animal and plant organisms. *Curr Drug Metab* 10, 369-94.

Passamonti, S., Vrhovsek, U., and Mattivi, F. (2002): The interaction of anthocyanins with bilitranslocase. *Biochem Biophys Res Commun* 296, 631-6.

Passamonti, S., Vrhovsek, U., Terdoslavich, M., Vanzo, A., Cocolo, A., Decorti, G., and Mattivi, F. (2003a): Hepatic uptake of dietary anthocyanins and the role of bilitranslocase. 1st International Conference on Polyphenols and Health, Vichy - France pp. 278.

Passamonti, S., Vrhovsek, U., Vanzo, A., and Mattivi, F. (2003b): The stomach as a site for anthocyanins absorption from food. *FEBS Letters* 544, 210-213.

Pierini, R., Gee, J. M., Belshaw, N. J., and Johnson, I. T. (2008): Flavonoids and intestinal cancers. *Br J Nutr* 99 E Suppl 1, ES53-9.

Prior, R. L., and Wu, X. (2006): Anthocyanins: structural characteristics that result in unique metabolic patterns and biological activities. *Free Radic Res* 40, 1014-28.

Pupa, S. M., Menard, S., Forti, S., and Tagliabue, E. (2002): New insights into the role of extracellular matrix during tumor onset and progression. *J Cell Physiol* 192, 259-67.

Ramos, A. M., and Aller, P. (2008): Quercetin decreases intracellular GSH content and potentiates the apoptotic action of the antileukemic drug arsenic trioxide in human leukemia cell lines. *Biochem Pharmacol* 75, 1912-23.

Rebollo, A., Gomez, J., Martinez de Aragon, A., Lastres, P., Silva, A., and Perez-Sala, D. (1995): Apoptosis induced by IL-2 withdrawal is associated with an intracellular acidification. *Exp Cell Res* 218, 581-5.

Reen, R. K., Nines, R., and Stoner, G. D. (2006): Modulation of N-nitrosomethylbenzylamine metabolism by black raspberries in the esophagus and liver of Fischer 344 rats. *Nutr Cancer* 54, 47-57.

Renis, M., Calandra, L., Scifo, C., Tomasello, B., Cardile, V., Vanella, L., Bei, R., La Fauci, L., and Galvano, F. (2008): Response of cell cycle/stress-related protein expression and DNA damage upon treatment of CaCo2 cells with anthocyanins. *Br J Nutr* 100, 27-35.

Reshkin, S. J., Bellizzi, A., Caldeira, S., Albarani, V., Malanchi, I., Poignee, M., Alunni-Fabbroni, M., Casavola, V., and Tommasino, M. (2000): Na+/H+ exchanger-dependent intracellular alkalinization is an early event in malignant transformation and plays an essential role in the development of subsequent transformation-associated phenotypes. *FASEB J* 14, 2185-97.

Rhee, I., Bachman, K. E., Park, B. H., Jair, K. W., Yen, R. W., Schuebel, K. E., Cui, H., Feinberg, A. P., Lengauer, C., Kinzler, K. W., Baylin, S. B., and Vogelstein, B. (2002): DNMT1 and DNMT3b cooperate to silence genes in human cancer cells. *Nature* 416, 552-6.

Rodriguez-Moranta, F., Salo, J., Arcusa, A., Boadas, J., Pinol, V., Bessa, X., Batiste-Alentorn, E., Lacy, A. M., Delgado, S., Maurel, J., Pique, J. M., and Castells, A. (2006): Postoperative surveillance in patients with colorectal cancer who have undergone curative resection: a prospective, multicenter, randomized, controlled trial. *J Clin Oncol* 24, 386-93.

Rose, P., Huang, Q., Ong, C. N., and Whiteman, M. (2005): Broccoli and watercress suppress matrix metalloproteinase-9 activity and invasiveness of human MDA-MB-231 breast cancer cells. *Toxicol Appl Pharmacol* 209, 105-13.

Ross, S. A. (2003): Diet and DNA methylation interactions in cancer prevention. *Ann N Y Acad Sci* 983, 197-207.

Rossi, M., Garavello, W., Talamini, R., La Vecchia, C., Franceschi, S., Lagiou, P., Zambon, P., Dal Maso, L., Bosetti, C., and Negri, E. (2007): Flavonoids and risk of squamous cell esophageal cancer. *Int J Cancer* 120, 1560-4.

Sablina, A. A., Budanov, A. V., Ilyinskaya, G. V., Agapova, L. S., Kravchenko, J. E., and Chumakov, P. M. (2005): The antioxidant function of the p53 tumor suppressor. *Nat Med* 11, 1306-13.

Samudio, I., Fiegl, M., and Andreeff, M. (2009): Mitochondrial uncoupling and the Warburg effect: molecular basis for the reprogramming of cancer cell metabolism. *Cancer Res* 69, 2163-6.

Seeram, N. P., Adams, L. S., Hardy, M. L., and Heber, D. (2004): Total cranberry extract versus its phytochemical constituents: antiproliferative and synergistic effects against human tumor cell lines. *J Agric Food Chem* 52, 2512-7.

Seeram, N. P., Bourquin, L. D., and Nair, M. G. (2001): Degradation products of cyanidin glycosides from tart cherries and their bioactivities. *J Agric Food Chem* 49, 4924-9.

Selma, M. V., Espin, J. C., and Tomas-Barberan, F. A. (2009): Interaction between phenolics and gut microbiota: role in human health. *J Agric Food Chem* 57, 6485-501.

Shih, P. H., Yeh, C. T., and Yen, G. C. (2005): Effects of anthocyanidin on the inhibition of proliferation and induction of apoptosis in human gastric adenocarcinoma cells. *Food Chem Toxicol* 43, 1557-66.

Shih, P. H., Yeh, C. T., and Yen, G. C. (2007): Anthocyanins induce the activation of phase II enzymes through the antioxidant response element pathway against oxidative stress-induced apoptosis. *J Agric Food Chem* 55, 9427-35.

Shin, D. Y., Lu, J. N., Kim, G. Y., Jung, J. M., Kang, H. S., Lee, W. S., and Choi, Y. H. (2011): Anti-invasive activities of anthocyanins through modulation of tight junctions and suppression of matrix metalloproteinase activities in HCT-116 human colon carcinoma cells. *Oncol Rep* 25, 567-72.

Sies, H. (1999): Glutathione and its role in cellular functions. *Free Radic Biol Med* 27, 916-21.

Singletary, K. W., Stansbury, M. J., Giusti, M., Van Breemen, R. B., Wallig, M., and Rimando, A. (2003): Inhibition of rat mammary tumorigenesis by concord grape juice constituents. *J Agric Food Chem* 51, 7280-6.

Sottocasa, G. L., Lunazzi, G. C., and Tiribelli, C. (1989): Isolation of bilitranslocase, the anion transporter from liver plasma membrane for bilirubin and other organic anions. *Methods Enzymol* 174, 50-7.

Srivastava, A., Akoh, C. C., Fischer, J., and Krewer, G. (2007): Effect of anthocyanin fractions from selected cultivars of Georgia-grown blueberries on apoptosis and phase II enzymes. *J Agric Food Chem* 55, 3180-5.

Stoner, G. D. (2009): Foodstuffs for preventing cancer: the preclinical and clinical development of berries. *Cancer Prev Res (Phila)* 2, 187-94.

Stoner, G. D., Wang, L. S., and Chen, T. (2007): Chemoprevention of esophageal squamous cell carcinoma. *Toxicol Appl Pharmacol* 224, 337-49.

Stresemann, C., Brueckner, B., Musch, T., Stopper, H., and Lyko, F. (2006): Functional diversity of DNA methyltransferase inhibitors in human cancer cell lines. *Cancer Res* 66, 2794-800.

Suda, I., Ishikawa, F., Hatakeyama, M., Miyawaki, M., Kudo, T., Hirano, K., Ito, A., Yamakawa, O., and Horiuchi, S. (2008): Intake of purple sweet potato beverage affects on serum hepatic biomarker levels of healthy adult men with borderline hepatitis. *Eur J Clin Nutr* 62, 60-7.

Szajdek, A., and Borowska, E. J. (2008): Bioactive compounds and health-promoting properties of berry fruits: a review. *Plant Foods Hum Nutr* 63, 147-56.

Takagaki, N., Sowa, Y., Oki, T., Nakanishi, R., Yogosawa, S., and Sakai, T. (2005): Apigenin induces cell cycle arrest and p21/WAF1 expression in a p53-independent pathway. *Int J Oncol* 26, 185-9.

Talavera, S., Felgines, C., Texier, O., Besson, C., Lamaison, J. L., and Remesy, C. (2003): Anthocyanins Are Efficiently Absorbed from the Stomach in Anesthetized Rats. *J Nutr* 133, 4178-4182.

Talavera, S., Felgines, C., Texier, O., Besson, C., Manach, C., Lamaison, J. L., and Remesy, C. (2004): Anthocyanins are efficiently absorbed from the small intestine in rats. *J Nutr* 134, 2275-9.

Thomasset, S., Berry, D. P., Cai, H., West, K., Marczylo, T. H., Marsden, D., Brown, K., Dennison, A., Garcea, G., Miller, A., Hemingway, D., Steward, W. P., and Gescher, A. J. (2009): Pilot study of oral anthocyanins for colorectal cancer chemoprevention. *Cancer Prev Res (Phila)* 2, 625-33.

Tol, J., and Punt, C. J. (2010): Monoclonal antibodies in the treatment of metastatic colorectal cancer: a review. *Clin Ther* 32, 437-53.

Trachootham, D., Zhou, Y., Zhang, H., Demizu, Y., Chen, Z., Pelicano, H., Chiao, P. J., Achanta, G., Arlinghaus, R. B., Liu, J., and Huang, P. (2006): Selective killing of oncogenically transformed cells through a ROS-mediated mechanism by beta-phenylethyl isothiocyanate. *Cancer Cell* 10, 241-52.

Underiner, T. L., Ruggeri, B., and Gingrich, D. E. (2004): Development of vascular endothelial growth factor receptor (VEGFR) kinase inhibitors as anti-angiogenic agents in cancer therapy. *Curr Med Chem* 11, 731-45.

Valle, A., Oliver, J., and Roca, P. (2010): Role of Uncoupling Proteins in Cancer. *Cancers* 2, 567-591.

Van Cutsem, E., Kohne, C. H., Hitre, E., Zaluski, J., Chang Chien, C. R., Makhson, A., D'Haens, G., Pinter, T., Lim, R., Bodoky, G., Roh, J. K., Folprecht, G., Ruff, P., Stroh, C., Tejpar, S., Schlichting, M., Nippgen, J., and Rougier, P. (2009): Cetuximab and chemotherapy as initial treatment for metastatic colorectal cancer. *N Engl J Med* 360, 1408-17.

van Duijnhoven, F. J. B., Bueno-De-Mesquita, H. B., Ferrari, P., Jenab, M., Boshuizen, H. C., Ros, M. M., Casagrande, C., Tjønneland, A., Olsen, A., Overvad, K., Thorlacius-Ussing, O., Clavel-Chapelon, F., Boutron-Ruault, M. C., Morois, S., Kaaks, R., Linseisen, J., Boeing, H., Nothlings, U., Trichopoulou, A., Trichopoulos, D., Misirli, G., Palli, D., Sieri, S., Panico, S., Tumino, R., Vineis, P., Peeters, P. H. M., van Gils, C. H., Ocke, M. C., Lund, E., Engeset, D., Skeie, G., Rodrıguez Suarez, L., Gonzalez, C. A., Sanchez, M. J., Dorronsoro, M., Navarro, C., Barricarte, A., Berglund, G., Manjer, J., Hallmans, G., Palmqvist, R., Bingham, S. A., Khaw, K. T., Key, T. J., Allen, N. E., Boffetta, P., Slimani, N., Rinaldi, S., Gallo, V., Norat, T., and Riboli, E. (2009): Fruit, vegetables, and colorectal cancer risk: the European Prospective Investigation into Cancer and Nutrition. *Am J Clin Nutr* 89, 1441-52.

Vander Heiden, M. G., Chandel, N. S., Schumacker, P. T., and Thompson, C. B. (1999): Bcl-xL prevents cell death following growth factor withdrawal by facilitating mitochondrial ATP/ADP exchange. *Mol Cell* 3, 159-67.

Vanzo, A., Vrhovsek, U., Tramer, F., Mattivi, F., and Passamonti, S. (2011): Exceptionally fast uptake and metabolism of cyanidin 3-glucoside by rat kidneys and liver. *J Nat Prod* 74, 1049-54.

Veigas, J. M., Shrivasthava, R., and Neelwarne, B. (2008): Efficient amelioration of carbon tetrachloride induced toxicity in isolated rat hepatocytes by Syzygium cumini Skeels extract. *Toxicol In Vitro* 22, 1440-6.

Venkatachalam, R., Ligtenberg, M. J., Hoogerbrugge, N., de Bruijn, D. R., Kuiper, R. P., and Geurts van Kessel, A. (2010): The epigenetics of (hereditary) colorectal cancer. *Cancer Genet Cytogenet* 203, 1-6.

Ververidis, F., Trantas, E., Douglas, C., Vollmer, G., Kretzschmar, G., and Panopoulos, N. (2007): Biotechnology of flavonoids and other phenylpropanoid-derived natural products. Part I: Chemical diversity, impacts on plant biology and human health. *Biotechnol J* 2, 1214-34.

Vitaglione, P., Donnarumma, G., Napolitano, A., Galvano, F., Gallo, A., Scalfi, L., and Fogliano, V. (2007): Protocatechuic acid is the major human metabolite of cyanidin-glucosides. *J Nutr* 137, 2043-8.

Wang, L. S., Sardo, C., Rocha, C. M., McIntyre, C. M., Frankel, W., Arnold, M., Martin, E., Lechner, J. F., and Stoner, G. D. (2007): Effect of freeze-dried black raspberries on human colorectal cancer lesions. AACR Special Conference in Cancer Research, Advances in Colon Cancer Research

Wang, L. S., and Stoner, G. D. (2008): Anthocyanins and their role in cancer prevention. *Cancer Lett* 269, 281-90.

Wang, S. Y., and Jiao, H. (2000): Scavenging capacity of berry crops on superoxide radicals, hydrogen peroxide, hydroxyl radicals, and singlet oxygen. *J Agric Food Chem* 48, 5677-84.

Warburg, O. (1956a): On respiratory impairment in cancer cells. *Science* 124, 269-70.

Warburg, O. (1956b): On the origin of cancer cells. *Science* 123, 309-14.

Weisel, T., Baum, M., Eisenbrand, G., Dietrich, H., Will, F., Stockis, J. P., Kulling, S., Rufer, C., Johannes, C., and Janzowski, C. (2006): An anthocyanin/polyphenolic-rich fruit juice reduces oxidative DNA damage and increases glutathione level in healthy probands. *Biotechnol J* 1, 388-97.

Wenzel, U., Nickel, A., and Daniel, H. (2005): Increased mitochondrial palmitoylcarnitine/carnitine countertransport by flavone causes oxidative stress and apoptosis in colon cancer cells. *Cell Mol Life Sci* 62, 3100-5.

Wolffram, S., Block, M., and Ader, P. (2002): Quercetin-3-glucoside is transported by the glucose carrier SGLT1 across the brush border membrane of rat small intestine. *J Nutr* 132, 630-5.

Wolter, F., Akoglu, B., Clausnitzer, A., and Stein, J. (2001): Downregulation of the cyclin D1/Cdk4 complex occurs during resveratrol-induced cell cycle arrest in colon cancer cell lines. *J Nutr* 131, 2197-203.

Won, K. Y., Lim, S. J., Kim, G. Y., Kim, Y. W., Han, S. A., Song, J. Y., and Lee, D. K. (2011): Regulatory role of p53 in cancer metabolism via SCO2 and TIGAR in human breast cancer. *Hum Pathol.*

Wu, G., Fang, Y. Z., Yang, S., Lupton, J. R., and Turner, N. D. (2004): Glutathione metabolism and its implications for health. *J Nutr* 134, 489-92.

Wu, Q. K., Koponen, J. M., Mykkanen, H. M., and Torronen, A. R. (2007): Berry phenolic extracts modulate the expression of p21(WAF1) and Bax but not Bcl-2 in HT-29 colon cancer cells. *J Agric Food Chem* 55, 1156-63.

Yao, H., Xu, W., Shi, X., and Zhang, Z. (2011): Dietary flavonoids as cancer prevention agents. *J Environ Sci Health C Environ Carcinog Ecotoxicol Rev* 29, 1-31.

Yasuda, S., Fujii, H., Nakahara, T., Nishiumi, N., Takahashi, W., Ide, M., and Shohtsu, A. (2001): 18F-FDG PET detection of colonic adenomas. *J Nucl Med* 42, 989-92.

Yasuzawa, T., Iida, T., Yoshida, M., Hirayama, N., Takahashi, M., Shirahata, K., and Sano, H. (1986): The structures of the novel protein kinase C inhibitors K-252a, b, c and d. *J Antibiot (Tokyo)* 39, 1072-8.

Yu, N. K., Baek, S. H., and Kaang, B. K. (2011): DNA methylation-mediated control of learning and memory. *Mol Brain* 4, 5.

Yun, J. W., Lee, W. S., Kim, M. J., Lu, J. N., Kang, M. H., Kim, H. G., Kim, D. C., Choi, E. J., Choi, J. Y., Lee, Y. K., Ryu, C. H., Kim, G., Choi, Y. H., Park, O. J., and Shin, S. C. (2010): Characterization of a profile of the anthocyanins isolated from Vitis coignetiae Pulliat and their anti-invasive activity on HT-29 human colon cancer cells. *Food Chem Toxicol* 48, 903-9.

Zhang, Y., Vareed, S. K., and Nair, M. G. (2005): Human tumor cell growth inhibition by nontoxic anthocyanidins, the pigments in fruits and vegetables. *Life Sci* 76, 1465-72.

Zhao, C., Giusti, M. M., Malik, M., Moyer, M. P., and Magnuson, B. A. (2004): Effects of commercial anthocyanin-rich extracts on colonic cancer and nontumorigenic colonic cell growth. *J Agric Food Chem* 52, 6122-8.

Ziberna, L., Lunder, M., Tramer, F., Drevensek, G., and Passamonti, S. (2011): The endothelial plasma membrane transporter bilitranslocase mediates rat aortic vasodilation induced by anthocyanins. *Nutr Metab Cardiovasc Dis*.

Zu, X. Y., Zhang, Z. Y., Zhang, X. W., Yoshioka, M., Yang, Y. N., and Li, J. (2010): Anthocyanins extracted from Chinese blueberry (Vaccinium uliginosum L.) and its anticancer effects on DLD-1 and COLO205 cells. *Chin Med J (Engl)* 123, 2714-9.

9

Colorectal Cancer and Alcohol

Seitz K. Helmut and Nils Homann

Department of Medicine (Gastroenterology & Hepatology), Salem Medical Centre,
Centre of Alcohol Research, University of Heidelberg,
Department of Gastroenterology, City Hospital Wolfsburg, Wolfsburg,
Germany

1. Introduction

Chronic alcohol consumption may lead to a variety of diseases and may deteriorate a great number of existing health problems. Among all these diseases the development of certain types of cancer is of major concern. Since decades it has been known that chronic alcohol consumption is a risk factor for cancer of the upper aerodigestive tract (oral cavity, pharynx, larynx and oesophagus), the liver and the female breast. Data with respect to alcohol and cancer concerning other organs do not show such clear correlations. In February 2007 an international group of epidemiologists and alcohol researchers met at the International Agency for Research on Cancer (IARC) in Lyon, France, to evaluate the role of alcohol and its first metabolite acetaldehyde as potential carcinogens in experimental animals and humans. The working group has concluded from the epidemiological data available that the occurrence of malignant tumours mentioned above is related to the consumption of alcoholic beverages. In addition, at this time epidemiologic and experimental data showed that alcohol is also a risk factor for colorectal cancer (Baan et al., 2007).

Worldwide a total of approximately 389,000 cases of cancer presenting 3.6 % of oral cancers (5.2 % in men and 1.7 % in women) derive from chronic alcohol consumption (Rehm et al., 2004). Besides the fact that alcohol is a co-carcinogen and may act as a promoter alcohol can also accelerate tumour spread as exemplified for liver metastases of colorectal cancer possibly due to immune suppression and induction of angiogenesis by the expression of vascular endothelial growth factor (VEGF) (Seitz & Stickel, 2010). In addition, it is important to know that ethanol also interacts with the metabolism of chemo-therapeutic drugs which can result in a decreased respond to medication and increased side-effects (De Bruijn & Slee, 1992).

This review focuses solely on the effect of chronic alcohol consumption on colorectal cancer, a cancer which is wide spread in Western societies and is No. 3 cancer in men and women in Germany. The present review will, therefore, discuss epidemiology of alcohol and colorectal cancer, will briefly address possible mechanism by which alcohol stimulates colorectal carcinogenesis and may finally give some suggestions and recommendations with respective to earlier detection and identification of high risk groups.

2. Epidemiology

An increased risk for the development of colorectal cancer associated with chronic alcohol ingestion has been considered for decades. In 1974 Breslow and Enstrom emphasized a correlation between beer consumption and rectal cancer occurrence (Breslow & Enstrom 1974). In 1992 Kune and Vitetta summarized the results of more than 50 epidemiologic studies between 1957 and 1991 including 7 correlational studies, more than 40 case control studies and 17 prospective cohort studies on the role of alcohol on the development of colorectal tumours (Kune & Vitetta 1992). Most of these studies reported a positive association of large bowel cancer with alcohol consumption. In addition a positive trend with respect to dose-response was found in 5 out of 10 case control studies and in all prospective cohort studies in which a dose-response analysis has been performed.

In the nineties of the last century another 12 epidemiological studies have been published with inconsistent results (Seitz et al., 2006). Most importantly a prospective cohort study in Japan reported a positive dose-response relationship between alcohol intake and colon cancer risk in men and women (N. Shimizu et al., 2003), while a Danish population based cohort study showed no association (Pedersen et al., 2003).

A panel of experts at a WHO consensus conference on nutrition and colorectal cancer reviewed in 1999 the epidemiology on alcohol and colorectal cancer and it was concluded that alcohol ingestion even in a low dose-intake between 10 and 40 grams especially consumed as beer resulted in a 1.5-fold increased risk for colorectal cancer and to a lesser extend for colonic cancer in both sexes but predominantly in men (Scheppach et al., 1999).

Cho et al showed in a meta-analysis of 8 cohort studies from the US and Europe a trend between the increased amount of alcohol intake and the risk for colorectal cancer. In this meta-analysis a consumption of more than 45 grams per day was associated with an increased risk of 45 % (Cho et al., 2004).

A huge prospective follow-up study of more than 10,000 US citizens concluded that alcohol consumption of one or more alcoholic beverages per day is associated with a 70 % greater risk of colonic cancer with a strong positive dose-response relationship (Su & Arab, 2004).

Most recently it was proposed that the alcohol colorectal cancer association is more apparent in Japanese than in Western populations. A pooled analysis of results from 5 cohort studies from Japan showed a strong and highly significant association between alcohol intake and colorectal cancer not only in men but also in women (Mizoue et al., 2008). Twenty five per cent of colorectal cancer cases in men were attributable to an alcohol intake of more than 23 grams per day. A recent meta analysis from the IARC of 34 case control and 7 cohort studies provides strong evidence for an association between alcohol consumption of more than 1 drink per day and the risk for colorectal cancer (Fedirko et al., 2011). Similar results were reported from the Netherlands (Bongaerts et al., 2008, 2010) and the US (Thygesen et al., 2008) but not from Great Britain (Park et al., 2009, 2010).

The accumulation of all these convincing epidemiologic data on alcohol and colorectal cancer resulted by the IARC that chronic alcohol consumption is a risk factor for colorectal cancer (Baan et al., 2007).

3. Animal experiments

Various animal experiments have been performed to study the effect of alcohol on chemically induced colorectal cancer. The results of these experiments depend on the experimental design, the type of carcinogen used, its time duration of exposure and dosage as well as the route of alcohol administration. While alcohol alone does not induce colorectal tumours, the administration of alcohol together with a colorectal carcinogen does under certain experimental conditions result in a stimulation of carcinogenesis (Seitz et al., 2006).

This is especially relevant when a carcinogen such as acetoxymethylmethylnitrosamine (AMMN) is locally applied to the rectal mucosa (Seitz et al., 1990). Some evidence exist that acetaldehyde (AA) is an important factor since inhibition of its degradation stimulates colorectal cancer (Seitz et al., 1990).

For a detailed summary of the animal experiments performed so far we refer to the following review article (Seitz et al., 2006).

4. Risk factors in alcohol mediated colorectal carcinogenesis

Various risk factors for ethanol-mediated colorectal carcinogenesis exist. Five out of 6 studies of the effect of alcohol on the occurrence of adenoma polyps in large intestine showed a positive association with alcohol (Kune et al., 1992; Seitz et al., 1998). In addition, also the occurrence of hyperplastic polyps is enhanced when more than 30 grams of alcohol per day were consumed. The relative risk for men was 1.8 and for women 2.5 (Kearney et al., 1995).

Alcohol affects the adenoma/carcinoma sequence at the different early steps (Boutron et al., 1995). High alcohol intake favours high risk polyps or colorectal cancer occurrence among patients with adenoma (Bardou et al., 2002). It has also been reported that a reduction in alcohol consumption for individuals with genetic predisposition for colorectal cancer had large beneficial effects on tumour incidence (Le Marchand et al., 1999). Thus, patients with tendency towards colorectal polyps have an increased risk to develop carcinoma when they consume additional alcohol.

Another additional risk is possibly the presence of ulcerative colitis, although the data are not completely clear. Alcohol by itself may additionally enhance inflammation and may thus favour carcinogenesis.

Another important factor is that alcohol reduces the availability of folate which results in a decrease of methylation and thus, a decrease of thymidine generation, DNA synthesis and cellular regeneration, in a situation of enhanced need. Therefore, folate, methionine and vitamin B6 deficiency are risk factors for ethanol mediated colorectal carcinogenesis (Giovannucci et al., 1995; Larsson et al., 2005; Schernhammer et al., 2008; Weinstein et al., 2008; Yamaji et al.; 2009; Figueiredo et al., 2009; Lee et al., 2010).

It is well known that tobacco smoking is associated with a higher risk for colonic adenoma and hyperplastic polyp formation as well as increased incidence of colorectal carcinoma (Seitz & Cho, 2009).

Age, another risk factor for colorectal cancer may also affect ethanol mediated cancer development in the large intestine. It has been shown in animal experiments that mucosal damage induced by chronic alcohol ingestion is more pronounced with advanced age compared to youth (Simanowski et al., 1994).

Finally, genetic risk factor with respect to alcohol metabolism and colorectal cancer has to be taken into consideration. Alcohol is metabolised by alcohol dehydrogenase (ADH) to AA. Seven different ADHs exist and two of them (ADH1B and ADH1C) reveal polymorphism. Among the two ADH1C is of considerable interest (see below) (Edenberg, 1997). Individuals with increase metabolism of ethanol via ADH1C due to homozygosity of the ADH1C*1 allele seem to have a significantly increased risk for colorectal cancer when they consume more than 30 grams alcohol per day (Homann et al., 2006).

5. Possible mechanisms of alcohol mediated colorectal carcinogenesis

5.1 Acetaldehyde (AA)

Most recently the IARC has identified AA as an important carcinogen for humans (Secretan et al., 2009). AA is produced from ethanol via ADH. In the gastrointestinal mucosa various ADHs are present and capable to produce AA from alcohol. In addition, gastrointestinal bacteria of the upper gastrointestinal tract and of the large intestine can metabolize ethanol to AA (Salaspuro, 2003) (Figure 1).

AA is highly toxic and carcinogenic and causes point mutations in the hypoxanthine-guanine phosphoribosyltransferase localized in human lymphocytes, induces sister chromatid exchanges and cross-chromosomal aberration (Seitz & Stickel, 2010). AA forms stable adducts with DNA. One of these adducts is especially generated in hyperregenerative tissues (in the presence of spermine and spermidine) such as the upper gastrointestinal tract and the colon where chronic alcohol consumption results in tissue hyperregenerativity. This propane DNA adduct is highly carcinogenic (Brooks & Thiruvathu, 2005). There is significant evidence that AA is responsible for the carcinogenic effect of alcohol in the upper gastrointestinal tract, oesophagus, larynx, pharynx and oral cavity (Baan et al., 2007; Seitz & Stickel, 2010). For more details about the role of AA on upper gastrointestinal cancer we refer to the following review article (Baan et al., 2007; Stickel et al., 2006).

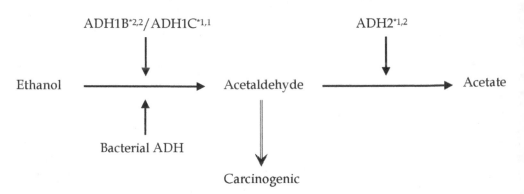

Fig. 1. Ethanol metabolism by mucosal enzymes and gastrointestinal bacteria. Ethanol is first metabolized by alcohol dehydrogenase (ADH) to acetaldehyde (AA) which is toxic and carcinogenic. AA is then further converted by acetaldehyde dehydrogenase (ALDH) to acetate which is non-toxic and is channelled into the intermediary metabolism of the cell. Accumulation of AA may either occur with rapid generation through ADH or slow degradation through ALDH. ADH1B and ADH1C are polymorphic. While the ADH1B*2 allele encodes for ADH enzymes approximately 40-fold more active as compared to the enzymes encoded by the ADH1B*2 allele, the ADH1C*1 allele encodes for an enzyme approximately 2.5-fold more active than the enzyme encoded by the ADH1C*2 allele. Thus, ADH1B*2,2 and ADH1C*1,1 homozygotes may accumulate AA. In addition, 40 % of Asians are heterozygote for the ALDH2 gene (ALDH2*1,2) encoding for an enzyme with very low ALDH activity resulting in AA accumulation.

In the colonic mucosa ADH1 and ADH3 are present and are involved in AA generation. On the other hand acetaldehyde dehydrogenase (ALDH), the enzyme responsible for AA degradation is detectable at relative low activities only (Seitz & Oneta, 1998). The net amount of AA present in the tissue may determine its toxic and carcinogenic action. Thus, individuals with an increased production and decreased degradation of AA are especially at risk for colorectal cancer development. It has been proposed that the ALDH activity of colonic mucosa may be sufficient for the removal of AA produced by colonic mucosal ADH during ethanol oxidation but it is insufficient for the removal of AA produced by intracolonic bacteria.

The most striking evidence of the causal role of AA in ethanol-associated carcinogenesis derives from genetic linkage studies in alcoholics and / or heavy drinkers. Individuals who accumulate AA due to polymorphism and / or mutation in the gene coding for enzymes responsible for AA generation and detoxification have been shown to have an increased cancer risk. In Japan as well as in other Asian countries a high percentage of individuals carry a mutation of the ALDH2 gene which codes for an enzyme with low activity leading to elevated AA levels after alcohol consumption. While homozygotes are completely protected against alcoholism and alcohol associated diseases due to the fact that they cannot tolerate alcohol even at very small doses, heterozygotes (ALDH2*1,2) have an increased risk for alimentary tract cancer including the colon and the rectum (Yokoyama et al., 1998) (Figure.1).

In addition, polymorphism of the ADH1C gene may also modulate AA levels. ADH1C*1 transcription leads to an ADH isoenzyme 2.5 times more active than that from ADH1C*2 (Figure1). We evaluated whether the associated between alcohol consumption and colorectal cancer development is modified by ADH1C polymorphism. We recruited 173 individuals with colorectal tumours diagnosed by coloscopy and 788 control individuals without colorectal tumours and determined their genotypes. Genotype ADH1C*1/1 was more frequent in patient with alcohol associated colorectal neoplasia compared to patients without cancer (Homann et al., 2006). In addition, only individuals drinking more than 30 grams ethanol per day with a genotype ADH1C*1/1 had an increased risk for colorectal tumours. These data identify ADH1C homozygosity as a genetic risk marker for colorectal tumours in individuals consuming more than 30 grams alcohol per day and emphasize further the role of AA as a carcinogenic agent in alcohol mediated colorectal carcinogenesis.

It has been shown that after alcohol administration, the amount of AA per gram of tissue is highest for the colonic mucosa compared to all other tissues in the body (Seitz et al., 1987). This is primarily due to the production of AA by the faecal bacteria. AA has toxic effects on the colon mucosa resulting in secondary compensatory hyperregeneration with increased crypt cell production rates and an extension of the proliferative compartment towards the lumen of the crypt (Simanowski et al., 1994, 2001). This change in crypt cell dynamics represents a condition associating with increased risk for colorectal cancer.

The alcohol associated hyperregeneration of the colonic mucosa is especially pronounced with increasing age (Simanowski et al., 1994). As already pointed out, this may have practical implications since age by itself is a risk factor for CRC.

High AA levels have been found after alcohol administration in the colon of rats and these concentrations were significantly lower in germ free animals as compared to the conventional rats suggesting that faecal bacteria are capable of producing AA (Seitz et al., 1990). Indeed, the reversed microbial ADH reaction produces under aerobic or microaerobic conditions striking amounts of AA when human colonic contents or some microbes representing normal colonic flora are incubated in vitro at 37°C with increasing ethanol concentrations (Jokelainen et al., 1996, 1994; Salaspuro et al., 1999). This reaction is already active at comparatively low ethanol concentrations (10-100 mg %) which exist in the colon following social drinking (Jokelainen et al., 1996). AA formation catalysed by microbial ADH takes place at a pH normally found in the colon and is rapidly reduced with decreasing pH (Jokelainen et al., 1994).

The administration of antibiotics to animals has significantly decreased colonic bacteria and colonic AA production (Jokelainen et al., 1997).

a. high AA levels occur in the colon due to bacterial and mucosal ethanol oxidation
b. animal experiments show an increased occurrence of colorectal tumours induced by the specific locally acting carcinogen AMMN when cyanamide, an ALDH inhibitor, is applied and AA levels are elevated,
c. crypt cell production rate correlates significantly with AA levels in the colonic mucosa, (d) colonic AA levels show a significant inverse relationship with mucosal folate concentration which supports in vitro data showing a destruction of folate by AA,
d. individuals with the inactive form of ALDH2 resulting in elevated AA concentrations exhibit an increased risk for CRC when they consume alcohol,
e. individuals homozygous for the ADH1C*1 allele coding for an enzyme with a 2.5 times higher AA production have also an increased risk for colorectal cancer, the action of AA seems the major mechanism of ethanol-mediated colorectal cancer development.

5.2 Oxidative stress

Chronic ethanol consumption results in the induction of cytochrome P4502E1 (CYP2E1) predominantly in the liver (Seitz & Stickel, 2010) but also in other tissues including the colorectal mucosa (Shimizu et al., 1990). This CYP2E1 induction is associated with an increased metabolism of ethanol through CYP2E1 and the generation of AA but also of reactive oxygen species (ROS). For more details we refer to the following review article (Seitz & Stickel, 2007). ROS may attack lipids and result in lipidperoxidation with the generation of lipidperoxidation products such as 4-hydroxy-nonenal or malondialdehyde. These lipidperoxidation products may bind to proteins but also to DNA and form exocyclic etheno DNA adducts with a high carcinogenic potency (Wang et al., 2009).

The effect of chronic ethanol consumption on the induction of CYP2E1 and the activation of procarcinogens has been convincingly demonstrated by the use of azoxymethane (AOM), a procarcinogen for the colon. The metabolism of AOM to its ultimate carcinogen has been inhibited in the presence of ethanol in the body since ethanol competes for the binding site at CYP2E1 but significantly enhanced when ethanol is withdrawn in a condition where CYP2E1 is induced and completely available for the metabolism of AOM (Sohn et al., 1987).

The induction of CYP2E1 in the colonic mucosa may lead to an enhanced activation of dietary (nitrosamines) and cigarette smoke derived (polycyclic hydrocarbons) procarcinogens and may be one mechanism by which ethanol enhances colorectal carcinogenesis (Seitz & Osswald, 1994).

In this context it is interesting that alpha tocopherol, a radical scavenger, prevents mucosal cell hyperproliferation induced by ethanol suggesting that ROS may be involved in this process (Vincon et al., 2003).

5.3 Epigenetics

There is increasing evidence that alcohol related epigenetic changes of DNA methylation and histone acetylation do occur which may potentially modulate tumour development (Stickel et al., 2006). Epidemiologic data have clearly shown that folate deficiency alone or together with methionine deficiency increases the risk for ethanol mediated colorectal cancer (Giovannucci et al., 1995; Larsson et al., 2005; Schernhammer et al., 2008; Weinstein et al., 2008; Yamaji et al., 2009; Figueiredo et al., 2009; Lee et al., 2010). Similarly, vitamin B6 deficiency also enhances tumour risk. All these factors are involved in methyl transfer. Their deficiency results in DNA hypomethylation, a condition relevant in carcinogenesis. In addition, histone acetylation is also favoured by chronic ethanol consumption (Kim & Shukla, 2006; Choudhury & Shukla, 2008) since ethanol metabolism leads to the accumulation of acetate on one hand and to a change in the intracellular redox potential with increasing concentrations of NADH and decreasing concentrations of NAD on the other hand. This change in redox potential also favours histone acetylation. In addition, histone deacetylation is blocked by ethanol through its inhibitory effect on histone deacetylase (HDA).

Indeed, animal experiments have shown DNA hypomethylation in the colon following chronic ethanol ingestion (Choi et al., 1999). However, site specific hypomethylation have not been demonstrated so far.

5.4 Other mechanisms

Other mechanisms of ethanol mediated carcinogenesis in the colon may including deficiency of retinoic acid (Wang X.D. & Seitz, 2004), effect of ethanol on intracellular signalling (Dunty, 2010) including various pathways such as Mitogenic signals (MAPK, RAS), Insensitivity to anti-growth signals (Rb and Cell cycle control, TGFβ), Apoptosis (p53, PTEN), Angiogenesis, Metastasis (ECM, Osteopontin, Wnt) and an ethanol effect on inflammation (Wang, J., 2010).

6. Summary, conclusion and recommendations

Chronic ethanol consumption at a dose of more than 30 grams ethanol per day is a risk factor for colorectal cancer. Chronic ethanol consumption also increases the risk for colorectal cancer in individuals with polyps and colorectal inflammation as well as in those with an ALDH mutation (ALDH2* 1,2, only Asians) and ADH1C*1 homozygosity since they accumulate AA following ethanol ingestion.

The mechanisms of ethanol mediated colorectal carcinogenesis may involve AA produced by mucosal ADH and intestinal bacteria. In addition, oxidative stress induced by ethanol may also play a role.

As a clinical consequence, chronic alcohol consumers should be screened earlier as the general population for colorectal cancer either by faecal blood test or colonoscopy depending on the methods available.

7. Acknowledgements

The authors wish to thank Mrs. Heike Grönebaum for typing the manuscript. Original research was supported by grants of the Manfred Lautenschläger- and Dietmar Hopp Foundation.

8. References

Baan, R.; Straif, K.; Grosse, Y.; Secretan, B.; El Ghissassi, F.; Bouvard, V.; et al. (2007) Carcinogenicity of alcoholic beverages. *Lancet Oncol.* Vol. 8: pp. 292-3

Bardou, M.; Montembault, S.; Giraud V.; Balian A.; Borotto E.; Houdayer C.; Capron F.; Chaput J.C. & Naveau S (2002). Excessive alcohol consumption favours high risk polyp or colorectal cancer occurrence among patients with adenomas: a case control study. *Gut* Vol. 50: pp. 38-42.

Bongaerts, B.W.; van den Brandt, P.A.; Goldbohm, R.A.; de Goeij, A.F. & Weijenberg, M.P. (2008). Alcohol consumption, type of alcoholic beverage and risk of colorectal cancer at specific subsites. *Int J Cancer* Vol. 123(10): pp. 2411-2417.

Bongaerts, B.W.; de Goeij, A.F.; Wouters, K.A.; van Engeland, M.; Gottschalk, R.W.; Van Schooten, F.J., et al.(2010) Alcohol consumption, alcohol dehydrogenase 1C (ADH1C) genotype, and risk of colorectal cancer in the Netherlands Cohort Study on diet and cancer. Alcohol (Epub ahead of printing) URL: *www.alcoholjournal.org*

Boutron, M.C.; Faivre, J.; Dop, M.C.; Quipourt, V. & Senesse, P. (1995). Tobacco, alcohol, and colorectal tumors: a multistep process. *Am J Epidemiol* Vol. 141: pp. 1038-1046.

Breslow, N.E. & Enstrom, J.E. (1974). Geographic correlations between mortality rates and alcohol, tobacco consumption in the United States. *J Natl Cancer Inst* Vol. 53: pp. 631-639.

Brooks, P.J. & Thiruvathu, J.A. (2005). DNA adducts from acetaldehyde: implications for alcohol-related carcinogenesis. *Alcohol* Vol. 35: pp. 187-193.

Cho, E.; Smith-Warner, S.A.; Ritz, J.; van den Brandt, P.A.; Colditz, G.A.; Folsom, A.R.; Freudenheim, J.L.; Giovannucci, E.; Goldbohm, R.A.; Graham, S.; Holmberg, L.; Kim, D.H.; Malila, N.; Miller, A.B.; Pietinen, P.; Rohan, T.E.; Sellers; T.A., Speizer, F.E.; Willett, W.C.; Wolk, A. & Hunter, D.J. (2004). Alcohol intake and colorectal cancer: a pooled analysis of 8 cohort studies. *Ann Intern Med* Vol. 140: pp. 603-613.

Choi, S.W.; Stickel, F.; Baik, H.W.; Kim, Y.I.; Seitz, H.K. & Mason, J.B. (1999). Chronic alcohol consumption induces genomic but not p53-specific DNA hypomethylation in rat colon. *J Nutr.* Vol. 129: pp. 1945-50.

Choudhury, M. & Shukla, S.D. (2008). Surrogate alcohols and their metabolites modify histone H3 acetylation: involvement of histone acetyl transferase and histone deacetylase. *Alcohol Clin Exp Res.* Vol. 32: pp. 829-39.

DeBruijn, E.A.; Slee, P.H.T.J. (1992) Alcohol effects on anticancer drug metabolism. In: *Alcohol and Cancer* (ed. R.R. Watson), CRC Press Boca Raton, Ann Arbor, London, Tokyo, pp. 135-150.

Dunty B. (2010) Alcohol, cancer genes, and signaling pathways. NIAAA Extramural Advisory Board 2010, *Alcohol and Cancer*, NIH June 8-9, 2010, pp. 69-93.

Edenberg, H.J. (2007). Role of alcohol dehydrogenase and aldehyde dehydrogenase variants. Alcohol Res Health Vol. 30: pp. 5-37.

Fedirko, V.; Tramacere, I.; Bagnardi, V.; Rota, M.; Scotti, L.; Islami, F.; Negri, E.; Straif, K.; Romieu, I.; La Vecchia, C. ; Boffetta, P. & Jenab, M. (2011). Alcohol drinking and colorectal cancer risk: an overall and dose-response meta-analysis of published studies. *Ann Oncol* (Epub ahead of print)

Figueiredo, J.C.; Grau, M.V.; Wallace, K.; Levine, A.J.; Shen, L.; Hamdan, R.; Chen, X.; Bresalier, R.S.; McKeown-Eyssen, G.; Haile, R.W.; Baron, J.A. & Issa, J.P.J. (2009). Global DNA hypomethylation (LINE-1) in the normal colon and lifestyle characteristics and dietary and genetic factors. *Cancer Epidemiol Biomarkers Prev* Vol. 18(4): pp. 1041-1049.

Giovannucci, E.; Rimm, E.B.; Ascherio, A.; Stampfer, M.J.; Colditz, G.A. & Willett, W.C. (1995). Alcohol, low-methionine – low folate diets, and risk of colon cancer in men. *J Natl Cancer Inst* Vol. 87: pp. 265-273.

Homann N; Stickel F; König IR; Jacobs A; Junghanns K; Benesova M; Schuppan D; Himsel S; Zuber-Jerger I; Hellerbrand C; Ludwig D; Caselmann WH; Seitz HK (2006). Alcohol dehydrogenase 1C*1 allele is a genetic marker for alcohol-associated cancer in heavy drinkers. *Int J Cancer* Vol. 118(8):pp. 1998-2002.

Jokelainen, K.; Roine, R.; Väänänen, H.; Salaspuro, M. (1994). In vitro acetaldehyde formation by human colonic bacteria. *Gut* Vol. 35: pp. 1271-1274.

Jokelainen, K.; Siitonen, A.; Jousimies-Somer, H. (1996). In vitro alcohol dehydrogenase-mediated acetaldehyde production by aerobic bacteria representing the normal colonic flora in man. *Alcohol Clin Exp Res* Vol. 20: pp. 967-972.

Jokelainen, K.; Matysiak-Budnik, T.; Mäkisalo, H.; Höckerstedt, K.; Salaspuro, M. (1996). High intracolonic acetaldehyde values produced by a bacteriocolonic pathway for ethanol oxidation in piglets. *Gut* Vol. 39: pp. 100-104.

Jokelainen K.; Nosova T.; Koivisto T.; Väkeväinen S.; Jousimies-Somer H.; Heine R.; Salaspuro M. (1997). Inhibition of bacteriocolonic pathway for ethanol oxidation by ciprofloxacin in rats. *Life Sci* Vol. 61: pp. 1755-1762.

Kearney, J.; Giovannucci, E.; Rimm, E.B.; Stampfer, M.J.; Colditz, G.A.; Ascherio, A.; Bleday, R. & Willett, W.C (1995). Diet, alcohol, and smoking and the occurrence of hyperplastic polyps of the colon and rectum (United States). *Cancer Causes Control* Vol. 6: pp. 45-56.

Kim, J.S. & Shukla, S.D. (2006) Acute in vivo effect of ethanol (binge drinking) on histone H3 modifications in rat tissues. *Alcohol Alcohol.* Vol. 41: pp. 126-32.

Kune, G.A. & Vitetta, L. (1992). Alcohol consumption and the etiology of colorectal cancer: a review of the scientific evidence from 1957 to 1991. *Nutr Cancer* Vol. 18: pp. 97-111.

Larsson, S.C.; Giovannucci, E. & Wolk, A. (2005). Vitamin B6 intake, alcohol consumption, and colorectal cancer: a longitudinal population-based cohort of women. *Gastroenterology* Vol. 128: pp. 1830-1837.

Lee, J.E.; Giovannucci, E.; Fuchs, C.S.; Willett, W.C.; Zeisel, S.H. & Cho, E. (2010). Choline and betaine intake and the risk of colorectal cancer in men. *Cancer Epidemiol Biomarkers Prev* Vol. 19(3): pp. 884-887.

Le Marchand, L.; Wilkens, L.R.; Hankin, J.H.; Kolonel, L.N. & Lyu, L.C. (1999). Independent and joint effects of family history and lifestyle on colorectal cancer risk: implications for prevention. *Cancer Epidemiol Biomarkers Prev* Vol. 8: pp. 45-851.

Mizoue, T.; Inoue, M.; Wakai, K.; Nagata, C.; Shimazu, T.; Tsuji, I.; Otani, T.; Tanaka, K.; Matsuo, K.; Tamakoshi, A.; Sasazuki, S. & Tsugane S. (2008). Alcohol drinking and colorectal cancer in Japanese: a pooled analysis of results from five cohort studies. *Am J Epidemiol* Vol. 167: pp. 1397-1406.

Park, J.Y.; Mitrou, P.N.; Dahm, C.C.; Luben, R.N.; Wareham, N.J.; Khaw, K.T. & Rodwell, S.A. (2009). Baseline alcohol consumption, type of alcoholic beverage and risk of colorectal cancer in the European Prospective Investigation into Cancer and Nutrition-Norfolk study. *Cancer Epidemiol* Vol. 33(5): pp. 347-354.

Park, J.Y.; Dahm, C.C.; Keogh, R.H.; Mitrou, P.N.; Cairns B.J.; Greenwood, D.C.; Spencer, E.A.; Fentiman, I.S.; Shipley, M.J.; Brunner, E.J.; Cade, J.E.; Burley, V.J.; Mishra, G.D.; Kuh, D.; Stephen, A.M.; White, I.R.; Luben, R.N.; Mulligan, A.A,; Khaw, K.T. & Rodwell, S.A. (2010). Alcohol intake and risk of colorectal cancer: results from the UK Dietary Cohort Consortium. *Br J Cancer* Vol. 24: pp.

Pedersen, A., Johansen, C. & Gronbaek, M. (2003). Relations between amount and type of alcohol and colon and rectal cancer in a Danish population based cohort study. *Gut* Vol. 52: pp. 861-867.

Rehm, J.; Room, R.; Monteiro, R.; Gmel, G.; Graham, K.; Rehn, T. (2004) Global and Regional Burden of Disease Attributable to Selected Major Risk Factors. In: *Comparative Quantification of Health Risks* Ezatti, M.; Murray, C.; Lopez, AD.; Rodgers, A.; Murray, C.; (Ed(s).), World Health Organisation , Geneva.

Salaspuro, V.; Nyfors, S.; Heine, R.; Siitonen, A.; Salaspuro, M.; Jousimies-Somer, H. (1999). Ethanol oxidation and acetaldehyde production in vitro by human intestinal strains of Eschericia coli under aerobic, microaerobic; and anaerobic conditions. *Scand J Gastroenterol* Vol. 34: pp. 967-973.

Salaspuro, M.; (2003). Acetaldehyde, microbes, and cancer of the digestive tract. *Critical reviews in Clinical Laboratory Science* Vol. 40: pp. 183-208.

Schernhammer, E.S.; Ogino, S. & Fuchs, C.S. (2008). Folate and vitamin B6 intake and risk of colon cancer in relation to p53 mutational status. *Gastroenterology* Vol. 135(3): pp 770-780.

Scheppach W.; Bingham, S.; Boutron-Ruault, M.C.; Gerhardsson de Verdier, M.; Moreno, V.; Nagengast, F.M.; Reifen, R.; Riboli, E.; Seitz, H.K. & Wahrendorf, J. (1999). WHO consensus statement on the role of nutrition in colorectal cancer. *Eur J Cancer Prev* Vol. 8: pp. 57-62.

Secretan B., Streif K., Baan R., Grosse Y., El Ghissassi F., Bouvard V., Benbrahin-Tallaa L, Guha N., Freeman C., Galichet L., et al. (2009) A review of human carcinogens – Part E: tobacco, areca nut, alcohol, coal smoke, and salted fish. Lancet Oncol. Vol. 10, pp. 1033-34.

Seitz, H.K. & Osswald, B. (1992) Effect of ethanol on procarcinogen activation. In: *Alcohol and Cancer* ,Watson, R. pp. 55-72, CRC Press, Boca Raton:;

Seitz, H.K. & Stickel, F. (2007) Molecular mechanisms of alcohol-mediated carcinogenesis. *Nat Rev Cancer* Vol. 7: pp. 599-612.

Seitz, H.K. & Stickel, F. (2010) Acetaldehyde as an underestimated risk factor for cancer development: role of genetics in ethanol metabolism. *Genes Nutr.* Vol. 5: pp. 121-128

Seitz, H.K., Cho, C.H. (2009) Contribution of Alcohol and Tobacco Use in Gastrointestinal Cancer Development . In: *Cancer Epidemiology, Vol. 2, Modifiable Factors*, Verma, M. pp. 217-241, Humana Press, New York

Seitz, H.K.; Pöschl, G.; Salaspuro, M. (2006) Alcohol and Cancer of the large intestine. In: *Alcohol Tobacco and Cancer*, Cho, C.H.; Purohit, V. pp. 63-77, Karger, Basel

Seitz, H.K.; Simanowski, U.A.; Garzon, F.T.; Peters, T.J. (1987). Alcohol and cancer (Letter to the Editor). *Hepatology* Vol. 7: pp. 616.

Seitz, H.K.; Oneta, C.M. (1998). Gastrointestinal alcohol dehydrogenases. *Nutr Rev* Vol. 56: pp. 52-60.

Seitz, H.K.; Pöschl, G. & Simanowski, U.A. (1998). Alcohol and cancer. *Recent Dev Alcohol* Vol. 14: pp. 67-95.

Seitz, H.K.; Simanowski, U.A.; Garzon, F.T.; Rideout, J.M.; Peters, T.J.; Koch, A.; Berger, M.R.; Einecke, H. & Maiwald, M. (1990). Possible role of acetaldehyde in ethanol-related rectal cocarcinogenesis in the rat. *Gastroenterology* Vol. 98: pp. 406-413.

Shimizu, M.; Lasker, J.M.; Tsutsumi, M.; Lieber, C.S. (1990). Immunohistochemical localization of ethanol inducible cytochrome P4502E1 in rat alimentary tract. *Gastroenterology* Vol. 93: pp. 1044-1050.

Shimizu, N.; Nagata, C.; Shimizu, H.; Kametani, M.; Takeyama, N.; Ohnuma, T. & Matsushita, S. (2003). Height, weight, and alcohol consumption in relation to the risk of colorectal cancer in Japan: a prospective study. *Br J Cancer* Vol. 88: pp. 1038-1043.

Simanowski, U.A.; Suter, P.; Russel, R.M.; Heller, M.; Waldherr, R.; Ward, R.; Peters, T.J.; Smith, D. & Seitz, H.K. (1994). Enhancement of ethanol induced rectal mucosal hyperregeneration with age in F244 rats. *Gut* Vol. 35: pp. 1102-1106.

Simanowski, U.A.; Homann, N.; Knühl, M.; Arce, C.; Waldherr, R.; Conradt, C.; Bosch, F.X.& Seitz, H.K. (2001). Increased rectal cell proliferation following alcohol abuse. *Gut* Vol. 49: pp. 418-422.

Sohn, O.A.; Fiala, E.S. & Puz, C. (1987). Enhancement of rat liver microsomal metabolism of azoxymethane to methylazoxymethanol by chronic ethanol administration: similarity to the microsomal metabolism of N-nitrosomethylamine. *Cancer Res* Vol. 47: pp. 3123-3129.

Stickel, F.; Herold, C. & Seitz, H.K. (2006). Alcohol and Methyl transfer: Implications for Alcohol-related Hepatocarcinogenesis

Su, L.J. & Arab, L. (2004). Alcohol consumption and risk of colon cancer: evidence from the national health and nutrition examination survey I epidemiologic follow-up study. *Nutr Cancer* Vol. 50: pp. 111-119.

Thygesen, L.C.; Wu, K.; Gronbaek, M.; Fuchs C.S.; Willett, W.C. & Giovannucci, E. (2008). Alcohol intake and colorectal cancer: a comparison of approaches for including repeated measures of alcohol consumption. *Epidemiology* Vol. 19(2): pp. 258-264.

Vincon, P.; Wunderer, J.; Simanowski, U.A.; Koll, M.; Preedy, V.R.; Peters,T.J.; Werner, J.; Waldherr, R.; Seitz, H.K. (2003). Effect of ethanol and vitamin E on cell regeneration and BCL-2 expression in the colorectal mucosa of rats. *Alcoholism Clin Exp Res* Vol. 27: pp. 100-106.

Wang J. (2010) Alcohol and inflammation in cancer development. NIAAA Extramural Advisory Board 2010, Alcohol and Cancer, NIH June 8-9,2010, pp. 134-148.

Wang, Y.; Millonig, G.; Nair, J.; Patsenker, E.; Stickel, F. & Mueller, S. (2009) Ethanol-induced cytochrome P4502E1 causes carcinogenic etheno-DNA lesions in alcoholic liver disease. *Hepatology*. Vol. 50: pp. 453-61.

Wang, X.D. & Seitz, H.K. (2004) Alcohol and Retinoid Interaction. In: *Nutrition and Alcohol: Linking nutrient interactions and dietary intake*. Watson RR, Preedy, V.R. (Ed(s).) pp. 313-321, CRC Press Boca Raton, London, New York, Washington.

Weinstein, S.J.; Albanes, D.; Selhub, J.; Graubard, B.; Lim, U.; Taylor, P.R.; Virtamo, J. & Stolzenberg-Solomon, R. (2008). One-carbon metabolism Biomarkers and risk of colon and rectal cancers. Cancer *Epidemiol Biomarkers Prev* Vol. 17(11): pp. 3233-3240.

Yamaji, T.; Iwasaki, M.; Sasazuki, S.; Sakamoto, H.; Yoshida, T. & Tsugane, S. (2009). Methionine synthase A2756G polymorphism interacts with alcohol and folate intake to influence the risk of colorectal adenoma. *Cancer Epidemiol Biomarkers Prev* Vol. 18(1): pp. 267-274.

Yokoyama, A.; Muramatsu, T.; Ohmori, T.; Yokoyama, T.; Okuyama, K.; Takahashi, H.; Hasegawa, Y.; Higuchi, S.; Maruyama, K.; Shirakura, K.; Ishii, H. (1998). Alcohol-related cancers and aldehydrogenase-2 in Japanese alcoholics. *Carcinogenesis* Vol. 19: pp. 1383-1387.

10

The Molecular Genetic Events in Colorectal Cancer and Diet

Adam Naguib[1], Laura J Gay[2], Panagiota N Mitrou[3] and Mark J Arends[4]

[1]Cold Spring Harbor Laboratory
[2]Queen Mary, University of London
[3]Medical Research Council Centre for Nutritional Epidemiology
in Cancer Prevention and Survival
[4]Department of Pathology, Addenbrooke's Hospital, University of Cambridge
[1]USA
[2,3,4]UK

1. Introduction

Compelling evidence suggests that dietary intakes directly influence colorectal cancer (CRC) risk. Initial observations that CRC incidence is not ubiquitous worldwide, with incidence rates varying up to twenty-five fold between populations (Parkin et al., 2005), indicate the large degree to which this cancer type is influenced by diet and environment. Additionally, observations that migration of individuals confers rapid (within one generation) adoption of the CRC incidence of the host population (Boyle & Langman, 2000; McMichael & Giles, 1988), suggest that dietary and environmental factors determine the risk of colorectal neoplasia to a degree similar to, or in excess of, genetic predisposition.

As diagnosis and treatment of CRC have improved, the study of the pathogenesis of colorectal neoplasia has increased. The most frequent precursor of CRC is the adenoma. As a proportion of adenomas, those of large size, with villous architecture and high grade dysplasia often progress to invasive adenocarcinoma, and this progression is associated with accumulation of mutations and other genetic and epigenetic changes. In the effort to understand the mechanisms and causes of colorectal cancer development, molecular genetic analyses have identified a variety of molecular changes and protein targets involved in colorectal tumourigenesis. The greater understanding of genetic, epigenetic and expression changes that occur during the development and progression of CRC has shown that these neoplasms do not comprise a single disease. Instead, colorectal cancers comprise a collection of distinct and independent neoplastic pathways, such as those pathways displaying chromosomal instability (CIN), microsatellite instability (MSI) or gene promoter activity changes due to the epigenetic phenomenon of methylation at CG dinucleotides (referred to as CIMP: CpG island methylation phenotype, whereby CpG describes dinucleotides of cytosine and guanosine, separated by the characteristic phosphate group in the DNA structure). Each pathway subtype is characterised by individual genetic and molecular characteristics (Poulogiannis,

Ichimura, Hamoudi, Luo, Leung, Yuen, Harrison, Wyllie & Arends, 2010; Poulogiannis, McIntyre, Dimitriadi, Apps, Wilson, Ichimura, Luo, Cantley, Wyllie, Adams & Arends, 2010). Dietary constituents have been studied in relation to the major genetic and molecular changes occurring in CRC development, including alterations in the proto-oncogenes, *K-RAS* and *BRAF* and the tumour suppressor genes *p53* and *APC*. Many studies have analysed a wide variety of dietary components in an effort to elucidate which, if any, dietary constituents may contribute to their mutation in CRC progression. Furthermore, in addition to these genetic lesions, the epigenetic phenomenon of CIMP and MSI have similarly been analysed in relation to dietary constituents.

This review is intended to summarise the currently available literature describing the associations between the molecular genetic changes seen most prevalently in colorectal cancer and dietary intakes. This report does not attempt to assess dietary associations with total CRC incidence. The objective is to highlight consensus observations, where several sources of data exist, suggestive of causative or protective effects of dietary constituents regarding specific molecular genetic changes frequently observed in colorectal neoplasia. Throughout, an emphasis is placed on the number of cases analysed in individual studies, but notably absent are descriptions of odds ratios, hazard ratios or p-values. Throughout, all associations discussed are statistically significant (all p≤0.05). However, due to the varying methodology of data collection and statistical analysis across studies, the inclusion of differing variables in adjusted models and the lack of consensus regarding the degree to which analyses should be adjusted following multiple statistical tests, detailed statistical aspects are not discussed. In order for an assessment to be made of the potential statistical power of each analysis, the number of cases involved in each study is instead highlighted when a statistically significant association is discussed. Full details of all statistical analyses can be found in the original reports, referenced in the text and listed at the end of the chapter.

2. Dietary influences on the major genetic and epigenetic perturbations leading to colorectal cancer development and progression

2.1 *K-RAS* and *BRAF* in colorectal cancer: the MAPK signalling pathway

Mitogen activated protein kinase (MAPK) signal transduction pathways are present in all eukaryotes, six versions of which have been distinguished in mammals (Robinson & Cobb, 1997). MAPK signal propagation is responsible for regulating a variety of cellular processes, which include potentially pro-tumourignenic properties such as proliferation, apoptosis and transformation (Arends et al., 1993; 1994; Peyssonnaux & Eychene, 2001; Robinson & Cobb, 1997). The best characterised of these pathways is the LIGAND RECEPTOR-RAS-RAF-MEK-ERK pathway (Figure 1), which consists of core modules including the RAS and RAF proteins. Although three *RAS* genes have been identified (*H-RAS*, *N-RAS* and *K-RAS*), the *K-RAS* gene is the only one mutated at significant frequency in CRC (Bos, 1989). Similarly, of the three *RAF* genes identified (*ARAF, BRAF* and *CRAF/RAF-1*), only the *BRAF* gene is mutated at significant frequencies in human cancers (Fransen et al., 2004). Experimental mouse models have provided direct evidence that mutated *K-RAS* genes expressed in the intestinal epithelium do not significantly initiate intestinal adenoma growth, but they can cooperate either with other mutant genes or carcinogens to accelerate intestinal tumour formation (Luo et al., 2007; 2009; Luo, Poulogiannis, Ye, Hamoudi & Arends, 2011;

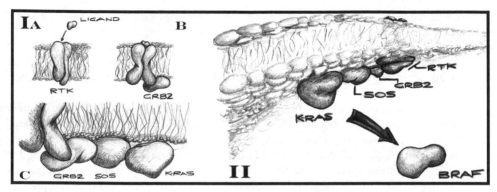

Fig. 1. **RAS, RAF and the MAPK signalling pathway: frequently perturbed in colorectal neoplasms.** Initially, RAS is inactive in a RAS-GTP bound state. **I:** Initiation of signalling through the MAPK pathway occurs at the plasma membrane. Upon extracellular ligand binding to membrane receptor tyrosine kinases (RTK), such as epidermal growth factor binding to the epidermal growth factor receptor (IA), receptor conformational change gives rise to receptor autophosphorylation. Subsequently, src-homology 2 (SH2) domains present in the GRB2 adaptor protein bind the phosphate moieties on the activated receptor (IB). Src-homology 3 (SH3) domains in GRB2 bind proline-rich motifs present in son of sevenless (SOS), localising SOS to the inner surface of the plasma membrane. SOS, a guanine nucleotide exchange factor (GEF) interacts with RAS proteins, catalysing the exchange of GDP for GTP, thus activating RAS to a RAS-GTP state (IC). **II:** Upon activation, RAS phosphorylates cytosolic RAF. The resulting activation of RAF in turn phosphorylates cytosolic MEK, which then phosphorylates ERK, leading to induction and repression of distinct transcription programmes, promoting cell proliferation and modulating cell death by apoptosis, among other processes. The vast majority of mutations in the *K-RAS* or *BRAF* genes are in distinct hotspot regions: *K-RAS* at codons 12 and 13, and also, but much more infrequently at codons 61 and 146 (Forbes et al., 2008). Additionally, mutations observed at lower prevalences at other sites in the gene have been described and their functional significance determined (Naguib, Wilson, Adams & Arends, 2011). Mutations in *BRAF* occur most frequently at codons 463-468 and codon 600 (Forbes et al., 2008). Activating mutations in the *K-RAS* and *BRAF* genes render their protein products constitutively active, leading to increased transduction through this signalling axis. Additionally, mutationally active *K-RAS* can also propogate signalling through other pathways, including the PI3K/AKT axis.

Luo, Poulogiannis, Ye, Hamoudi, Zhang, Dong & Arends, 2011). *K-RAS* mutations are observed 20-50% of sporadic human CRC and *BRAF* mutations are observed in 5-15% of CRC (Forbes et al., 2008). The high frequencies at which *K-RAS* and *BRAF* mutations are observed in CRC has prompted several analyses of dietary intakes in relation to these genetic lesions.

2.1.1 *K-RAS* mutation and meat consumption

Specific types of meat consumption have been identified as associated with general CRC incidence (Norat et al., 2005; Santarelli et al., 2008) with plausible mechanisms postulated as to the manner in which these consumptions may influence colorectal carcinogenesis (Kuhnle & Bingham, 2007; Kuhnle et al., 2007). Consequently, several studies have attempted to identify the nature of these associations in relation to *K-RAS* mutations. Some reports have identified associations with meat consumption and *K-RAS* mutation, although not all.

A single study analysing 390 *K-RAS* wildtype and 218 *K-RAS* mutated CRC identified an increased consumption of beef with higher incidence of *K-RAS* wildtype colonic cancers (Brink, Weijenberg, de Goeij, Roemen, Lentjes, de Bruïne, Goldbohm & van den Brandt, 2005). In this same report, a reduction in pork consumption was found to be linked to reduced frequency of both colonic and rectal cancers harbouring mutated *K-RAS*. Another report, assessing *K-RAS* mutations and diet in 155 *K-RAS* wildtype and 41 *K-RAS* mutated CRC, identified an increased white meat consumption associated with higher incidence of *K-RAS* mutated CRC (Naguib et al., 2010). Although positive associations were identified in these two analyses, there appears to be little consistency between these independent findings. The report by Naguib and colleagues also analysed red and processed meat consumption in relation to mutation status and found no statistically significant association between the two, although, beef consumption was not tested independently of other meat types, as in the report by Brink and co-workers. The study by Naguib and colleagues did not test pork consumption in isolation: this meat type was included in the 'red' or 'processed' meat categories. Similarly, Brink and coworkers did not identify an association between white meat and increased incidence of *K-RAS* mutations. This analysis tested the consumption of chicken in isolation, not in a combined 'white meat' category containing other meat types, such as turkey etc.

Notwithstanding the identified statistically significant associations between meat consumption and *K-RAS* mutation status described above, the majority of studies which have attempted to address this question have failed to identify any link between meat intake and the mutation status of this gene. An analysis testing 67 *K-RAS* wildtype and 39 *K-RAS* mutated CRC assessed animal protein intake and found no link between this and *K-RAS* mutation status (Bautista et al., 1997) although clearly, 'animal protein' as a variable makes no distinction between meat types and is an assessment of protein, not animal product, consumption. A large analysis testing 971 *K-RAS* wildtype and 457 *K-RAS* mutated CRC (Slattery et al., 2000) identified no assocaition between total *K-RAS* mutations and meat intake. A small study (28 wildtype, 15 mutated rectal cancers) failed to identify an association between red meat intake and *K-RAS* mutation (O'Brien et al., 2000). An assessment of a larger cohort of rectal cancers (535 *K-RAS* wildtype and 215 *K-RAS* mutated) corroborated this observation of lack of association with red meat intake and rectal cancer (Slattery, Curtin, Wolff, Herrick, Caan & Samowitz, 2010).

In addition to colorectal cancers, pre-cancerous adenomas have also been tested in order to identify dietary assocaitions with *K-RAS* mutation status in the early stages of colorectal neoplasia. An assessment of 558 *K-RAS* wildtype and 120 *K-RAS* mutated adenomas failed to identify an association between red meat intake and mutation status (Martínez et al., 1999). Another study, testing 453 *K-RAS* wildtype and 81 *K-RAS* mutated adenomas also failed to identify a statistically significant association between red meat, processed meat or poultry and *K-RAS* mutation status (Wark et al., 2006).

Published reports assessing *K-RAS* mutation status in CRC in relation to meat intakes provide limited evidence to suggest that total *K-RAS* mutations are either positively or negatively associated with meat consumption. The majority of studies have categorised meat types according to shared properties (such as haem content or preservation methods) and have generally failed to identify links between these groups and *K-RAS* mutation status. It is

Study	K-RAS WT CRC/RC/adenomas	K-RAS mutated CRC/RC/adenomas	dietary association
Bautista *et al* 1997	CRC: 67	CRC: 39	↑ MUFA with *K-RAS* mutation, ↓ calcium with *K-RAS* mutation
Bongaerts *et al* 2006	CRC: 385	CRC: 193	no association between alcohol and *K-RAS* mutated or wildtype cancers
Brink *et al* 2004	CRC: 390	CRC: 218	↑ PUFA (specifically linoleic acid) with *K-RAS* mutated colonic, but not rectal, cancers
Brink *et al* 2005	CRC: 390	CRC: 218	↑ folate reduced risk of *K-RAS* mutated rectal, not colonic, cancer in men only
Brink *et al* 2005	CRC: 390	CRC: 218	↑ beef, ↓ pork with *K-RAS* wildtype colonic tumours, ↓ pork with *K-RAS* wildtype rectal tumours
Laso *et al* 2004	CRC: 68	CRC: 49	*K-RAS* codon 12 mutation was associated with ↓ vitamin A, B1, D and iron
Martinez *et al* 1999	Adenomas: 558	Adenomas: 120	↑ folate reduced risk of developing *K-RAS* mutated adenomas
Naguib *et al* 2010	CRC: 155	CRC: 41	↑ white meat consumption with *K-RAS* mutation
O'Brien *et al* 2000	RC: 28	RC: 15	no association between red meat consumption and *K-RAS* mutation
Schernhammer *et al* 2008	CRC: 427	CRC: 242	no association between folate intake and prevalence of *K-RAS* mutated or wildtype cancers
Slattery *et al* 2000	CRC: 971	CRC: 457	↓ cruciferous vegetables with reduced risk of *K-RAS* mutation
Slattery *et al* 2010	RC: 535	RC: 215	no association between calcium and vitamin D and *K-RAS* mutation
Slattery *et al* 2010	RC: 535	RC: 215	↑ vegetables and dietary fibre with a reduced risk of *K-RAS* mutations
Wark *et al* 2006	Adenomas: 453	Adenomas: 81	↓ MUFA and ↑ vitamin B2 associated with *K-RAS* mutation

Table 1. Summarised description of literature analysing *K-RAS* mutations in colorectal neoplasms (case numbers provided) in relation to dietary intakes and the statistically significant findings described. *WT*: wildtype, *CRC*: colorectal cancer, *RC*: rectal cancer, *MUFA*: monunsaturated fatty acid, *PUFA*: polyunsaturated fatty acid, ↑ and ↓ denote an increase or decrease in consumption respectively.

plausible that if specific meat types, as suggested in at least one study (Brink, Weijenberg, de Goeij, Roemen, Lentjes, de Bruïne, Goldbohm & van den Brandt, 2005), are linked to the incidence of *K-RAS* mutated CRC, that grouping of meat types together may have failed to identify associations where they existed. However, in practical terms, it should be noted that similarities in the composition of meat types, such as in terms of haem content, a postulated carcinogen intermediate (Kuhnle & Bingham, 2007), justify a grouping of types in order to minimise multiple statistical testing and to test consumption levels large enough to be likely to affect bowel carcinogenesis.

Several reports have analysed the relationship between base changes at specific positions in the *K-RAS* gene, types of mutations (i.e. transition *versus* transversion) or specific types of base changes (i.e. G→A) in relation to meat intakes. It is entirely plausible that the nature of the mutation, not the gene in which it arises, is linked to dietary constituents. However, due to the very limited number of studies instigated with objectives of such an analysis, and the often low numbers of different mutation subgroups existent in the studies which do attempt such an assessment rendering lower statistical power, such analyses are not discussed in this review.

2.1.2 *K-RAS* mutation and folate consumption

Several studies have described an association between folate intake and the prevalence of *K-RAS* mutations in CRC. A report analysing 390 *K-RAS* wildtype and 218 *K-RAS* mutated CRC identified an increased consumption of folate associated with a reduced prevalence of *K-RAS* mutated rectal, but not colonic, cancers in males only (Brink, Weijenberg, de Goeij, Roemen, Lentjes, de Bruïne, van Engeland, Goldbohm & van den Brandt, 2005). Testing in this study demonstrated that in the male participants of this cohort, increased intake of folate was linked to reduced prevalence of rectal cancer incidence, however, this link, when considering mutation status, seemed only to reduce the risk of *K-RAS* mutated rectal cancers. A large analysis of colorectal adenomas (558 wildtype, 120 *K-RAS* mutated) also identified increased folate intake associated with a reduced incidence of *K-RAS* mutation (Martínez et al., 1999). However, in addition to these positive associations in relatively large cohorts, several other studies have failed to identify a link between folate intake and *K-RAS* mutation status in colorectal neoplasms. Reports describing the testing of 67 K-RAS wildtype and 39 K-RAS mutated CRC (Bautista et al., 1997), 68 K-RAS wildtype, 49 K-RAS mutated CRC (Laso et al., 2004), 155 K-RAS wildtype, 41 K-RAS mutated CRC (Naguib et al., 2010), 427 K-RAS wildtype, 242 K-RAS mutated CRC (Schernhammer, Giovannuccci, Fuchs & Ogino, 2008), 971 K-RAS wildtype 457 K-RAS mutated CRC (Slattery et al., 2000) and 453 K-RAS wildtype, 81 K-RAS mutated adenomas (Wark et al., 2006) failed to identify folate intake as associated with K-RAS mutation status.

Increased consumption of folate offering some degree of protection against K-RAS mutation was observed in two independent studies. The failure to confirm this link in many other reports may potentially be explained several ways. Firstly, many of the studies described which identified no link between K-RAS mutation and folate intake contained relatively few mutated samples (<100). It is plausible that in these instances too few cases were analysed to detect any association, although this does not explain the studies which failed to identify a link using relatively large sample sets (Schernhammer, Giovannuccci, Fuchs & Ogino, 2008; Slattery et al., 2000). Secondly, some dietary constituents have been described to affect folate utilisation, such as alcohol (Eichholzer et al., 2001; Freudenheim et al., 1991). It may be possible that the protective effect of folate against K-RAS mutation is only prevalent in the context of certain dietary patterns, possibly explaining why associations are not observed in all epidemiological studies. Finally, Martinez and colleagues identified an increased protective effect against K-RAS mutation as provided by supplement derived intake relative to natural dietary intake of this macronutrient (Martínez et al., 1999). The nature of folate consumption, i.e. bioavailablilty, may also determine the degree to which it offers a protective effect in colorectal carcinogenesis.

Although not observed in every analysis, increased intake of folate is associated with a reduced prevalence of total CRC incidence, which is observed in approximately half of the analyses testing this link (Eichholzer et al., 2001). It is probable, that at least to a limited degree and in certain circumstances, that this may be due to the ability of folate to protect against K-RAS mutation during development of colorectal neoplasia.

2.1.3 *K-RAS* mutation and fat consumption

Consumption of several forms of fat intake have been described to affect the prevalence of K-RAS mutations in CRC. However, there is no consensus in the literature to date, regarding both the manner of the association and type of fat involved. Independent studies have identified monounsaturated fatty acid (MUFA) consumption as associated with the prevalence of K-RAS mutations in CRC. One report, analysing 67 K-RAS wildtype and 39 K-RAS mutated CRC, identified an increased MUFA consumption as linked to an increased prevalence of K-RAS mutated CRC (Bautista et al., 1997). MUFA, mostly derived from olive oil in this population, reduced the risk of CRC harbouring wildtype K-RAS, but offered no protection against K-RAS mutated cancers. However, contradictory findings of an increased MUFA consumption being associated with a higher prevalence of K-RAS wildtype neoplasia in a study assessing adenomas (453 wildtype, 81 mutated) (Wark et al., 2006) challenges the observation made by Bautista and co-workers. Other published reports have failed to identify any link between K-RAS mutation status and MUFA intake (Brink et al., 2004; Laso et al., 2004; Naguib et al., 2010; Slattery et al., 2000; Slattery, Curtin, Wolff, Herrick, Caan & Samowitz, 2010).

In addition to these observations, one report describes an increase in polyunsaturated fatty acids (PUFA), specifically linoleic acid, as associated with increased prevalence of *K-RAS* mutated colonic, but not rectal, cancers (Brink et al., 2004). However, this association with PUFA has not been identifed in any other report (Bautista et al., 1997; Laso et al., 2004; Naguib et al., 2010; Slattery et al., 2000; Slattery, Curtin, Wolff, Herrick, Caan & Samowitz, 2010; Wark et al., 2006).

Taken together, the published data describing the association of dietary fats with *K-RAS* mutations have failed to identify a convincing association, and have generated conflicting results. Presently, the evidence suggesting that the *K-RAS* mutation status of colorectal neoplasia may be affected by fat intakes is weak: the limited data available suggest that the mutation status of this gene is largely independent of this dietary consumption. It should be noted however, that although fat intake itself is probably not associated with this mutation type, increased body mass index (BMI), which may be associated with fat intake, is associated with overall CRC risk.

2.1.4 *K-RAS* mutation and other dietary constituents

The mutation status of *K-RAS* in CRC has also been linked to several other dietary variables in addition to meat, folate and fat. Testing of 971 *K-RAS* wildtype and 457 *K-RAS* mutated CRC identified an increased risk of *K-RAS* mutations with reduced consumption of cruciferous vegetables (Slattery et al., 2000). Another analysis of rectal cancers (535 wildtype, 215 mutated) identified a reduced incidence of *K-RAS* mutated rectal cancers with increased vegetable and fibre intake (Slattery, Curtin, Wolff, Herrick, Caan & Samowitz, 2010). Although corroborative, these two analyses were performed on the same test cohort and are yet to be identified in other independent populations. In this cohort at least, the data of Slattery and colleagues suggest that increased vegetable intake reduced the prevalence of *K-RAS* mutations in CRC, with an overt association identified in rectally located neoplasia.

Increased vitamin B2 intake has been identified to reduce the prevalence of adenomas harbouring *K-RAS* mutations. In an analysis of 453 *K-RAS* mutated and 81 *K-RAS* wildtype pre-cancerous adenomas an inverse association suggested a protective effect against *K-RAS* mutated adenomas. This protection was not found in relation to the prevalence of *K-RAS* wildtype adenomas (Wark et al., 2006). This association has not been identified in cohorts testing colorectal cancers.

Some dietary intakes have been repeatedly tested with no link to the prevalence of *K-RAS* mutation in CRC having been identified, notably alcohol. Many studies have included assessment of this dietary factor, with some studies analysing alcohol consumption independent of any other dietary factors (Bongaerts et al., 2006).

In summary, current literature describing the assessment of *K-RAS* mutation status in colorectal neoplasia has identified many associations with dietary intakes (summarised in Table 1). Very few of these associations have been repeatedly identified in independent cohorts, making assessment of their general validity challenging. Presently, few dietary components seem to be strongly linked to *K-RAS* mutation status in CRC across many populations, environments and genetic backgrounds. Furthermore, it is problematic to directly compare different studies. Other than folate, which has been described by the World Cancer Research Fund as having a 'limited' protective effect against CRC, which may impart this limited protection through reduced prevalence of *K-RAS* mutation, there is a lack of strong evidence to firmly suggest any other dietary intakes affect the prevalence of *K-RAS* mutations in CRC.

2.1.5 *BRAF* mutations and dietary associations

Relative to *K-RAS*, far fewer data exist describing the association between *BRAF* mutations in CRC and dietary influences. A prospective study involving 186 colorectal cancers, of which 29 harboured *BRAF* mutations, analysing meat, fruit and vegetable, fat, vitamin and macronutrient intakes identified no potential dietary associations with *BRAF* mutation in CRC (Naguib et al., 2010).

Other analyses have centred on analysing dietary constituents which may act as methyl group donors, such as folate, or vitamins, such as B6 and B2, which function as co-factors in the pathway responsible for DNA methylation (de Vogel et al., 2008; Kim, 2005). Based on observations that *BRAF* mutation has been linked previously to the CIMP phenotype (Lee et al., 2008; Samowitz et al., 2005; Velho et al., 2008) and has been linked to 60-80% of CRC demonstrating the highest levels of CIMP with concurrent MSI (Kambara et al., 2004; Samowitz et al., 2005), this mutation type may be influenced by dietary factors thought to influence DNA methylation. One such analysis used data and tissue samples from 648 individuals, of which 101 harboured CRC with mutations in the *BRAF* gene. This report identified a positive association between *BRAF* mutation in males and the highest tertile of folate consumption (de Vogel et al., 2008). This same report also identified an inverse correlation between methionine intake, as well as no association between vitamin B2 and alcohol consumption and *BRAF* mutations in the male portion of the cohort. In the female cohort members, no dietary consumptions were identified which were associated with *BRAF* mutations. An additional assessment of 86 *BRAF* mutated and 300 *BRAF* wildtype colonic cancers failed to identify an association between alcohol, folate, vitamins B6 and B12 or methionine consumption and *BRAF* mutation status (Schernhammer et al., 2011).

Another study population, of which 1108 cases of CRC were assessed for the presence of *BRAF* mutations, identified no associations between the 114 cancers harbouring this genetic lesion and intake of either vitamins B6, B12, folate, methionine or fibre consumptions, when compared with non-cancerous controls (Slattery et al., 2007). Similarly, the determination of *BRAF* mutation status in 189 CRC cases in another study cohort identified no associations between mutations in this gene and plasma levels of folate, vitamin B12 and homocysteine (Van Guelpen et al., 2010).

At present, few analyses of dietary intake in relation to the incidence of *BRAF* mutations in CRC have been attempted, and the majority of the limited data which do exist generally fail to identify strong associations between CRC harbouring *BRAF* mutations and any dietary constituent. In only one study to date, limited, sex specific dietary associations with *BRAF* mutation have been identified (de Vogel et al., 2008), but these observations are yet to be validated and corroborated in other studies.

The lack of identification of any of dietary component associated with *BRAF* mutation in CRC may have several causes. Primarily, only one study, analysing a very limited number of *BRAF* mutated tumours (n=29) has attempted a broad analysis of many dietary factors (Naguib et al., 2010). The remaining limited data has involved anlaysis of only a selected spectrum of dietary components hypothesised to be involved in the DNA methylation process. The limited scope of these studies in terms of dietary factors tested does not exclude the possibility that other dietary factors may be associated with *BRAF* mutated CRC. Secondly, *BRAF* is identified at higher frequency in CRC demonstrating CIMP and MSI. Definitive evidence is yet to be provided describing the order in which tumours displaying CIMP and MSI acquire these instabilities and when *BRAF* mutations are acquired during progression. It is plausible that mutation in the *BRAF* gene is secondary to the acquisition of these global genomic alterations. As such, the question of diet and any relationships with this mutation may be redundant, if following the acquisition of CIMP and MSI status, *BRAF* mutation may arise independent of dietary influences. Thirdly, the limited number of studies available addressing the question of dietary associations and *BRAF* mutation may be too few in number to identify any dietary associations with this lesion, or, the majority of the studies performed are correct and that in this instance, dietary components do not affect the prevalence of *BRAF* mutations in CRC.

2.2 *p53* mutations in colorectal cancer

The *p53* tumour suppressor gene is the most commonly mutated gene in all human cancers, mutated in approximately 50% of human malignancies, including 50-60% of CRC (Forbes et al., 2008). Subsequent to its activation following DNA damage, oxidative stress or other cellular insults, wildtype p53 protein accumulates in the cell nucleus and acts as a transcription factor, capable of activating and suppressing transcription programmes leading to cell cycle arrest, DNA damage repair and apoptosis (Aylon & Oren, 2011; Bourdon et al., 2003). As such, perturbation of the normal role of p53 is highly selected for in cancer cells. The high prevalence of *p53* mutation in CRC, notably in later stage cancers, has led to various studies of mutations of this gene in the context of dietary consumptions.

2.2.1 *p53* mutations and dietary associations

Mutations in the *p53* gene have been linked to a variety of dietary intakes. Low folate and vitamin B6 intakes have been linked to p53 over-expressing cancers (Schernhammer, Ogino & Fuchs, 2008). This report, analysing 143 p53 over-expressing and 256 colonic cancers demonstrating low or absent p53 expression used an immunohistochemical (IHC) analysis to assess p53 accumulation following mutation. p53 over-expression or accumulation is the result of reduced protein degradation, mostly due to point mutations in the *p53* gene, greatly increasing the half-life of the gene's protein product (Melhem et al., 1995). This fast method of assessment of a range of activating *p53* mutations should be interpreted with some caution however, as less commonly observed mutations giving rise to truncated protein, such as those introducing premature *stop* codons, are not identified using this method. The observation linking low folate intake to an increased prevalence of cancers of the colon exhibiting over-expression of p53 is yet to be corroborated. Two reports using DNA sequencing, testing 62 *p53* mutated and 123 *p53* wildtype CRC (Park et al., 2010) and 686 *p53* mutated and 772 *p53* wildtype colonic cancers (Slattery et al., 2002), identified no link between p53 status and folate intakes. Little or no apparent other data exist describing vitamin B6 intakes and possible relationships with *p53* mutation status.

Specific meat intakes have been linked to *p53* mutation status in several independent studies. One report by Park and colleagues identified an increased consumption of red and total meat (all types, including poultry) as associated with increased prevalence of *p53* mutations in CRC, however, this was only present in advanced stage CRC (Dukes' C or D), not in those of less advanced stages (Dukes' A or B) (Park et al., 2010). In addition to this, an assessment by

Slattery and co-workers identified high glycaemic load, increased red meat, increased fast food and increased trans fatty acid intakes as associated with increased prevalence of *p53* mutations in colonic cancers (Slattery et al., 2002). These two independent studies suggest that red meat in particular may promote mutations in *p53* in neoplasia of the large intestine. However, these data do not completely overlap: the study by Park and colleagues only found this association in advanced stage cancers and the report by Slattery and co-workers assessed only colonic, not rectal cancers. Opposed to the above observations of meat intakes promoting *p53* mutations in CRC, an IHC based analysis (73 p53 over-expressing, 90 p53 absent CRC) identified increased beef consumption as associated with reduced prevalence of p53 over-expressing cancers (Freedman et al., 1996). Further data are needed to evaluate the potential association of meat, and meat types, with *p53* mutations in CRC, with particular emphasis on cancer location and stage.

In a study of colonic cancers assessing both p53 expression and *p53* gene mutations, total and saturated fats were identified as linked to tumours not over-expressing p53 or harbouring gene mutations (Voskuil et al., 1999). Of the 185 colonic cancers tested in this study, 81 displayed p53 overexpression by IHC, of which 59 were found to harbour mutations in the sequenced region (exons 5-8) of these cancers. Mutations in *p53* were not found to be linked to total fat intake in other reports assessing either CRC as a general subgroup (Park et al., 2010) or rectal cancers in particular (Slattery, Curtin, Wolff, Herrick, Caan & Samowitz, 2010). An analysis of 340 *p53* mutated and 410 *p53* wildtype rectal cancers reported an increased consumption of vegetables, whole grains and fibre associated with reduced prevalence of *p53* mutation (Slattery, Curtin, Wolff, Herrick, Caan & Samowitz, 2010). Conversely, a high intake of refined grains was found to increase the prevalence of rectal cancer harbouring *p53* mutations. Increased intakes of cruciferous vegetables have also been described to be associated with reduced prevalence of p53 over-expressing CRC (73 p53 over-expressing CRC, 90 p53 absent CRC) (Freedman et al., 1996). The observation of increased vegetable intakes associated with reduced frequency of *p53* mutations in CRC was not observed in another study analysing general CRC (Park et al., 2010). Fibre was not observed to be associated with a protective effect in analyses combining colonic and rectal cancers (Park et al., 2010) or assessing colonic cancers in isolation (Slattery et al., 2002; Voskuil et al., 1999).

Alcohol intakes and *p53* mutation status in CRC have been assessed in several reports. A study analysing 340 *p53* mutated and 410 *p53* wildtype rectal cancers identified increased beer consumption as being associated with higher prevalence of *p53* mutations when compared with non-beer drinkers (Slattery, Wolff, Herrick, Curtin, Caan & Samowitz, 2010). No associations between alcohol intakes and *p53* mutation status have been identified in several analyses of colonic cancers (Schernhammer, Ogino & Fuchs, 2008; Voskuil et al., 1999), however, neither of these studies assessed specific alcoholic beverages, just total alcohol intake. Total alcohol intake was found to be linked to increased prevalence of *p53* mutations in CRC of advanced Dukes' stage (C and D), but not in CRC of less advanced stage (Dukes' A or B) (Park et al., 2010). Another report analysing Dukes' stage C cancers by IHC (42 p53 over-expressing CRC, 65 p53 absent CRC) did not identify total alcohol intake as linked to p53 expression status (Zhang et al., 1995).

Presently, the limited data on *p53* mutation status in CRC and dietary intakes are inconsistent. As a result, several consumptions have been linked to *p53* mutation status but none have been corroborated by other studies performing a similar assessment in an independent cohort.

Further evidence is needed to substantiate these isolated observations. Future studies should focus on the analysis of the potential association of vegetable and meat intakes in relation to p53 status as several data exist suggesting a possible link between these intakes and p53 aberrations, although contrary observations have been published.

2.3 *APC* mutations in colorectal cancer

The *adenomatous polyposis coli* (*APC*) gene is one of the most frequently mutated genes in colorectal cancer (Sjöblom et al., 2006; Wood et al., 2007), with some studies reporting 50-80% of CRC harbouring mutations in this gene (Forbes et al., 2008). The majority of mutations identified in CRC in the *APC* gene are located in exon 15 in the central third of the coding sequence, the *mutation cluster region*, which corresponds to the β-catenin-binding region of the protein (Goss & Groden, 2000). Mutations in *APC* most frequently result in truncation of the protein, corresponding with a reduction in the ability of APC to bind β-catenin (Figure 2). In addition to its role as a modulator of WNT pathway signalling, APC also has a role in mitosis and cytokinesis: cells harbouring truncated APC undergo abnormal chromosomal segregation and may develop aneuploidy (Ceol et al., 2007). Wildtype APC functions as a regulator of apoptosis, differentiation and migration and functions during cell division (Ceol et al., 2007; Fodde et al., 2001; Goss & Groden, 2000).

Although mutations in other genes, such as *p53*, may be almost as frequent as those in *APC* in CRC, *APC* mutations seem to be particularly prevalent from the earliest stages of CRC initiation and progression. Dysplastic aberrant crypt foci (ACF), monocryptal or oligocryptal adenomas, which are the lesions considered to be the earliest forms of colorectal neoplasia, frequently display *APC* mutations (Jen et al., 1994) and can develop into CRC through the adenoma-carcinoma sequence (Suehiro & Hinoda, 2008; Takayama et al., 1998). Intriguingly, the more frequently occurring heteroplastic ACF, which possess limited, if any, potential to develop to malignancy, very rarely harbour *APC* mutations but frequently exhibit *K-RAS* mutations (Jen et al., 1994). These data suggest that initiating genetic lesions in CRC determine malignant potential, and that if the initial mutations occur in the *APC* gene, there is a high probability of subsequent adenoma formation. In concordance with observations in dysplastic ACF, *APC* mutations are very frequently observed in colorectal adenomas (Kinzler & Vogelstein, 1996) and when inherited as germline *APC* mutations allow formation of hundreds of colorectal adenomas in the Familial Adenomatous Polyposis Coli syndrome. Hence, there have been several analyses of APC mutations in CRC relation to dietary intakes, with the purpose of identifying links between this early genetic lesion and dietary carcinogens.

2.3.1 *APC* mutations and dietary associations

APC mutations have been linked to several dietary constituents. One report, analysing 121 *APC* wildtype and 63 *APC* mutated colonic cancers, identified alcohol as inversely associated with *APC* mutated and positively associated with *APC* wildtype cancers (Diergaarde, van Geloof, van Muijen, Kok & Kampman, 2003). Additionally, red meat, fish and fat, notably unsaturated fat, were shown to be associated with development of *APC* mutated colonic cancers. Conversely, another report assessing 347 *APC* wildtype CRC and 184 *APC* mutated CRC identified increased consumption of saturated fat, but not unsaturated fats, as associated with *APC* mutated rectal cancers (Weijenberg et al., 2007). Furthermore, the analysis by

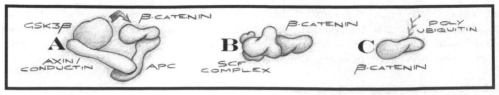

Fig. 2. **APC and the WNT signalling pathway**. **A:** In the absence of WNT signal, free β-catenin is bound by APC, in a complex with axin/conductin and glycogen synthase kinase 3β (GSK3β) and this complex acts as a scaffold, bringing β-catenin into close proximity with GSK3β. This results in GSK3β mediated phosphorylation of β catenin. **B:** Phosphorylated β-catenin is recognised by the SCF complex and is polyubiquitinated. **C:** Polyubiquitinated β-catenin is recognised by the proteasome and degraded. In the absence of WNT signalling, β-catenin is largely degraded, thus preventing β-catenin nuclear accumulation and subsequent co-activation of transcription programs. Upon binding of WNT ligand to membrane-located receptors, a subsequent signalling cascade prevents formation of the APC-axin-conductin-GSK3β complex. As a result, β-catenin avoids degradation and can translocate to the nucleus where it co-activates transcription of target genes, such as *c-myc*.

Weijenberg and co-workers identified specific types of *APC* wildtype CRC (i.e. those harbouring *K-RAS* mutations and showing no loss of MLH1 expression [see 2.4.2]) as being linked to increased intake of linoleic acid, a polyunsaturated fatty acid.

A further study has identified increased consumption of folate associated with reduced prevalence of *APC* wildtype colonic cancer, but increased prevalence of *APC* mutated colonic cancers in males (de Vogel et al., 2006). These associations were not observed in rectal cancers of men or in either colonic or rectal female cancer cases. This analysis, studying 347 *APC* wildtype CRC and 182 *APC* mutated CRC, also identified increased vitamin B2 and iron intakes in men associated with colonic cancers harbouring *APC* mutations compared with those men with colonic cancer not harbouring *APC* mutations.

These analyses are difficult to compare, notably as Diergaarde and colleagues did not stratify cases by sex or cancer location, which may possibly explain the lack of association between folate intake and *APC* mutation status in their report. The study by Diergaarde and co-workers did not analyse iron or vitamin B2, and de Vogel and colleagues did not assess meat and fish intakes. Alcohol association with *APC* mutation status was not observed in the testing by de Vogel and co-workers. Assessed in conjunction, these studies do not corroborate each other as direct comparisons are difficult to make.

Further analysis of *APC* mutation status has been performed in the context of specific meat intakes. In a study of 347 *APC* wildtype CRC and 184 *APC* mutated CRC, increased processed meat consumption was linked to an increased prevalence of *APC* mutated colonic cancers (Lüchtenborg et al., 2005). Additionally, increased beef consumption was linked to increased frequency of *APC* wildtype colonic cancers. Rectal cancers without *APC* mutations were found to be more prevalent amongst those with increased consumption of other meat types, which included horsemeats, lamb and mutton among other products. This detailed analysis of *APC* mutation status in the context of very specific meat types, with both positive and negative associations having been identified, is yet to be corroborated by similarly detailed meat-type subgroups testing in additional studies. This report does suggest however, that meat classification is important when testing for associations with *APC* mutations. In this context, these observations partially confirm the increased consumption of general red meat that was observed to be associated with an increased risk of *APC* mutated CRC in the report by Diergaarde and co-workers.

In addition to reports assessing *APC* mutation status relative to dietary intakes in CRC, a single study has assessed these relationships in colorectal adenomas (Diergaarde et al., 2005). This analysis of 117 *APC* wildtype adenomas and 161 *APC* mutated colorectal adenomas identified a high intake of red meat and fat as associated with increased prevalence of *APC* wildtype adenomas. These observations are intriguing as identification of increased consumptions of certain red meat types being specifically associated with certain *APC* wildtype CRC has been described previously (Lüchtenborg et al., 2005).

Taken together, the available data describing *APC* mutations in CRC in relation to dietary intakes are too few and inconsistent to draw any strong conclusions. However, several analyses have identified certain meat consumptions as linked to either colonic or rectal cancers with a particular *APC* mutation status. These observations, although not in full agreement, indicate that certain red meat types, determined by both animal origin and preparation method, may affect the prevalence of mutation in *APC* in CRC. Further assessment of these particular dietary associations are warranted to determine the relationship between *APC* mutation status and specific red meat consumptions. Based on these somewhat conflicting data, some associations do seem plausible.

2.4 Microsatellite instability (MSI) and CpG island methylator phenotype (CIMP) in colorectal cancer

2.4.1 MSI and CIMP as genomic instabilities in colorectal cancer

Acquired variation in length of repetitive DNA sequences (microsatellites) can be detected as microsatellite instability (MSI) and is prevalent in approximately 15% of sporadic CRC and in almost all CRC in Lynch/Hereditary Non-Polyposis Colorectal Cancer syndrome (Soreide et al., 2006). MSI arises as a result of DNA replication errors that produce a change in length of repetitive sequences, which if not repaired (by the DNA mismatch repair (MMR) system), accumulate with increasing frequency (Martin et al., 2010; Soreide et al., 2006). In sporadic CRC, the most frequent inactivating cause of MMR is the methylation of the *MLH1* promoter on one or both alleles (Herman et al., 1998; Wheeler et al., 2000).

The MMR process is responsible for the correction of DNA replication errors which result in small insertions or deletions in the genome; these are especially prevalent at microsatellites due to increased frequency of DNA polymerase slippage at repetitive sequences. In humans, two major components comprise the MMR pathway: MutS (which is present in two heterodimers of MSH2/MSH6 and MSH2/MSH3) and MutL (which is also present in several heterodimer forms:- MLH1/PMS2, MLH1/PMS1 and MLH1/MLH3) (Martin et al., 2010). Disruption of the formation of the MutS and MutL dimers (by abrogation of the component proteins due to acquired promoter methylation or mutation) leads to a limited or defective MMR pathway, giving rise to genomic instability whereby DNA regions, most frequently repetitive sequences, increase or decrease in length (MSI). Such instability can lead to gene mutations, frequently of frameshift type, which can contribute to cancer progression.

CIMP is observed in 30-40% of proximal colonic and 3-12% of distal/rectal cancers (Curtin et al., 2011; Ibrahim et al., 2011). The exact causes of excessive methylation in DNA regions harbouring high levels of adjacent cytosine and guanine bases (CpG islands) are unknown, although some evidence exists which suggest that such an increase in methyl group incorporation at these sites occurs during ageing in normal epithelial cells in the gut, and this is elevated in cancer (Toyota et al., 1999). Hypermethylation of gene promotors, in addition to or independent of methylation of other local DNA sequences, leads to transcriptional silencing of those genes. Such transcriptional silencing can be considered as one mechanism by which genes can be 'knocked out', in addition to mutation and deletion, in Knudson's model of tumour suppressor gene inactivation (Kondo & Issa, 2004). In this way, the aberrant methylation of genes can contribute to their inactivation in cancer epigenetically, such that in the absence of inactivating genetic changes tumour suppressor gene activity can be lost, leading to cancer progression.

2.4.2 MSI and dietary associations

MSI in CRC has been assessed in relation to dietary intakes in several reports, many of which did not identify a link between this type of genomic instability in CRC and specific dietary intakes (Chang et al., 2007; de Vogel et al., 2008; Jensen et al., 2008; Schernhammer, Giovannuccci, Fuchs & Ogino, 2008) (Table 2). However, a limited number of studies have described links between dietary intakes and MSI in colorectal neoplasms. An analysis of 144 microsatellite stable (MSS) and 40 MSI colonic cancers described an increased intake of red meat as associated with increased prevalence of MSS cancers (Diergaarde, Braam, van Muijen, Ligtenberg, Kok & Kampman, 2003). However, an assessment of 437 MSS and 49 MSI colonic cancers, failed to identify a similar association with red meat and MSS status (Satia et al., 2005). Additionally, a further report, testing 238 MSS and 35 MSI colonic cancers also failed to identify red meat intake as associated with MSI or MSS status (Wu et al., 2001). However, in the study performed by Wu and colleagues, heterocyclic amines were found to be associated with increased prevalence of MSI CRC. Heterocyclic amines can be produced during certain high-temperature methods of cooking of meats (Santarelli et al., 2008). Consequently, it is plausible that cooking method, independent of, or in conjunction with, certain meat types, may be associated with MSI status in CRC, potentially explaining the inconsistent observations between MSI and meat intakes.

Alcohol intake has been described as associated with MSI status in CRC. One report, analysing 1337 MSS and 227 MSI CRC identified increased alcohol intake as associated with a higher prevalence of MSS cancers (Poynter et al., 2009). Discordantly, a second analysis of 1244 MSS and 266 MSI colonic cancers identified increased alcohol consumption as linked to increased prevalence of MSI cancers (Slattery et al., 2001).

Folate intake has also been assessed relative to MSI status in CRC. Increased levels of plasma folate were associated with MSI cancer prevalence in a report assessing 166 MSS and 24 MSI CRC (Van Guelpen et al., 2010). However, assessment of dietary intake of folate in studies testing 179 MSS and 16 MSI CRC (Chang et al., 2007), 572 MSS and 76 MSI CRC (de Vogel et al., 2008), 111 MSS and 19 MSI CRC (Jensen et al., 2008) and 542 MSS and 127 MSI colonic cancers (Schernhammer, Giovannuccci, Fuchs & Ogino, 2008) all identified no association between folate intake and MSI status in CRC.

Presently, the data describing dietary associations and MSI status in CRC are contradictory and difficult to interpret. No strong associations have been identified and corroborated in independent cohorts. The difficulty in identification of plausible dietary constituents which may affect MSI prevalence in CRC may be due to the lack of such a relationship existing. It

Study	MSS/MSI-low CRC/CC	MSI/MSI-high CRC/CC	dietary association
Chang et al 2007	CRC: 179	CRC: 16	no statistically significant association between folate or vitamin B12 and MSI status
de Vogel et al 2008	CRC: 572	CRC: 76	no statistically significant association between folate, vitamin B2, methionine or alcohol and MSI status
Diergaarde et al 2003	CC: 144	CC: 40	↑ red meat associated with MSS cancers
Jensen et al 2008	CRC: 111	CRC: 19	no association between MSI and folate or vitamin B12
Poynter et al 2009	CRC: 1337	CRC: 227	↑ alcohol associated with MSS cancers
Satia et al 2005	CC: 437	CC: 49	no association between diet and MSI status [some associations comparing MSI/MSS cases vs controls]
Schernhammer et al 2008	CC: 542	CC: 127	no statistically significant association between folate, vitamin B6, B12, methionine or alcohol and MSI status
Slattery et al 2001	CC: 1244	CC: 266	↑ alcohol associated with MSI cancers
Van Guelpen et al 2010	CRC: 166	CRC: 24	Increased levels of plasma folate associated with MSI cancers
Wu et al 2001	CC: 238	CC: 35	↑ heterocyclic aromatic amines associated with MSI cancers

Table 2. Summarised description of literature analysing microsatellite instability (MSI) in colorectal neoplasia in relation to dietary intakes with the statistically significant associations described. *MSS*: microsatellite stability, *WT*: wildtype, *CRC*: colorectal cancer, *CC*: colonic cancer, ↑ and ↓ denote an increase or decrease in consumption respectively.

may also be plausible that such relationships exist and are particularly subtle. Methylation of the *MLH1* promoter, leading to gene silencing and subsequent DNA MMR deficiency, occurs in the vast majority, but not all, of MSI CRC (Kuismanen et al., 2000); suggesting that other components of the MMR system can be disrupted, such as mutations to the *MSH2* or *MSH6* genes, and that MSI may develop from a group of distinct initial aberrations in a small proportion of CRC. Furthermore, subsequent instability at microsatellites as a result may depend on other promoting factors. As such, it appears that a series of molecular events takes place leading to the MSI phenotype, which may arise from different epigenetic silencing or mutational events in different cancers. The multiple causes of MSI, and the different associated factors, may explain, at least in part, the lack of consistently identified dietary constituents which have been associated with this type of genomic instability. Alternatively, age-related susceptibility to promoter methylation, including the MLH1 promoter, may be the predominant risk factor for MSI in CRC rather than dietary factors.

2.4.3 CIMP and dietary associations

Studies assessing dietary associations with CIMP in CRC have centred largely on testing intakes of those compounds which may act as methyl group donors, or which function in the biochemical pathways responsible for methylation processes. Vitamin B6 has been described as associated with an increased prevalence of CIMP in CRC in one study assessing 496 CIMP-low/absent and 152 CIMP-high cancers (de Vogel et al., 2008). However, several other reports, assessing 288 CIMP-low/absent and 87 CIMP-high (Schernhammer et al., 2011) and 824 CIMP-low/absent and 330 CIMP-high (Slattery et al., 2007) colonic cancers failed to identify a similar association.

A similar lack of consensus has been observed when assessing vitamin B12. A single study assessing 107 CIMP-low/absent and 44 CIMP-high colonic cancers described an increased serum vitamin B12 concentration as associated with CIMP in this cohort (Mokarram et al., 2008). Schernhammer and colleagues (Schernhammer et al., 2011) and Slattery and co-workers (Slattery et al., 2007) did not identify a similar association in their studies. A report assessing 163 CIMP-low/absent and 27 CIMP-high CRC also identified no association between vitamin B12 intakes and CIMP status (Van Guelpen et al., 2010). Assessment of folate intake in relation to CIMP status has consistently failed to identify associations between the two in both colorectal and colonic cancer studies (Schernhammer et al., 2011; Slattery et al., 2007; Van Guelpen et al., 2010).

A single report, assessing 167 CIMP-low/negative and 17 CIMP-high colonic cancers identified reduced fruit intake as associated with an increased prevalence of CIMP-high colonic cancer (Diergaarde, Braam, van Muijen, Ligtenberg, Kok & Kampman, 2003). In an independent study, reduced consumption of vitamin A was identified as associated with increased prevalence of CIMP-high CRC (98 CIMP-low/absent CRC and 22 CIMP-high CRC) (Mas et al., 2007). These observations are yet to be corroborated in other studies. An additional report, assessing 776 CIMP-low/absent and 74 CIMP-high rectal cancers (Slattery, Curtin, Wolff, Herrick, Caan & Samowitz, 2010) failed to identify fruit intakes as associated with CIMP-high rectal cancer prevalence. Little additional data exists describing vitamin A intakes relative to CIMP status in CRC.

A limited number of additional associations have been observed relating CIMP status to certain dietary patterns. One report, assessing broad dietary patterns in addition to specific nutrient and foodstuff intakes identified increased fat-rich dairy products and omega-3 fatty acid consumption as associated with increased frequency of CIMP-high rectal cancers (776 CIMP-low/absent cancers and 74 CIMP-high cancers) (Slattery, Curtin, Wolff, Herrick, Caan & Samowitz, 2010). In an additional analysis, using this same patient cohort, long-term liquor/spirit intake was also found to be associated with an increased prevalence of CIMP-high status (Slattery, Wolff, Herrick, Curtin, Caan & Samowitz, 2010). Very few studies have assessed alcohol intake in terms of beverage consumed, as such, this observation awaits confirmation in an independent study. Additional data do not exist at present which validate the observed associations between increased consumption of fat-rich dairy products and omega-3 fatty acid with CIMP-high status.

There is no dietary intake which has been identified in several cohorts as associated with CIMP-high colorectal neoplasia. This may be due to the variety of methodologies used to assess CIMP status and the different criteria used to define CIMP-high status in these cancers, with no consensus method and definition having been used across studies (see Table 3). Furthermore, CIMP itself is the resulting phenotype of precursor genetic and epigenetic aberrations. As such, it may be plausible that this CRC subtype may not be linked to dietary risk factors, but instead diet may be linked to the causative precursor events, such as *MLH1* promoter methylation and MSI. Assessment of large study cohorts, in which CIMP-high cancers are categorised by causative lesions or processes, would in part help to understand dietary intakes and causation in the context of this phenotype.

3. Review limitations

This review has attempted to assess the available data describing the relationship between dietary factors and the molecular genetic events occurring during the development and progression of CRC. Published analyses have been summarised and where consensus between studies exists, this has been highlighted. Although providing a synopsis of the available information, several limitations are inherent in such a general discussion.

No detailed analysis or discussion of the methods of statistical analysis in each report has been provided. The wide range of methodology employed for this purpose across studies makes such a discussion in the present chapter impractical. Opinions on statistical methods vary across reports in terms of adjustment for multiple testing, inclusion of confounding variables in statistical models and the requirement for power calculations. In this context, no discussion or comparison of statistical methods has been attempted; notably, hazard and odds

Study	CIMP-low/absent CRC/CC/RC	CIMP-high CRC/CC/RC	dietary association
de Vogel et al 2008	CRC: 496*	CRC: 152*	↑ vitamin B6 associated with MLH1 promoter methylation in males only
Diergaarde et al 2003	CC: 167**	CC: 17**	↓ fruit associated with MLH1 promoter methylation and concurrent absence of MLH1 protein
Mas et al 2007	CRC: 98*	CRC: 22*	↓ vitamin A associated with MLH1 promoter methylation
Mokarram et al 2008	CC: 107∓	CC: 44∓	increased levels of serum B12 associated with CIMP
Schernhammer et al 2011	CC: 288†	CC: 87†	no association between folate, vitamin B6, B12, methionine or alcohol consumption and CIMP
Slattery et al 2007	CC: 824††	CC: 330††	no association between folate, vitamin B6, B12, methionine or alcohol consumption and CIMP
Slattery et al 2010	RC: 776††	RC: 74††	no association between calcium and vitamin D consumption and CIMP
Slattery et al 2010	RC: 776††	RC: 74††	↑ fat-rich dairy products and ↑ omega-3 fatty acids associated with CIMP
Slattery et al 2010	RC: 776††	RC: 74††	long-term ↑ spirits/liquor with CIMP
Van Guelpen et al 2010	CRC: 163‡	CRC: 27‡	no association between plasma folate or plasma vitamin B12 and CIMP

Table 3. Summarised description of literature analysing CpG island methylator phenotype (CIMP) in colorectal neoplasia in relation to dietary intakes with the statistically significant associations described. WT: wildtype, CRC: colorectal cancer, CC: colonic cancer, RC: rectal cancer, ↑ and ↓ denote an increase or decrease in consumption respectively. * CIMP positive status defined by MLH1 promoter methylation. ** CIMP positive status defined by MLH1 promoter methylation and concurrent loss of MLH1 expression as determined by immunohistochemistry. ∓ CIMP positive status defined by methylation of one or more of the p16, MLH1 or MSH2 promoters. † CIMP positive status defined by methylation at 11 of 16 tested markers. †† CIMP positive status defined by methylation at 2 of 5 tested markers. ‡ CIMP positive status defined by methylation at 6 of 8 tested markers.

ratios should be further analysed in order to interpret the relative 'strength' of the associations highlighted here.

In addition to statistical methods, the methodology of dietary assessment in each individual report has not been discussed. Dietary intakes can be measured in a variety of ways, including person-to-person interview, food frequency questionnaires, food diaries and biomarker assessment. Such an assessment is beyond the scope of this chapter. Outside of this review, several specific reports have been published describing the merits, limits and practicality of some of the available options for dietary assessment (Bingham et al., 1995; Day et al., 2001). To fully interpret dietary associations identified in different studies, although not discussed herein, an appreciation of dietary assessment methodology, and the relative accuracy of such techniques, should be taken into account.

Further to the limits inherent in the compilation of this review, consideration of the nature of assessment of dietary intakes relative to characteristics of colorectal cancers is required. For example, considerably more data exist describing the relationship between mutations in K-RAS and diet than for APC. An 'assessment bias' exists, presumably due to the significantly simpler task of examining hotspot mutation regions of the K-RAS proto-oncogene compared with the longer lengths of sequencing required for mutational assessment of tumour suppressor genes. As a result, the molecular genetic changes which occur during CRC development have not been assessed at equal frequencies. Such 'assessment bias' should be noted when considering such a broad view, as presented in this chapter. This should be particularly considered when trying to interpret the genetic or molecular changes which have been tested in relation to diet in only a small number of studies.

It should also be understood that in many reports assessing dietary associations in CRC broad definitions are employed, in order to maintain the practicality and feasibility of studies. For example, often reports describing mutations in BRAF are actually describing mutations only in exons 11 and 15; reports describing p53 mutations are frequently only describing mutational analyses of exons 5-8. Such limited analyses of coding regions is justified, with the significant majority of mutations in these examples being present in the regions described.

Furthermore, such limitations increase the practicality of these studies, in terms of both financial support and time investments required. Additionally, these limited regions of analyses are frequently selected based on biological evidence. Although justified, the limited extent to which genes are searched for the presence of mutations should be appreciated, and such variability between studies may in part explain inconsistent observations. In conjunction with this, different methods of mutational assessment provide different levels of sensitivity. For example, hotspot mutational assessment has been demonstrated to be more sensitively performed using pyrosequencing compared with dideoxysequencing (Naguib et al., 2010; Ogino et al., 2005). Such discrepancies between different reports were not discussed in this chapter, but should be considered when making side-by-side comparisons of studies.

In addition to the genetic and epigenetic changes giving rise to CRC development and progression described in this chapter, additional events occur during progression of these neoplasms. Furthermore, these events may be associated with dietary intakes, and data exist describing their associations with dietary consumptions; for example, loss of PTEN expression has also been tested for association with dietary intakes in CRC (Naguib, Cooke, Happerfield, Kerr, Gay, Luben, Ball, Mitrou, McTaggart & Arends, 2011). Studies of genetic and epigentic events beyond those discussed here were omitted due to the current low number of studies assessing their relationship with diet.

4. Future directions of the field

Next generation sequencing technology now affords the practical and accurate sequencing of entire genomes, with such strategies being employed to assess the genetic changes in several cancer types (Stratton et al., 2009). Furthermore, genomewide single nucleotide polymorphism analyses are being employed in a variety of settings. With these tools it is now possible to ask different questions relating diet to cancer. Are certain chemicals in the diet associated with an increased prevalence of any type of base change across the genome? Are transitions or transversions associated with intakes of specific compounds? The prospect of such investigations greatly expand the potential to understand the biochemical implications of certain dietary intakes, and provide an attractive avenue by which the identification of initiating factors in colorectal carcinogenesis might be pursued.

At present, a moderate number of studies have attempted to assess what impact, if any, dietary factors may have on CRC and the molecular subtypes of tumours which comprise this disease. With new technologies becoming available which have the power to expand this field of study, the underlying question of the purpose of such analyses should be clarified. Simply identifying dietary links to disease is only of limited use: how can this understanding be employed to reduce cancer-related mortality? It may be unrealistic to expect that if dietary constituents can be shown to be associated with increased prevalence of any particular molecular subtypes of colorectal cancer that these may be eliminated from the diet. The overwhelming evidence describing the strong association between tobacco use and cancer mortality fails to deter a significant number of smokers; although, the identification of such a link has undoubtedly provided individuals with knowledge upon which informed decisions have been made to refrain from tobacco use. Instead, a more 'protective' approach might be endorsed, such that dietary constituents which are found to confer protection against certain types of CRC might be promoted. This may be particularly useful in the attempt to lower the number of diagnoses of the molecular subtypes of CRC which confer a poor prognosis. Some have suggested that excessive administration of dietary advice may prove to be counterproductive: advice should be administered sparsely and where the greatest potential to reduce cancer-related deaths exists. It is in this context that the understanding of diet and the molecular subtypes of CRC has the greatest potential and will provide the greatest impact in the effort to reduce the number of CRC-related deaths.

5. Conclusions and summary

At present, although data exist describing the association of particular dietary factors with the specific molecular genetic changes in CRC, very few consistently reproducible associations have been described. Several factors may contribute to this, including variations in study methodologies (dietary intake assessment, sequencing strategies), statistical assessment (variation in the statistical power/number of samples, inclusion of different confounding variables in models) and features of study design.

Assessment of the presently available data do describe some associations which warrant further study: *K-RAS* mutation appears to be less frequent in CRC in individuals consuming a high folate diet. Furthermore, *APC* mutation appears to be associated with meat intakes to some degree, although this exact relationship is unclear.

At present, the study of diet in relation to the specific subtypes of CRC is at an exciting stage. Sequencing technology advancements now provide an avenue by which the total genetic composition of CRC, and the specific molecular subtypes, can be assessed. Using such tools, detailed understanding of genomewide events can be correlated with dietary intakes. Such modern approaches, coupled with renewed efforts to improve, validate and employ the most reliable and accurate methods of dietary intake assessment, provide the keys to the success of this field, which will help to provide the sought after end goal of a reduction in the number of CRC-related deaths.

6. Acknowledgments

This work was supported by EPIC Norfolk and the Medical Research Council Centre for Nutritional Epidemiology in Cancer Prevention and Survival. Furthermore, the dedication and support of Professor Kay-Tee Khaw and the late Professor Sheila Bingham were essential in the completion of this chapter.

7. References

Arends, M. J., McGregor, A. H., Toft, N. J., Brown, E. J. & Wyllie, A. H. (1993). Susceptibility to apoptosis is differentially regulated by c-myc and mutated Ha-ras oncogenes and is associated with endonuclease availability, *Br J Cancer* 68(6): 1127–1133.

Arends, M. J., McGregor, A. H. & Wyllie, A. H. (1994). Apoptosis is inversely related to necrosis and determines net growth in tumors bearing constitutively expressed myc, ras, and HPV oncogenes, *Am J Pathol* 144(5): 1045–1057.

Aylon, Y. & Oren, M. (2011). New plays in the p53 theater, *Curr Opin Genet Dev* 21(1): 86–92.

Bautista, D., Obrador, A., Moreno, V., Cabeza, E., Canet, R., Benito, E., Bosch, X. & Costa, J. (1997). Ki-ras mutation modifies the protective effect of dietary monounsaturated fat and calcium on sporadic colorectal cancer, *Cancer Epidemiol Biomarkers Prev* 6(1): 57–61.

Bingham, S. A., Cassidy, A., Cole, T. J., Welch, A., Runswick, S. A., Black, A. E., Thurnham, D., Bates, C., Khaw, K. T. & Key, T. J. (1995). Validation of weighed records and other methods of dietary assessment using the 24 h urine nitrogen technique and other biological markers, *Br J Nutr* 73(4): 531–550.

Bongaerts, B. W. C., de Goeij, A. F. P. M., van den Brandt, P. A. & Weijenberg, M. P. (2006). Alcohol and the risk of colon and rectal cancer with mutations in the K-ras gene, *Alcohol* 38(3): 147–154.

Bos, J. L. (1989). Ras oncogenes in human cancer: a review., *Cancer Res* 49(17): 4682–4689.

Bourdon, J. C., Laurenzi, V. D., Melino, G. & Lane, D. (2003). p53: 25 years of research and more questions to answer., *Cell Death Differ* 10(4): 397–399.

Boyle, P. & Langman, J. S. (2000). ABC of colorectal cancer: Epidemiology., *BMJ* 321(7264): 805–808.

Brink, M., Weijenberg, M. P., de Goeij, A. F. P. M., Roemen, G. M. J. M., Lentjes, M. H. F. M., de Bruïne, A. P., Goldbohm, R. A. & van den Brandt, P. A. (2005). Meat consumption and K-ras mutations in sporadic colon and rectal cancer in The Netherlands Cohort Study, *Br J Cancer* 92(7): 1310–1320.

Brink, M., Weijenberg, M. P., de Goeij, A. F. P. M., Roemen, G. M. J. M., Lentjes, M. H. F. M., de Bruïne, A. P., van Engeland, M., Goldbohm, R. A. & van den Brandt, P. A. (2005). Dietary folate intake and k-ras mutations in sporadic colon and rectal cancer in The Netherlands Cohort Study, *Int J Cancer* 114(5): 824–830.

Brink, M., Weijenberg, M. P., De Goeij, A. F. P. M., Schouten, L. J., Koedijk, F. D. H., Roemen, G. M. J. M., Lentjes, M. H. F. M., De Bruïne, A. P., Goldbohm, R. A. & Van Den Brandt, P. A. (2004). Fat and K-ras mutations in sporadic colorectal cancer in The Netherlands Cohort Study, *Carcinogenesis* 25(9): 1619–1628.

Ceol, C. J., Pellman, D. & Zon, L. I. (2007). APC and colon cancer: two hits for one., *Nat Med* 13(11): 1286–1287.

Chang, S.-C., Lin, P.-C., Lin, J.-K., Yang, S.-H., Wang, H.-S. & Li, A. F.-Y. (2007). Role of MTHFR polymorphisms and folate levels in different phenotypes of sporadic colorectal cancers, *Int J Colorectal Dis* 22(5): 483–489.

Curtin, K., Slattery, M. L. & Samowitz, W. S. (2011). CpG island methylation in colorectal cancer: past, present and future, *Patholog Res Int* 2011: 902674.

Day, N., McKeown, N., Wong, M., Welch, A. & Bingham, S. (2001). Epidemiological assessment of diet: a comparison of a 7-day diary with a food frequency questionnaire using urinary markers of nitrogen, potassium and sodium, *Int J Epidemiol* 30(2): 309–317.

de Vogel, S., Bongaerts, B. W. C., Wouters, K. A. D., Kester, A. D. M., Schouten, L. J., de Goeij, A. F. P. M., de Bruïne, A. P., Goldbohm, R. A., van den Brandt, P. A., van Engeland, M. & Weijenberg, M. P. (2008). Associations of dietary methyl donor intake with MLH1 promoter hypermethylation and related molecular phenotypes in sporadic colorectal cancer, *Carcinogenesis* 29(9): 1765–1773.

de Vogel, S., van Engeland, M., Lüchtenborg, M., de Bruïne, A. P., Roemen, G. M. J. M., Lentjes, M. H. F. M., Goldbohm, R. A., van den Brandt, P. A., de Goeij, A. F. P. M.

& Weijenberg, M. P. (2006). Dietary folate and APC mutations in sporadic colorectal cancer, *J Nutr* 136(12): 3015–3021.

Diergaarde, B., Braam, H., van Muijen, G. N. P., Ligtenberg, M. J. L., Kok, F. J. & Kampman, E. (2003). Dietary factors and microsatellite instability in sporadic colon carcinomas, *Cancer Epidemiol Biomarkers Prev* 12(11 Pt 1): 1130–1136.

Diergaarde, B., Tiemersma, E. W., Braam, H., van Muijen, G. N. P., Nagengast, F. M., Kok, F. J. & Kampman, E. (2005). Dietary factors and truncating APC mutations in sporadic colorectal adenomas, *Int J Cancer* 113(1): 126–132.

Diergaarde, B., van Geloof, W. L., van Muijen, G. N. P., Kok, F. J. & Kampman, E. (2003). Dietary factors and the occurrence of truncating APC mutations in sporadic colon carcinomas: a Dutch population-based study, *Carcinogenesis* 24(2): 283–290.

Eichholzer, M., Luthy, J., Moser, U. & Fowler, B. (2001). Folate and the risk of colorectal, breast and cervix cancer: the epidemiological evidence., *Swiss Med Wkly* 131(37-38): 539–549.

Fodde, R., Smits, R. & Clevers, H. (2001). APC, signal transduction and genetic instability in colorectal cancer., *Nat Rev Cancer* 1(1): 55–67.

Forbes, S. A., Bhamra, G., Bamford, S., Dawson, E., Kok, C., Clements, J., Menzies, A., Teague, J. W., Futreal, P. A. & Stratton, M. R. (2008). The Catalogue of Somatic Mutations in Cancer (COSMIC), *Curr Protoc Hum Genet* Chapter 10: Unit 10.11.

Fransen, K., Klintenas, M., Osterstrom, A., Dimberg, J., Monstein, H.-J. & Soderkvist, P. (2004). Mutation analysis of the BRAF, ARAF and RAF-1 genes in human colorectal adenocarcinomas., *Carcinogenesis* 25(4): 527–533.

Freedman, A. N., Michalek, A. M., Marshall, J. R., Mettlin, C. J., Petrelli, N. J., Black, J. D., Zhang, Z. F., Satchidanand, S. & Asirwatham, J. E. (1996). Familial and nutritional risk factors for p53 overexpression in colorectal cancer, *Cancer Epidemiol Biomarkers Prev* 5(4): 285–291.

Freudenheim, J. L., Graham, S., Marshall, J. R., Haughey, B. P., Cholewinski, S. & Wilkinson, G. (1991). Folate intake and carcinogenesis of the colon and rectum., *Int J Epidemiol* 20(2): 368–374.

Goss, K. H. & Groden, J. (2000). Biology of the adenomatous polyposis coli tumor suppressor, *J Clin Oncol* 18(9): 1967–1979.

Herman, J. G., Umar, A., Polyak, K., Graff, J. R., Ahuja, N., Issa, J. P., Markowitz, S., Willson, J. K., Hamilton, S. R., Kinzler, K. W., Kane, M. F., Kolodner, R. D., Vogelstein, B., Kunkel, T. A. & Baylin, S. B. (1998). Incidence and functional consequences of hMLH1 promoter hypermethylation in colorectal carcinoma, *Proc Natl Acad Sci U S A* 95(12): 6870–6875.

Ibrahim, A. E. K., Arends, M. J., Silva, A.-L., Wyllie, A. H., Greger, L., Ito, Y., Vowler, S. L., Huang, T. H.-M., Tavaré, S., Murrell, A. & Brenton, J. D. (2011). Sequential DNA methylation changes are associated with DNMT3B overexpression in colorectal neoplastic progression, *Gut* 60(4): 499–508.

Jen, J., Powell, S. M., Papadopoulos, N., Smith, K. J., Hamilton, S. R., Vogelstein, B. & Kinzler, K. W. (1994). Molecular determinants of dysplasia in colorectal lesions., *Cancer Res* 54(21): 5523–5526.

Jensen, L. H., Lindebjerg, J., Crüger, D. G., Brandslund, I., Jakobsen, A., Kolvraa, S. & Nielsen, J. N. (2008). Microsatellite instability and the association with plasma homocysteine and thymidylate synthase in colorectal cancer, *Cancer Invest* 26(6): 583–589.

Kambara, T., Simms, L. A., Whitehall, V. L., Spring, K. J., Wynter, C. V., Walsh, M. D., Barker, M. A., Arnold, S., McGivern, A., Matsubara, N., Tanaka, N., Higuchi, T., Young, J., Jass, J. R. & Leggett, B. A. (2004). BRAF mutation is associated with DNA methylation in serrated polyps and cancers of the colorectum, *Gut* 53(8): 1137–1144.

Kim, Y.-I. (2005). Nutritional epigenetics: impact of folate deficiency on DNA methylation and colon cancer susceptibility, *J Nutr* 135(11): 2703–2709.

Kinzler, K. W. & Vogelstein, B. (1996). Lessons from hereditary colorectal cancer, *Cell* 87(2): 159–170.

Kondo, Y. & Issa, J.-P. J. (2004). Epigenetic changes in colorectal cancer, *Cancer Metastasis Rev* 23(1-2): 29–39.

Kuhnle, G. G. & Bingham, S. A. (2007). Dietary meat, endogenous nitrosation and colorectal cancer, *Biochem Soc Trans* 35(Pt 5): 1355–1357.

Kuhnle, G. G. C., Story, G. W., Reda, T., Mani, A. R., Moore, K. P., Lunn, J. C. & Bingham, S. A. (2007). Diet-induced endogenous formation of nitroso compounds in the GI tract., *Free Radic Biol Med* 43(7): 1040–1047.

Kuismanen, S. A., Holmberg, M. T., Salovaara, R., de la Chapelle, A. & Peltomäki, P. (2000). Genetic and epigenetic modification of MLH1 accounts for a major share of microsatellite-unstable colorectal cancers, *Am J Pathol* 156(5): 1773–1779.

Laso, N., Mas, S., Jose Lafuente, M., Casterad, X., Trias, M., Ballesta, A., Molina, R., Salas, J., Ascaso, C., Zheng, S., Wiencke, J. K. & Lafuente, A. (2004). Decrease in specific micronutrient intake in colorectal cancer patients with tumors presenting Ki-ras mutation, *Anticancer Res* 24(3b): 2011–2020.

Lee, S., Cho, N. Y., Choi, M., Yoo, E. J., Kim, J. H. & Kang, G. H. (2008). Clinicopathological features of CpG island methylator phenotype-positive colorectal cancer and its adverse prognosis in relation to KRAS/BRAF mutation, *Pathol Int* 58(2): 104–113.

Lüchtenborg, M., Weijenberg, M. P., de Goeij, A. F. P. M., Wark, P. A., Brink, M., Roemen, G. M. J. M., Lentjes, M. H. F. M., de Bruïne, A. P., Goldbohm, R. A., van 't Veer, P. & van den Brandt, P. A. (2005). Meat and fish consumption, APC gene mutations and hMLH1 expression in colon and rectal cancer: a prospective cohort study (The Netherlands), *Cancer Causes Control* 16(9): 1041–1054.

Luo, F., Brooks, D. G., Ye, H., Hamoudi, R., Poulogiannis, G., Patek, C. E., Winton, D. J. & Arends, M. J. (2007). Conditional expression of mutated K-ras accelerates intestinal tumorigenesis in Msh2-deficient mice, *Oncogene* 26(30): 4415–4427.

Luo, F., Brooks, D. G., Ye, H., Hamoudi, R., Poulogiannis, G., Patek, C. E., Winton, D. J. & Arends, M. J. (2009). Mutated K-ras(Asp12) promotes tumourigenesis in Apc(Min) mice more in the large than the small intestines, with synergistic effects between K-ras and Wnt pathways, *Int J Exp Pathol* 90(5): 558–574.

Luo, F., Poulogiannis, G., Ye, H., Hamoudi, R. & Arends, M. J. (2011). Synergism between K-rasVal12 and mutant Apc accelerates murine large intestinal tumourigenesis, *Oncol Rep* 26(1): 125–133.

Luo, F., Poulogiannis, G., Ye, H., Hamoudi, R., Zhang, W., Dong, G. & Arends, M. J. (2011). Mutant K-ras promotes carcinogen-induced murine colorectal tumourigenesis, but does not alter tumour chromosome stability, *J Pathol* 223(3): 390–399.

Martin, S. A., Lord, C. J. & Ashworth, A. (2010). Therapeutic targeting of the DNA mismatch repair pathway, *Clin Cancer Res* 16(21): 5107–5113.

Martínez, M. E., Maltzman, T., Marshall, J. R., Einspahr, J., Reid, M. E., Sampliner, R., Ahnen, D. J., Hamilton, S. R. & Alberts, D. S. (1999). Risk factors for Ki-ras protooncogene mutation in sporadic colorectal adenomas, *Cancer Res* 59(20): 5181–5185.

Mas, S., Lafuente, M. J., Crescenti, A., Trias, M., Ballesta, A., Molina, R., Zheng, S., Wiencke, J. K. & Lafuente, A. (2007). Lower specific micronutrient intake in colorectal cancer patients with tumors presenting promoter hypermethylation in p16(INK4a), p4(ARF) and hMLH1, *Anticancer Res* 27(2): 1151–1156.

McMichael, A. J. & Giles, G. G. (1988). Cancer in migrants to Australia: extending the descriptive epidemiological data., *Cancer Res* 48(3): 751–756.

Melhem, M. F., Law, J. C., el Ashmawy, L., Johnson, J. T., Landreneau, R. J., Srivastava, S. & Whiteside, T. L. (1995). Assessment of sensitivity and specificity of immunohistochemical staining of p53 in lung and head and neck cancers, *Am J Pathol* 146(5): 1170–1177.

Mokarram, P., Naghibalhossaini, F., Saberi Firoozi, M., Hosseini, S. V., Izadpanah, A., Salahi, H., Malek-Hosseini, S. A., Talei, A. & Mojallal, M. (2008). Methylenetetrahydrofolate reductase C677T genotype affects promoter methylation of tumor-specific genes in sporadic colorectal cancer through an interaction with folate/vitamin B12 status, *World J Gastroenterol* 14(23): 3662–3671.

Naguib, A., Cooke, J. C., Happerfield, L., Kerr, L., Gay, L. J., Luben, R. N., Ball, R. Y., Mitrou, P. N., McTaggart, A. & Arends, M. J. (2011). Alterations in PTEN and PIK3CA in colorectal cancers in the EPIC Norfolk study: associations with clinicopathological and dietary factors, *BMC Cancer* 11: 123.

Naguib, A., Mitrou, P. N., Gay, L. J., Cooke, J. C., Luben, R. N., Ball, R. Y., McTaggart, A., Arends, M. J. & Rodwell, S. A. (2010). Dietary, lifestyle and clinicopathological factors associated with BRAF and K-ras mutations arising in distinct subsets of colorectal cancers in the EPIC Norfolk study, *BMC Cancer* 10: 99.

Naguib, A., Wilson, C. H., Adams, D. J. & Arends, M. J. (2011). Activation of K-RAS by co-mutation of codons 19 and 20 is transforming, *J Mol Signal* 6: 2.

Norat, T., Bingham, S., Ferrari, P., Slimani, N., Jenab, M., Mazuir, M., Overvad, K., Olsen, A., Tjonneland, A., Clavel, F., Boutron-Ruault, M.-C., Kesse, E., Boeing, H., Bergmann, M. M., Nieters, A., Linseisen, J., Trichopoulou, A., Trichopoulos, D., Tountas, Y., Berrino, F., Palli, D., Panico, S., Tumino, R., Vineis, P., Bueno-de Mesquita, H. B., Peeters, P. H. M., Engeset, D., Lund, E., Skeie, G., Ardanaz, E., Gonzalez, C., Navarro, C., Quiros, J. R., Sanchez, M.-J., Berglund, G., Mattisson, I., Hallmans, G., Palmqvist, R., Day, N. E., Khaw, K.-T., Key, T. J., San Joaquin, M., Hemon, B., Saracci, R., Kaaks, R. & Riboli, E. (2005). Meat, fish, and colorectal cancer risk: the European Prospective Investigation into cancer and nutrition., *J Natl Cancer Inst* 97(12): 906–916.

O'Brien, H., Matthew, J. A., Gee, J. M., Watson, M., Rhodes, M., Speakman, C. T., Stebbings, W. S., Kennedy, H. J. & Johnson, I. T. (2000). K-ras mutations, rectal crypt cells proliferation, and meat consumption in patients with left-sided colorectal carcinoma, *Eur J Cancer Prev* 9(1): 41–47.

Ogino, S., Kawasaki, T., Brahmandam, M., Yan, L., Cantor, M., Namgyal, C., Mino-Kenudson, M., Lauwers, G. Y., Loda, M. & Fuchs, C. S. (2005). Sensitive sequencing method for KRAS mutation detection by Pyrosequencing., *J Mol Diagn* 7(3): 413–421.

Park, J. Y., Mitrou, P. N., Keen, J., Dahm, C. C., Gay, L. J., Luben, R. N., McTaggart, A., Khaw, K.-T., Ball, R. Y., Arends, M. J. & Rodwell, S. A. (2010). Lifestyle factors and p53 mutation patterns in colorectal cancer patients in the EPIC-Norfolk study, *Mutagenesis* 25(4): 351–358.

Parkin, D. M., Bray, F., Ferlay, J. & Pisani, P. (2005). Global cancer statistics, 2002., *CA Cancer J Clin* 55(2): 74–108.

Peyssonnaux, C. & Eychene, A. (2001). The Raf/MEK/ERK pathway: new concepts of activation, *Biol Cell* 93(1-2): 53–62.

Poulogiannis, G., Ichimura, K., Hamoudi, R. A., Luo, F., Leung, S. Y., Yuen, S. T., Harrison, D. J., Wyllie, A. H. & Arends, M. J. (2010). Prognostic relevance of DNA copy number changes in colorectal cancer, *J Pathol* 220(3): 338–347.

Poulogiannis, G., McIntyre, R. E., Dimitriadi, M., Apps, J. R., Wilson, C. H., Ichimura, K., Luo, F., Cantley, L. C., Wyllie, A. H., Adams, D. J. & Arends, M. J. (2010). PARK2 deletions occur frequently in sporadic colorectal cancer and accelerate adenoma development in Apc mutant mice, *Proc Natl Acad Sci U S A* 107(34): 15145–15150.

Poynter, J. N., Haile, R. W., Siegmund, K. D., Campbell, P. T., Figueiredo, J. C., Limburg, P., Young, J., Le Marchand, L., Potter, J. D., Cotterchio, M., Casey, G., Hopper, J. L., Jenkins, M. A., Thibodeau, S. N., Newcomb, P. A., Baron, J. A. & Colon Cancer Family Registry (2009). Associations between smoking, alcohol consumption, and colorectal cancer, overall and by tumor microsatellite instability status, *Cancer Epidemiol Biomarkers Prev* 18(10): 2745–2750.

Robinson, M. J. & Cobb, M. H. (1997). Mitogen-activated protein kinase pathways, *Curr Opin Cell Biol* 9(2): 180–186.

Samowitz, W. S., Albertsen, H., Herrick, J., Levin, T. R., Sweeney, C., Murtaugh, M. A., Wolff, R. K. & Slattery, M. L. (2005). Evaluation of a large, population-based sample supports a CpG island methylator phenotype in colon cancer, *Gastroenterology* 129(3): 837–845.

Santarelli, R. L., Pierre, F. & Corpet, D. E. (2008). Processed meat and colorectal cancer: a review of epidemiologic and experimental evidence, *Nutr Cancer* 60(2): 131–144.

Satia, J. A., Keku, T., Galanko, J. A., Martin, C., Doctolero, R. T., Tajima, A., Sandler, R. S. & Carethers, J. M. (2005). Diet, lifestyle, and genomic instability in the North Carolina Colon Cancer Study, *Cancer Epidemiol Biomarkers Prev* 14(2): 429–436.

Schernhammer, E. S., Giovannuccci, E., Fuchs, C. S. & Ogino, S. (2008). A prospective study of dietary folate and vitamin B and colon cancer according to microsatellite instability and KRAS mutational status, *Cancer Epidemiol Biomarkers Prev* 17(10): 2895–2898.

Schernhammer, E. S., Giovannucci, E., Baba, Y., Fuchs, C. S. & Ogino, S. (2011). B vitamins, methionine and alcohol intake and risk of colon cancer in relation to BRAF mutation and CpG island methylator phenotype (CIMP), *PLoS One* 6(6): e21102.

Schernhammer, E. S., Ogino, S. & Fuchs, C. S. (2008). Folate and vitamin B6 intake and risk of colon cancer in relation to p53 expression, *Gastroenterology* 135(3): 770–780.

Sjöblom, T., Jones, S., Wood, L. D., Parsons, D. W., Lin, J., Barber, T. D., Mandelker, D., Leary, R. J., Ptak, J., Silliman, N., Szabo, S., Buckhaults, P., Farrell, C., Meeh, P., Markowitz, S. D., Willis, J., Dawson, D., Willson, J. K. V., Gazdar, A. F., Hartigan, J., Wu, L., Liu, C., Parmigiani, G., Park, B. H., Bachman, K. E., Papadopoulos, N., Vogelstein, B., Kinzler, K. W. & Velculescu, V. E. (2006). The consensus coding sequences of human breast and colorectal cancers, *Science* 314(5797): 268–274.

Slattery, M. L., Anderson, K., Curtin, K., Ma, K. N., Schaffer, D. & Samowitz, W. (2001). Dietary intake and microsatellite instability in colon tumors, *Int J Cancer* 93(4): 601–607.

Slattery, M. L., Curtin, K., Anderson, K., Ma, K. N., Edwards, S., Leppert, M., Potter, J., Schaffer, D. & Samowitz, W. S. (2000). Associations between dietary intake and Ki-ras mutations in colon tumors: a population-based study, *Cancer Res* 60(24): 6935–6941.

Slattery, M. L., Curtin, K., Ma, K., Edwards, S., Schaffer, D., Anderson, K. & Samowitz, W. (2002). Diet activity, and lifestyle associations with p53 mutations in colon tumors., *Cancer Epidemiol Biomarkers Prev* 11(6): 541–548.

Slattery, M. L., Curtin, K., Sweeney, C., Levin, T. R., Potter, J., Wolff, R. K., Albertsen, H. & Samowitz, W. S. (2007). Diet and lifestyle factor associations with CpG island methylator phenotype and BRAF mutations in colon cancer, *Int J Cancer* 120(3): 656–663.

Slattery, M. L., Curtin, K., Wolff, R. K., Herrick, J. S., Caan, B. J. & Samowitz, W. (2010). Diet, physical activity, and body size associations with rectal tumor mutations and epigenetic changes, *Cancer Causes Control* 21(8): 1237–1245.

Slattery, M. L., Wolff, R. K., Herrick, J. S., Curtin, K., Caan, B. J. & Samowitz, W. (2010). Alcohol consumption and rectal tumor mutations and epigenetic changes, *Dis Colon Rectum* 53(8): 1182–1189.

Soreide, K., Janssen, E. A., Soiland, H., Korner, H. & Baak, J. P. (2006). Microsatellite instability in colorectal cancer, *Br J Surg* 93(4): 395–406.

Stratton, M. R., Campbell, P. J. & Futreal, P. A. (2009). The cancer genome, *Nature* 458(7239): 719–724.

Suehiro, Y. & Hinoda, Y. (2008). Genetic and epigenetic changes in aberrant crypt foci and serrated polyps., *Cancer Sci* 99(6): 1071–1076.

Takayama, T., Katsuki, S., Takahashi, Y., Ohi, M., Nojiri, S., Sakamaki, S., Kato, J., Kogawa, K., Miyake, H. & Niitsu, Y. (1998). Aberrant crypt foci of the colon as precursors of adenoma and cancer., *N Engl J Med* 339(18): 1277–1284.

Toyota, M., Ahuja, N., Ohe-Toyota, M., Herman, J. G., Baylin, S. B. & Issa, J. P. (1999). CpG island methylator phenotype in colorectal cancer, *Proc Natl Acad Sci U S A* 96(15): 8681–8686.

Van Guelpen, B., Dahlin, A. M., Hultdin, J., Eklöf, V., Johansson, I., Henriksson, M. L., Cullman, I., Hallmans, G. & Palmqvist, R. (2010). One-carbon metabolism and CpG island methylator phenotype status in incident colorectal cancer: a nested case-referent study, *Cancer Causes Control* 21(4): 557–566.

Velho, S., Moutinho, C., Cirnes, L., Albuquerque, C., Hamelin, R., Schmitt, F., Carneiro, F., Oliveira, C. & Seruca, R. (2008). BRAF, KRAS and PIK3CA mutations in colorectal serrated polyps and cancer: primary or secondary genetic events in colorectal carcinogenesis?, *BMC Cancer* 8: 255.

Voskuil, D. W., Kampman, E., van Kraats, A. A., Balder, H. F., van Muijen, G. N., Goldbohm, R. A. & van't Veer, P. (1999). p53 over-expression and p53 mutations in colon carcinomas: relation to dietary risk factors, *Int J Cancer* 81(5): 675–681.

Wark, P. A., Van der Kuil, W., Ploemacher, J., Van Muijen, G. N. P., Mulder, C. J. J., Weijenberg, M. P., Kok, F. J. & Kampman, E. (2006). Diet, lifestyle and risk of K-ras mutation-positive and -negative colorectal adenomas, *Int J Cancer* 119(2): 398–405.

Weijenberg, M. P., Luchtenborg, M., de Goeij, A. F., Brink, M., van Muijen, G. N., de Bruine, A. P., Goldbohm, R. A. & van den Brandt, P. A. (2007). Dietary fat and risk of colon and rectal cancer with aberrant MLH1 expression, APC or KRAS genes, *Cancer Causes Control* 18(8): 865–879.

Wheeler, J. M., Loukola, A., Aaltonen, L. A., Mortensen, N. J. & Bodmer, W. F. (2000). The role of hypermethylation of the hMLH1 promoter region in HNPCC versus MSI+ sporadic colorectal cancers, *J Med Genet* 37(8): 588–592.

Wood, L. D., Parsons, D. W., Jones, S., Lin, J., Sjoblom, T., Leary, R. J., Shen, D., Boca, S. M., Barber, T., Ptak, J., Silliman, N., Szabo, S., Dezso, Z., Ustyanksky, V., Nikolskaya, T., Nikolsky, Y., Karchin, R., Wilson, P. A., Kaminker, J. S., Zhang, Z., Croshaw, R., Willis, J., Dawson, D., Shipitsin, M., Willson, J. K., Sukumar, S., Polyak, K., Park, B. H., Pethiyagoda, C. L., Pant, P. V., Ballinger, D. G., Sparks, A. B., Hartigan, J., Smith, D. R., Suh, E., Papadopoulos, N., Buckhaults, P., Markowitz, S. D., Parmigiani, G., Kinzler, K. W., Velculescu, V. E. & Vogelstein, B. (2007). The genomic landscapes of human breast and colorectal cancers, *Science* 318(5853): 1108–1113.

Wu, A. H., Shibata, D., Yu, M. C., Lai, M. Y. & Ross, R. K. (2001). Dietary heterocyclic amines and microsatellite instability in colon adenocarcinomas, *Carcinogenesis* 22(10): 1681–1684.

Zhang, Z. F., Zeng, Z. S., Sarkis, A. S., Klimstra, D. S., Charytonowicz, E., Pollack, D., Vena, J., Guillem, J., Marshall, J. R., Cordon-Cardo, C., Cohen, A. M. & Begg, C. B. (1995). Family history of cancer, body weight, and p53 nuclear overexpression in Duke's C colorectal cancer, *Br J Cancer* 71(4): 888–893.

11

Effects of Dietary Counseling on Patients with Colorectal Cancer

Renata Dobrila-Dintinjana[1], Dragan Trivanović[2],
Marijan Dintinjana[3], Jelena Vukelic[4] and Nenad Vanis[5]
*[1]Department of Radiation Oncology, Clinical Hospital Center Rijeka,
University of Rijeka, School of Medicine,
[2]General Hospital Pula, Department of Internal Medicine,
[3]Clinic of General Medicine Dr Dintinjana,
[4]Department of Speech and Hearing Disorders Diagnostics and Rehabilitation,
Clinical Hospital Center Rijeka,
[5]Division for Gastroenterology and Hepatology, Clinical Center University of Sarajevo,
Faculty of Medicine, University of Sarajevo,
[1,2,3,4]Croatia
[5]Bosnia and Herzegovina*

1. Introduction

Cancers of the colon and rectum together are second most common tumor type worldwide. The prognosis for the survival after disease progression is usually poor (1). Cancer anorexia-cachexia syndrome is highly prevalent among patients with colorectal cancer, and has a large impact on morbidity and mortality, and on patient quality of life. Early intervention with nutritional supplementation has been shown to halt malnutrition, and may improve outcome in some patients (2).

The etiology of cancer-associated malnutrition appears to be related to the pathological loss of inhibitory control of catabolic pathways, whose increased activities are not counterbalanced by the increased central and peripheral anabolic drive (3).

The goals of nutritional support in patients with colorectal cancer are to improve nutritional status to allow initiation and completion of active anticancer therapies (chemotherapy and or radiotherapy) and improve quality of life (3, 4).

Cancer growth and dissemination but also cancer treatments, including surgery, chemotherapy, and radiation therapy, interfere with taste, ingestion, swallowing, and digest food which leads to hypophagia. Also, chemotherapy agents may cause nausea and diarrhea (3, 4). Although many new agents are on the market to combat these symptoms, prevalence of colorectal cancer is still high (1).

We studied the influence of nutritional support (counseling, nutritional supplements, megestrol acetate) on physical status and symptoms in patients with colorectal cancer during chemotherapy. The study was designed to investigate whether dietary counseling or oral nutrition commercial supplements during chemotherapy and/or BSC affected nutritional status and influence survival status prevalence in patients with colorectal cancer.

Results: Three hundred and eighty-eight colorectal cancer patients were included in the study. Nottingham Screening Tool Questionnaire, Appetite Loss Scale and Karnofsky Performance Status were taken to evaluate the nutritive status of patients. Group I consisted of 215 patients who were monitored prospectively and were given nutritional support and in this group weight gain of 1,5 kg (0,6-2,8 kg) and appetite improvement was observed in patients with colorectal cancer. In both groups Karnofsky Performance Status didn't change significantly reflecting the impact of the disease itself.

Nutritional counseling, supplemental feeding and pharmacological support do temporarily stop weight loss and improve appetite, QoL and social life, but this improvement has no implications on patients KPS and course of their disease.

Conclusion: These results encourage further studies with more specific nutritional supplementation in patients with colorectal cancer and probably in gastrointestinal oncology.

2. Colorectal cancer

The incidence and mortality rates for cancers of the colon and rectum are among the highest of all malignancies worldwide (1, 2). Colorectal cancer is second in global cancer incidence and it is the most common cause of cancer death among non-smokers. US and EU incidence figures exceed global averages, which is consistent with an increased risk in industrialized nations (2). Factors associated with increased risk of colorectal cancer are host susceptibility and a sequence of different carcinogenic exposures. Specific etiology for sporadic colorectal cancer is still elusive but predisposing hereditary and environmental factors have been clearly identified (5).

2.1 Etiology of colorectal cancer

Important causes of colorectal cancers are uncommon genetic syndromes. A small percentage of "sporadic" colon cancers cluster in families. Relatives of people with colorectal cancer have increased risk for colorectal cancer, and risk varies depending on the number of relatives affected and the age at which cancer occurred (5).

Colorectal cancer is a heterogeneous disease that can develop through only partly known complex series of molecular changes. It is a long-term, gradual process which, besides external factors (carcinogens), also involves ever more recognized hereditary factors that cause genetic changes capable of triggering the uncontrolled mucosal (epithelial) growth (1, 5). The sequence of events that leads to the development of disease are passage from normal mucosa to adenoma – malignantly transformed adenoma and invasive carcinoma is associated with a series of genetic events occurring over long periods (5-7 years), the knowledge of which keeps expanding for the past ten years (1). In other words, the malignant transformation of cells requires various types of genetic damage in the form of gene mutation, deletion, amplification or expression disorder (1). In the 1990-ies, Fearon and Vogelstein first developed an algorithm for genetic events in colorectal cancer. According to their model, sporadic colon cancer arises as a result of a series of genetic changes that affect the process progression from enhanced epithelial proliferation to metastatic disease. The ultimate outcome of the process depends more on the number of accumulated changes than on their chronology.

The syndromes of colorectal cancer are inherited in an autosomal dominant fashion and are categorized by phenotypic, histological and genetic findings. Familial adenomatous polyposis, hereditary nonpolyposis colorectal cancer, Peutz-Jeghers disease, juvenile polyposis, Cowden disease are rare conditions (6, 7).

Ulcerative colitis, among other diseases in the medical history, is the top risk factor. The longer the disease and the segment of the colon affected, the higher the risk. The risk is also increased in individuals with Crohn's disease. The patient undergoing surgery for colorectal cancer has three times the risk of cancer recurrence (9).

The inheritance determines individual susceptibility to sporadic cancer but the lifestyle and environmental exposures are necessary for cancer expression. Colorectal cancer incidence varies between different geographic regions and incidence and mortality rates have been highest in developed western nations (10, 11). The basic argument that environment plays a huge role in colorectal cancer expression we get from observational studies in migrant populations. Migrants from low-incident regions to the high-incident regions of North America within one generation accept the incidence of the host country. Yet, studies with migrants also suggest that geographic variation in colorectal cancer incidences is due to environmental exposures and not due to the inherent predisposition (racial and ethnic group) (1, 10, 11).

Population based investigations have found many dietary and other environmental factors associated with colorectal cancer incidence (2). Most of these studies have methodologic limitations and therefore the interpretation of such studies has to be made with caution. Many studies have been conducted to investigate external factors that may increase or diminish the incidence of colorectal cancer. Many authors recognize four risk factor categories: epidemiological, intestinal, dietetic and mixed. The most frequently reported factors, among these shown to increase the risk of developing the disease, are diets rich in meat and animal fats (bile salts), physical inactivity, smoking and alcohol consumption (1, 2, 12). Between other diets ingested, consumption of red meat has the strongest correlation with colorectal cancer; over 30 case control studies report increased risk of colorectal cancer with higher red meat intake. Especially fried, barbecued and well-done meat is associated with colorectal cancer risk. Obesity and high caloric intake are the independent risk factors for colorectal cancer, excessive body mass gives a two fold increase in colorectal cancer, and this association in more expressed in men than women (12). Although studies carried out in humans and animal models have shown a positive correlation between the saturated fats/red meat consumption and the development of colorectal cancer, only a few of them are confirmed to be statistically significant. The total amount of fat in terms of daily caloric intake (>40%) and their form appears to have special significance. The conversion of dietary phospholipids to diacylglycerol by intestinal bacteria is assumed to be a potential mechanism of carcinogenesis. Diacylglycerol can enter the epithelial cell directly and by stimulating protein kinase C, it evokes intracellular signal transduction or mucosal proliferation. Another important mechanism is the formation of free radicals during fat metabolism and the mucosal damage induced by the secondary bile acids (lithocholic acid). Nitroso compounds, heat-generated heterocyclic amines and high protein intake (accelerated epithelial proliferation) have potential carcinogenic consequencies (12, 13).

Among the factors mentioned to reduce the risk are diet high in plant fibers and calcium, antioxidants (vitamin E, selenium etc.), menopausal hormone replacement therapy and administration of nonsteroidal anti-inflammatory drugs (12). In 1990 more than 13 studies showed significant reductions in colorectal cancer risk comparing the group with higher vs group with lower fibre intake. Some of the potential benefit mechanisms are: increased stool weight, dilution of potential carcinogens and increased colon transit rate. But other studies did not confirm such results, and today in this field we have inconclusive and controversial results (12, 13).

A complex interaction between inherited predispositions and external factors is responsible for the development of colorectal cancer (Table 1).

RISK FACTORS FOR COLORECTAL CANCER	
Genetic factors	- inherited polyposis syndrome - syndromes: Gardner, Turcot - Peutz-Jeghers, juvenile polyposis
Family factors	- inherited colorectal cancer syndrome - hereditary adenocarcinomatosis syndrome - family history of colorectal cancer
Pre-existing diseases	- ulcerative colitis, Crohn's disease - colorectal cancer - radiation therapy to the small pelvis - colorectal polyps
External factors	- diet rich in meat and animal fat - physical activity - smoking
Other factors	- age over 40 years

Table 1. Risk factors for colorectal cancer development

2.2 Pathology

Molecular basis of disease are genetic mutations of somatic cells and the inner innervation of the colon is important in carcinoma pathogenesis and spread. According to their macroscopic appearance, colorectal cancers are divided into exophytic, ulcerative and stenosing tumors. Exophytic tumors are most often located in the right half of the colon, while stenosing tumors are mostly found in its left half. The majority (up to 75%) of colorectal cancer occur within the descending colon, sigmoid colon and rectum, 15% of cases are located in the cecum and ascending colon, and only 10% in the transverse colon (13, 14, 15). Adenocarcinoma accounts for more than 95% of colorectal cancer cases. The prognosis of the disease is associated with the depth of tumor invasion through the colonic wall, peripheral lymph node involvement and absence or presence of distant metastases. The Dukes staging system (Table 2) as used in clinical practice divides this cancer into three stages, depending on the depth of cancer invasion into the colorectal wall (16, 17).

DUKES A	- tumor confined within the colorectal wall
DUKES B	- tumor invaded through the colorectal wall B1-tumor limited to muscular mucosa B2-tumor protruding in/trough serosa
DUKES C	- metastases to lymph nodes

Table 2. The Dukes staging system for colorectal cancer

2.3 Clinical signs and diagnostic procedures

The symptoms of colorectal carcinoma depend on the anatomical location and size of the tumor. The tumor located in the cecoascendent portion will not necessarily produce obstruction since in this portion the stool has a liquid consistency, and the colonic lumen is wider than in the other parts. Patients complain of weakness, subfebrile temperature and blunt pain in the right lower hemiabdomen, and their laboratory tests show a high sedimentation rate and sideropenic anemia (1, 13).

Tumors of the transverse colon and on the left side of the half usually invade the colonic wall in a ring-shaped pattern mainly producing symptoms of the obstructive nature (cramping pain after meal, meteorism, change in stool form, occasional sudden ileus development and even bowel perforation). Symptoms of tumors confined to the rectosigmoid portion are most often false and/or painful urge to defecate (tenesmus), narrow stool and hematochezia (13).

The patient with suspicion of colorectal cancer should undergo a complete physical examination which must include digital rectal examination. In a large number of patients, the digital rectal examination already shows a hard lump inside the rectum, bleeding on touch. Colonoscopy is a procedure for visualizing colonic mucosa and obtaining samples for pathohistological analysis. Colonoscopy is the gold standard for detecting colorectal cancer. If for technical difficulties colonoscopy cannot be done, double-contrast irrigography may be considered although only 70-80% of lesions are detected by this method. Virtual colonoscopy and MR colonoscopy are also more and more often used. These radiology techniques use high-speed spiral CT and magnetic resonance imaging, and sophisticated software to process endoluminal images of the air-filled colon. Diagnostic techniques show a sensitivity of about 90% for tumors larger than 10 mm. Disadvantage is an inability to take biopsy samples and perform interventions available during colonoscopy. 'Colon capsule' for minutely detailed inspection of the colonic mucosa is also being gradually introduced, although this technique has the same disadvantage as the above mentioned techniques, and that is its inability to obtain biopsy samples (1, 13). Endoscopic ultrasound of the lower digestive tract is capable of providing assessment of tumor invasion into muscles and adjacent structures, as well as assessment of regional lymph node enlargement. The technique is employed to determine the extent of the spread of rectal tumors. Diagnosis of the spread of the disease involves imaging techniques (US, CT/MSCT/MRI of the abdomen and small pelvis, and CT/MSCT of the thorax). Serum CEA has limitations in sensitivity and specificity but was recommended for detection of recurrence. Molecular detection of tumor cells in circulation may prove to be more sensitive and specific than CEA (13, 18).

2.4 Treatment

Treatment for colorectal cancer depends on the extent of cancer spread. Surgery is the method of choice for treatment of localized tumors. Colon resection surgery for colorectal cancer must be as radical as possible. Chemotherapy, immunotherapy and radiotherapy used may be adjuvant, neo-adjuvant, curative or palliative in nature. Adjuvant chemotherapy aims to destroy micrometastases following surgery, and neo-adjuvant chemotherapy is aimed at reducing the tumor mass to allow surgery for either the primary tumor or distant metastases (usually to the liver or lungs) (1, 13). Systemic therapy for disseminated disease has been gaining popularity over the past few years. Treatment options for colorectal cancer include a variety of chemotherapy and immunotherapy regimens, with 5-fluorouracil/leucovorin, which may be added irinotecan and/or oxaliplatin, and bevacizumab, cetuximab and panitumumab as biological therapy, still remaining the mainstay for the management of patients with disseminated disease (3). The addition of this molecularly targeted therapy to standard chemotherapy improves treatment response, prolongs both the time to disease progression and eventually, median survival for disseminated or metastatic colorectal cancer, which currently is over 30 months (3, 19). In the future, prognostic and predictive factors will allow individual identification of patients who may benefit most from adjuvant chemotherapy, and which therapy should be used for the treatment of disseminated disease (personalized medicine). Therapy of rectal cancer includes adjuvant chemotherapy combined with radiation therapy (19).

Despite huge advances in diagnostic and surgery and despite global and national programs of prevention, about 50% of colorectal carcinomas are diagnosed in advanced stage (11). Advanced disease is largely refractory to conventional therapy and 5 years survival is still poor. Patients with advanced disease suffer from many stress symptoms (pain, vomiting, diarrhea, anorexia-cachexia syndrome, and etc.) and the therapeutic goal for them is maintenance of quality of life (QoL) (13). Many of those symptoms have implications for diagnostic and therapeutic procedures and can heavily disturb the process of chemo-immunotherapy and radiotherapy (3).

3. Anorexia-cachexia syndrome

3.1 Pathophysiology of anorexia-cachexia syndrome

Anorexia is defined as an unintentional reduction in food intake and anticipated cachexia. Cachexia develops as a result of progressive wasting of skeletal muscle mass and to a lesser extent adipose tissue (20). In cachexia, progressive wasting of skeletal muscle mass is replaced with adipose tissue and this occurs even before weight loss. Anorexia-cachexia syndrome is highly prevalent among patients with malignant diseases. Depending on primary tumor site anorexia-cachexia syndrome is present in 8-88% of cancer patients. Tumors of head and neck, stomach and pancreas have highest percentage of cachexia (21). At the time of diagnosis weight loss is present in about 50% of patients. Weight loss is independent predictive factor of survival (21). Cachexia-anorexia syndrome includes clinical features which are associated with growth of cancer. In addition, it has a large impact on morbidity, mortality and on patients' quality of life. Cancer cachexia develops in a majority of patients with advanced disease (22) (70 %) and directly causes death in 20% of cancer patients. Clinical signs of cancer cachexia are anorexia and weight loss. Abnormalities in carbohydrates, fat, protein and energy metabolism are clinically manifested as weakness, fatigue, malaise, loss of skeletal muscle and adipose tissue. In serum chemistry and haematology tests we can find anaemia, hypertrigliceridaemia, hypoproteinaemia with low albumines, hyperlacticacidaemia and glucose intolerance (insulin resistence) (23). Metabolic aberration in cancer cells and cells and microenvironment (inadequate energy intake, increased energy expenditure, mucositis, nausea, vomiting, change in taste or psychological problems as reaction to cancer disease) cause primary cancer cachexia. There are several conditions that can contribute decreased food intake (gastrointestinal obstruction, post-chemotherapy nausea and vomiting, pain and etc) and cause secondary cancer cachexia (24, 25). Anorexia-cachexia syndrome often occurs or worsens after the administration of chemotherapy. Chemotherapeutic agents are toxic to malignant tissue, and also to the quickly proliferating cells. This group of cells also includes cells of the gastrointestinal mucosa. Consequently, the absorption of nutrients is reduced. Some chemotherapeutics may affect the digestive system causing severe nausea, vomiting, abdominal pain, stomatitis and aversion to food. It should be noted that, in addition to the above mechanism for development of this syndrome, some chemotherapeutic agents also affect the taste buds of the tongue resulting in a changed and reduced sense of taste. It may also lead to reduced saliva production (26).

Sometimes we cannot find a reason for anorexia and weight loss may be unrelated to nutritional intake. In this cases weight loss is reflection of elevated resting energy expenditures and over expression of pro-inflammatory cytokines (27). The most common factors to stimulate the production of proinflammatory cytokines include: TNF-alpha, interleukins, interferon gamma and leukemia inhibitory factor. It should be noted that, due to such complex mechanism, energy supplementation in cachectic patients does not result in an increased body mass index (28).

The pathophysiologic mechanism is correlated with the production of catabolic factors either by the tumor or via factors produced by the host. Cancer cachexia differ from starvation. It is an unquestionable fact today that cancer cachexia is pro-inflammatory condition. The pathophysiology of cachexia involves very complex pathways; cachexia is caused with numerous metabolic changes mediated with pro-inflammatory cytokines. The most known mediators are tumor necrosis factor α, interleukin-1 (IL-1), interleukin 6 (IL-6), interferon-Y (from patients mononuclears) and molecules from tumor cells as lipid mobilisation factor (LMF) and proteolysis inducing factor (PIF). PIF is stimulating adenosine-triphosphate ubiquitin proteolitic pathway that is important in degradation of muscle mass and its stimulating synthesis of C-reactive protein (28, 29).

The result of these changes is impairment of immune functions, quality of life, and performance status. The worst consequence is inability of patient to endure chemo, immunotherapy and radiotherapy. Cachexia decreases response to therapy due to frequent toxicity and severe complications, what leads to shortened survival time (3, 20).

3.2 Nutritional support

Although increasing nutritional intake is insufficient to prevent the development of cachexia, nutritional support (taking into account the specific needs of the patient group), is required to reduce the consequences of nutritional decline and to improve quality of life and possibility to support the anticancer therapy (30). However, data from published studies are divided; some studies suggest that aggressive nutritional support can improve response to the antitumor treatment and decrease complications, but some deny any impact of nutritional support on tumor response, chemotherapy toxicity and survival (3, 30). Aggressive nutritional therapy does not significantly influence the outcome of patients with advanced cancer; „super"nutrition alone cannot reverse cachexia. But its use is still warranted because the patients QoL is significantly improved (3). The pharmacological treatments of cachexia antagonize the main symptoms (anorexia and chronic nausea) and improve the muscle metabolism. A significant number of studies (many uncontrolled) have suggested that anorexia and asthenia can be alleviated in cancer patient under corticosteroid treatment; also, the feeling of well-being is observed (31).

We must not underestimate advantage of nutritional treatment in improvement of asthenia and patients body image. Oral nutrition (after nutritional counseling) is ideal for cancer patients with a functional bowel. Enteral nutrition is useful in patients with advanced head and neck cancers or esophageal and gastric cancer and the use of parenteral nutrition (due to high costs and morbidity of 15%) with exception of high selected cases has no major role in care of cancer patients, especially in terminal disease (30, 31). In patients with colorectal cancer, enteral nutrition is usually provided by administration of food and/or commercial nutrient solutions and formulas (32). They either supplement daily diet or provide basic nutritional needs to patients who are unable to ingest sufficient amounts of food. The baseline requirements to administer such feeding include preserved swallowing function and the ability of the esophagus and stomach. There is a wide range of enteral nutrition formulas available for everyday use (33). Enteral nutrition formulas are classified into the following categories: monomeric (elementary) formulas, oligomeric formulas, polymeric formulas (32, 34, 35). The essential difference between them is in their size and/or the amount and type of molecules present. Accordingly, formulas containing a larger number of molecules that are also shorter at the same time, have a higher osmolality and can therefore cause side effects, such as diarrhea. The osmolality of an enteral formula depends on the type and amount of carbohydrates. Polysaccharides account for the vast majority of carbohydrate types present in the enteral feeding formulas. According to their solubility, fibers in the digestive system are divided into two categories: soluble and insoluble. Soluble fiber absorbs water in the intestinal lumen and increase the volume of the stool. They thus help regulate bowel motility. Soluble fibers are fermented by bowel bacteria using the aerobic pathway. Pectin slows down the emptying of the stomach and prolongs the passage of contents through the colon resulting in formation of the stool of satisfactory consistency even in tube fed patients (37). Normal metabolism requires daily protein intake of 0.8-1.0 g/kg body weight, and in the hypercatabolic state daily protein needs range from 1.2 to 1.6 g/kg body weight. According to the presence of nitrogen-containing compounds the diet may be divided into three groups: polymeric diet (includes natural proteins), oligomeric diet (includes small peptides), elementary diet (containing amino acids). Patients with the preserved gastrointestinal function require a diet in which complete proteins prevail (38). In case of compromised digestion, peptides should be the most represented. Among the amino acids, glutamine should be singled out. Glutamine helps maintain normal intestinal integrity by stimulating RNA, DNA and protein synthesis, resulting in an increase in the number and size of intestinal villi. Glutamine also prevents damage to intestinal permeability, preserves mucosal structure and prevents translocation of bacteria and toxins in the intestine. Glutamine is an important nutritional substrate for the intestinal cell line. In catabolic conditions including colorectal cancer, the intestinal system's requirements for glutamine are increased. The deficiency can be compensated for by addition of glutamine to the enteral nutrition formula (39). Arginine is another amino acid that plays a significant role in the immune events. It stimulates nitrogen oxide (NO) synthesis and the CD4/CD8 ratio, as well as the release of insulin, glucagon, prolactin and somatostatin (40, 41). The use of arginine requires caution as increased NO synthesis may accelerate the synthesis of proinflammatory cytokines and thereby cause a number of side effects. The main role of lipids in enteral formulas is to ensure large amounts of energy stored in relatively small volumes and sufficient amount of essential fatty acids which are a vital component of cell membranes and organelles. Corn oil and soybean oil used in enteral formulas provide long-chain triglycerides (LCT), while coconut and palm oil provide medium-chain triglycerides (MCT). These products have a favorable effect on: 1) growth, differentiation and function of lymphocytes, macrophages and granulocytes; 2) release of trophic hormones or growth factors; 3) function of NK cells; 4) IL-2 synthesis; 5) improvement of mesenteric blood flow;

6) reduction of skeletal and visceral muscle proteolysis; 7) prevention of bacterial translocation; 8) reduction in the frequency and severity of infectious complications and 9) shortening hospital stay (42). Fatty acids are thus formed providing a basic substrate for the colonic mucosa. Formulas containing omega-3 fatty acids from fish oil have been recently introduced. Omega-3 fatty acids reduce the synthesis of immunosuppressive and proinflammatory mediators. Meta-analyses of several studies have shown that immunomodulatory formulas do not significantly reduce mortality compared with standard enteral formulas. Their administration, however, achieves a lower rate of infection and septic complications, reduces dependency on assisted ventilation and shortens length of hospital treatment (43).

Omega-3 polyunsaturated fatty acid, eicosapentaenoic acid (EPA) can down-regulate the production of pro-inflammatory cytokines such as IL-6, IL-1 and TNF in patients with cancer and in healthy individuals. EPA can also inhibit the effects of proteolysis inducing factor (PIF). EPA normalizes metabolic pathways changed due to malignant disease and stabilize weight gain through the competitive metabolism with arachidonic acid. EPA metabolites have lower inflammatory and immunosuppressive effect versus arachidonic acid metabolites. Especially interestingly is inhibitory effect of EPA on pancreatic and colorectal cancer cell line growth observed „in vitro" (44, 45). Wigmor and Bruera, like many other investigators, showed that EPA can stabilize body weight in cancer patients (46). We investigated if dietary counseling and oral nutrition supplement during chemotherapy affected nutritional status and symptom prevalence in our first study on 388 patients with colorectal cancer receiving chemotherapy for advanced disease (FOLFIRI/XELIRI/FOLFOX) (47, 48).

Megestrol acetate is a type of medicine that comes in suspension form recommended in treatment guidelines for appetite and body weight loss in patients with malignant diseases. The drug belongs to a group of steroid hormones - progesterone. Its empirical formula is $C_{24}H_{32}O_4$. Progestational derivate megestrol acetate has been evaluated in many studies; conclusion is that megestrol acetate significantly increases appetite, caloric intake and nutritional status with mild side effects as edema and hypercalcaemia. It is not completely clear through which mechanisms megestrol is acting. It is assumed that megestrol acetate changes the cytokines which are inhibiting TNF effects. Stimulation of appetite is due to stimulation neuropeptide Y in lateral hypothalamus. Megestrol acetate enhances appetite and increases food intake, enables the administration of specific treatments, and improves both patient treatment tolerance and their quality of life. Implementation of megestrol acetate in nutritional support plan is necessary; according to the highlights of the 2004 Cachexia Cancer Conference anorexia preceding to weight loss and orexigenics are necessary even when weight loss is absent. Furthermore, patients with cancer cachexia do not react on isolated over caloric food intake. Mild side effects (edema) are not enough pronounced over the social benefits caused by appetite stimulation; patients do not withdraw megestrol acetate therapy (49). Therefore, the International Association for Hospice and Palliative Care, NCCN Guidellines and European Palliative Care Research Collaborative Group recommend megestrol acetate as a mandatory drug for treatment cancer cachexia (50). The recommended starting dose is 400 mg (10 ml) once a day. The dose may be increased up to 800 mg (20 ml) / day. The most common side effects of megestrol acetate include edemas, insomnia, impaired libido, and very rarely thromboembolic complications (48, 50).

The choice of enteral route depends on the underlying pathology, anticipated duration of enteral feeding and patient's preferences (30). In addition to the oral route of nutrition administration the transnasal route can also be considered. Indications for transnasal tube feeding include conditions or illnesses where normal feeding cannot be provided, and where the gastrointestinal tract maintains its function. For this purpose, nasogastric, nasoduodenal and nasojejunal types of tubes may be used. The tubes are usually placed 'blindly', however they may be placed by radiological and endoscopic means. The tubes are used when it is anticipated that tube feeding will be needed for up to 4 weeks. If enteral feeding is likely to be needed for more than 4 weeks, percutaneous endoscopic gastrostomy tubes or percutaneous endoscopic jejunostomies may be placed via an endoscopic access. The surgical placement of the gastrostomy or jejunostomy tube may also be taken into consideration. Two types of feeding can be used for patients requiring tube feeding: bolus (6 to 10 doses a day, each ranging from 50 to 200 ml, given over 5 to 30 minutes) or continuous feeding(20 to 150 ml per hour during 16-18 hours). The method of 'bolus feeding' is more frequently reported to cause side effects than continuous feedings (30, 35).

In some clinical situations, enteral feeding may be unsafe or contraindicated. Reasons for postponing enteral nutrition administration are as follows: persistent nausea/vomiting, intensive postprandial pain, diarrhea, mechanical obstruction, diminished bowel motility, malabsorption, gastrointestinal bleeding. In mentioned situations, parenteral feeding is used. Parenteral feeding may be administered by peripheral or central vein access. Risk-benefit assessment of parenteral nutrition is necessary for each patient (30, 31, 35).

We can evaluate nutritional status of the cancer patient with quick screening methods (NRS-2002, NSTQ, ect) or more detailed examination (laboratory findings, anthropometric measurement, body composition measurement, BMI). Nottingham Screening Tool Questionnaire is simple, quick, and proper for re-evaluating. Another simple model (Fearon) is suggested for quick evaluation: if patient unintentionally decrease in weight gain more than 5% in 3 to 6 months, if caloric intake is less than 1500 kcal/day and C-reactive protein value is 10 and higher. Based on these data we can assume that cancer cachexia is developing (34, 35, 36, 43, 46, 50)

3.3 Study results

Our study was conducted at the Gastrointestinal Oncology Department, Clinic for Internal Medicine, University Hospital Center Rijeka, from January 2001 to December 2007. The aim of the study was to evaluate the effect of nutritional support in patients with colorectal cancer. The follow-up included 338 patients divided into two groups. Group I: patients receiving nutritional support (215 patients), and group II patients who did not receive nutritional support (173 patients); retrospectively collected data. Visit 0 took place one week before initiation of chemotherapy. The nutritional status was evaluated according to body weight change. The body mass index (BMI) was calculated for all patients and all patients were also evaluated through three questionnaires: Nottingham Screening Tool (Table 3), Appetite Loss Scale and Karnofsky Performance Status. The reassessments were done at control visits, each visit taking place before the next chemotherapy course. There were, in total, 12 visits performed. The aim of the study was to assess the effects of nutritional support in colorectal cancer patients on chemotherapy. For all patients, the following parameters were monitored and statistically evaluated: selection of nutritional support regimen in group I, BMI in groups I and II, at visit 0 and visit 12, Nottingham Screening Tool Questionnaire in groups I and II, at visit 0 and visit 12, Appetite Loss Scale in groups I and II, at visit 0 and visit 1, Weight loss in groups I and II , at visit 0 and visit 12, Karnofsky Performance Status in groups I and II, at visit 0 and visit 12, side effects of megestrol acetate. Evaluating the initial risk measurement according to BMI, decrease in weight gain and NST, we did not find any significant difference between the two groups. We performed 12 visits in follow-up according to chemotherapy schedule. Before initiation of chemotherapy, we re-evaluated nutritional status of our patients using evaluation tools. After chemotherapy was completed, in group I (consisted of 215 patients who were monitored prospectively and were given nutritional support) we observed weight gain of 1.5 kg (0.6-2.8 kg) and appetite improvement, the most commonly seen result after 4 weeks of therapy with megestrol acetate. The appetite also improved on Appetite Loss Scale from 3.1 (pre-chemotherapy) to 4.7 (post-chemotherapy). But KPS did not change significantly (74.2% before chemo versus 80.4% after chemo respectively) reflecting the impact of the disease itself. The most common side effects in patients receiving enteral nutrition were diarrhea (12% of patients) , abdominal pain (9%) and altered taste sensation(5%). The most frequently reported side effect in patients receiving megestrol acetate was the occurrence of edema (20% of patients).

This clinical study is ongoing and preliminary results from more than 600 patients are similar to this one.

BMI	Score
>20	0
18-20	1
<18	2

Has the patient unintentionally lost weight during last 3 months?	Score
No	0
A little, up to 3 kg	1
A lot, more than 3 kg	2

Table 3. Nottingham Screening Tool Questionnaire

Score: 0-2 Patient is not in nutritive risk and does not need nutritional support

3-4 Patient need re-evaluation weekly

≥ 5 Patient is in nutritive risk and needs nutritive support

4. Discussion

Anorexia-cachexia syndrome often occurs in patients with gastrointestinal cancers. Malnutrition has huge impact on outcome in patients who underwent major surgical resections, and also in patients who have chemo/radiotherapy treatment (3, 22).

Although manifestations of chemotherapy injury on nutritional status is well-known, the potential role of nutritional supplementing is still not explored in detail. When treating cancer patients with chemotherapy we observed two problems and one of them is general failure in recognition of the weight loss early enough to perform nutritional support (30).

But if we know that patients will undergo to stress-full procedure which can have impact on his nutritional status (diagnostic procedures, colonoscopy for example, major gastrointestinal surgery) we have to give adequate nutritional support according to different clinical algorithms (3).

Adequate substitution with metabolites, increased caloric intake, inhibition of catabolic and inflammatory mediators leads to decrease of surgery, chemo and radiotherapy complications, but still has no significant impact on survival. Nutritional counseling, supplemental feeding and pharmacological support do temporarily stop weight loss and improve appetite, QoL and social life but this improvement has no implications on patient´s KPS and course of their disease. An improved knowledge of the pathophysiology of cancer induced cachexia will lead to development of more effective treatments (26).

In clinical practice, the role of nutrition therapy is often assumed to be less important than role of chemo, immunotherapy and radiotherapy as outcomes are less clear in literature (22, 26, 30). Our study showed that early nutritional intervention can decrease course of weight deterioration in the early course or locally advanced or metastatic colorectal cancer. Karnofsky Performance Status did not change significantly, what we expected.

Taking food is not only a physiologic necessity, but also cultural and a social event reflecting life and religious philosophy. Nutritive support can facilitate life of oncology patienta, their family support and caregivers understand (1). Therefore we have to recognize nutrition-related issues and to implement strategies that will lead to a better outcome for patient and his caregivers. In the end of the life the wish of dying patient is most important factor regarding enteral/parenteral nutrition. The interaction between major syndromes in terminal disease (pain, cachexia, cognitive failure) should be better established because it seems that severity of them has impact on the others. If we improve pain and depression we can expect impact on cachexia syndrome (3, 21).

5. Conclusion

The role of nutritional therapy in oncology patients has been neglected. This mainly results from failure to recognize malnutrition and untimely introduction of nutritional support.

Our study shows that early introduction of nutritional support can decrease weight loss and in some cases even enable weight gain in patients with locally advanced and metastatic colorectal cancer.

To achieve better treatment results for patients with colorectal cancer, nutritional therapy should be considered as a highly important part of their treatment and more attention should be paid to timely recognition of malnutrition and introduction of nutritional support. Patients with anorexia-cachexia syndrome should undergo to individualized nutritional intervention where nutrition counseling is base for improvement of nutritional status, quality of life and social life. Anorectic patients have changes in taste and smell and do not support high-fat food and therefore frequent but small meals are highly recommended (20).

Future perspectives:

Cancer patients have increased level of growth hormone (GH), low serum concentrations of insulin growth factor-1 (IGF-1) and insulin resistence. Loss of lean mass and inflammatory processes are closely connected to the action of three signaling molecules: insulin, growth hormone and insulin growth factor-1 is essential (51). Basic stimuli of insulin, IGF-1 and GH does not provide response in muscle cells in cachexia, its reasonable to target post-receptor pathways or using alternative pathways in muscle cells. A number of molecules exhibiting anti cytokines activity have been tested without significant clinical data (20). Ghrelin is a hormone that stimulates the release of GH and increases appetite. In a phase II clinical study, ghrelin agonist anamorelin produced an improvement in total body mass (52).

Despite cachexia is very common condition in cancers, there are still very few trials of drug therapies to reduce weight loss in cancer cachexia. Cachexia remains poorly studied and often undertreated condition that causes severe impairment of quality of life and increases mortality.

6. References

[1] Brkić M, Grgić T. Kolorektalni karcinom. Medicus 15 (1): 89-97, 2006.

[2] Heavey PM, McKenna D, Rowland IR. Colorectal cancer and the relationship between genes and the environment. Nutr Cancer, 48 (124), 2004.

[3] Dobrila-Dintinjana R, Guina T, Krznarić Ž, Radić M, Dobrila M. Effects of Nutritional Support in Patients with Colorectal Cancer during Chemotherapy. Collegium Antropologicum 32: 737–740, 2008.

[4] Markman B, Rodríguez-Freixinos V, Tabernero J. Biomarkers in colorectal cancer. Clin Transl Oncol. 2010;12:261-70.

[5] Sobczak A, Wawrzyn-Sobczak K, Sobaniec-Lotowska M. [The colorectal carcinoma risk factors]. Pol Merkuriusz Lek, 19:808, 2005.

[6] Gala M, Chung DC. Hereditary colon cancer syndromes. Semin Oncol. 2011;38:490-9.

[7] Migliore L, Migheli F, Spisni R, Coppedè F. Genetics, cytogenetics, and epigenetics of colorectal cancer. J Biomed Biotechnol. 2011;2011:792362.

[8] Hans F.A. Vasen, Patrice Watson, Jukka–Pekka Mecklin, Henry T. Lynch and the ICG–HNPCC. New clinical criteria for hereditary nonpolyposis colorectal cancer (HNPCC, Lynch syndrome) proposed by the International Collaborative Group on HNPCC. Gastroenterology 1999;116:1453-1456.

[9] Billioud V, Allen PB, Peyrin-Biroulet L. Update on Crohn's disease and ulcerative colitis. Expert Rev Gastroenterol Hepatol. 2011;5:311-4.

[10] Watson AJ, Collins PD. Colon cancer: a civilization disorder. Dig Dis. 2011;29:222-8.

[11] Kujundžić M, Banić M, Bokun T. Epidemiologija kolorektalnog karcinoma. Medix 75/76: 70-76, 2008

[12] Sung MK, Bae YJ. Linking obesity to colorectal cancer: application of nutrigenomics. Biotechnol J. 2010;5:930-41.

[13] Wactawski-Wende J, Kotchen JM, Anderson GL. Calcium plus vitamin D supplementation and the risk of colorectal cancer. N. Engl. J. Med. 2006; **354** (7): 684–96.

[14] Astin, M; Griffin, T, Neal, RD, Rose, P, Hamilton, W . The diagnostic value of symptoms for colorectal cancer in primary care: a systematic review. The British journal of general practice : the journal of the Royal College of General Practitioners 2011;**61** (586): 231–43.

[15] Cervera P, Fléjou JF. Changing pathology with changing drugs: tumors of the gastrointestinal tract. Pathobiology. 2011;78:76-89.

[16] Kyriakos M: The President cancer, the Dukes classification, and confusion, Arch Pathol Lab Med 109:1063, 1985.

[17] Dukes CE. The classification of cancer of the rectum. Journal of Pathological Bacteriology 1932;35:323.

[18] Astin M, Griffin T, Neal RD, Rose P, Hamilton W. The diagnostic value of symptoms for colorectal cancer in primary care: a systematic review. Br J Gen Pract. 2011;61:e231-43.

[19] Orbell J, West NJ. Improving detection of colorectal cancer. Practitioner. 2010;254:17-21, 2-3.

[20] Laviano A, Meguid MM, Inui A, Muscaritoli M, Rossi-Fanelli F. Therapy insight: Cancer anorexia-cachexia syndrome--when all you can eat is yourself. Nat Clin Pract Oncol. 2:158, 2005.

[21] Penet MF, Winnard PT Jr, Jacobs MA, Bhujwalla Understanding cancer-induced cachexia: imaging the flame and its fuel. Curr Opin Support Palliat Care. 2011.

[22] Van Cutsem E, Arends The causes and consequences of cancer-associated malnutrition. J. Eur J Oncol Nurs, 9:51, 2005.

[23] Bing C. Lipid Mobilization in cachexia: mechanisms and mediators. Curr Opin Support Palliat Care. 2011; 5(4):356-360.

[24] Inui A. Nippon Ronen Igakkai Zasshi, [Pathogenesis and treatment of cancer anorexia-cachexia, with special emphasis on aged patients]. Nihon Ronen Igakkai Zasshi. 20;4:460-7.

[25] Esper DH, Harb WA. The cancer cachexia syndrome: a review of metabolic and clinical manifestations. Nutr Clin Pract, 20:369.2005.

[26] Van Cutsem E, Arends J. The causes and consequences of cancer-associated malnutrition. Eur J Oncol Nurs. 2005;9 Suppl 2:S51-63.

[27] Scheede-Bergdahl C, Watt HL, Trutschnigg B, Kilgour RD, Haggarty A, Lucar E, Vigano A Is IL-6 the best pro-inflammatory biomarker of clinical outcomes of cancer cachexia? Clin Nutr. 2011.

[28] Ravasco P, Monteiro-Grillo I, Camilo M How relevant are cytokines in colorectal cancer wasting? Cancer J. 2007;13:392-8.

[29] Shibata M, Nezu T, Kanou H, Abe H, Takekawa M, Fukuzawa M. Decreased production of interleukin-12 and type 2 immune responses are marked in cachectic patients with colorectal and gastric cancer. J Clin Gastroenterol. 2002;34:416-20.

[30] Krznarić Ž: Klinička prehrana u gastroenterologiji. Medicus 15: 169-181, 2006.

[31] Bozzetti F. Guidelines on Artificial Nutrition versus Hydratation in terminal cancer patients.Nutrition 12:163-167, 1996.

[32] Mirhosseini N, Fainsinger RL, Baracos V. Parenteral nutrition in advanced cancer: indications and clinical practice guidelines. J Palliat Med, 8:914. 2005.

[33] Ries A, Trottenberg P, Elsner F, Stiel S, Haugen D, Kaasa S, Radbruch L. A systematic review on the role of fish oil for the treatment of cachexia in advanced cancer: An EPCRC cachexia guidelines project. Palliat Med. 2011.

[34] Ockenga J, Valentini L. Anorexia and cachexia in gastrointestinal cancer. Aliment Pharmacol Ther. 2005, 22(7):583-594.

[35] Coss CC, Bohl CE, Dalton JT. Curr Opin Clin Nutr Metab Care. Cancer cachexia therapy: a key weapon in the fight against cancer. 2011 May;14:268-73 Aliment Pharmacol Ther. 22: 583. 2005.

[36] Mattox TW, Treatment of unintentional weight loss in patients with cancer. Nutr Clin Pract, 20:400, 2005.

[37] Klosterbuer A, Roughead ZF, Slavin J. Benefits of dietary fiber in clinical nutrition. Nutr Clin Pract. 201.26:625-35.

[38] Blum D, Strasser F. Cachexia assessment tools. Curr Opin Support Palliat Care. 2011, 5(4):350-355.

[39] Evans MA, Shronts EP. Intestinal fuels: glutamine, short-chain fatty acids, and dietary fiber. J Am Diet Assoc. 1992;92:1239-46,1249.

[40] Jobgen WS, Fried SK, Fu WJ, Meininger CJ, Wu G. J Nutr Biochem.Regulatory role for the arginine-nitric oxide pathway in metabolism of energy substrates. 2006;17:571-88.

[41] Parry RV, Ward SG. Protein arginine methylation: a new handle on T lymphocytes? Trends Immunol. 2010;31:164-9.

[42] Swails WS, Kenler AS, Driscoll DF, DeMichele SJ, Babineau TJ, Utsunamiya T, Chavali S, Forse RA, Bistrian BR. Effect of a fish oil structured lipid-based diet on prostaglandin release from mononuclear cells in cancer patients after surgery. JPEN J Parenter Enteral Nutr. 1997;21:266-74.

[43] Mantovani G, Maccio A, Madeddu C, Gramignano G, Serpe R, Massa E, Dessi M, Tanca FM, Sanna E, Deiana L, Panzone F, Contu P, Floris C. Randomized phase III clinical trial of five different arms of treatment for patients with cancer cachexia: interim results. Nutrition, 24:305, 2008.

[44] Calder PC. Immunomodulation by omega-3 fatty acids. Prostaglandins Leukot Essent Fatty Acids. 2007;77:327-35.

[45] La Guardia M, Giammanco S, Di Majo D, Tabacchi G, Tripoli E, Giammanco M. Omega 3 fatty acids: biological activity and effects on human health. Panminerva Med. 2005;47:245-57.

[46] Wigmore SJ, Ross JA, Falconer JS, Plester CE, Tisdale MJ, Carter DC, Fearon KC. The effect of polyunsaturated fatty acids on the progress of cachexia in patients with pancreatic cancer. Nutrition. 1996;12(1 Suppl):S27-30

[47] Dintinjana RD, Guina T, Krznarić Z, Radić M, Dintinjana M. Effects of nutritional support in patients with colorectal cancer during chemotherapy. Coll Antropol. 2008 ; 32:737-40.

[48] Krznarić Ž, Juretić A, Šamija M, Dintinjana-Dobrila R, Vrdoljak E, Samaržija M, Kolaček S, Vrbanec D, Prgomet D, Ivkić M, Zelić M. [Croatian guidelines for use of eicosapentaenoic acid and megestrol acetate in cancer cachexia syndrome]. Lijec Vjesn, 129:381, 2007.

[49] Loprinzi CL, Kugler JW, Sloan JA, Mailliard JA, Krook JE, wilwerding MB, Rowland KM, Camoriano JK, Novotny PJ, Christensen BJ. Randomised Comparison of Megestrole Acetate Versus Dexamethasone Versus Fluoxymestrone for the Treatment of Cancer Anorexia/Cachexia . JCO 1999(17);10:3299-3306.

[50] Evans JW. Megestrol Acetate Use for Weight Gain should be Carefully Considered. The Journal of Endocrinology and Metabolism 2007(92);2:420-421.

[51] Trobec K, Haehling S, Anker SD, Lainscak M. Growth hormone, insulin-like growth factor 1, and insulin signaling-a pharmacological target in body wasting and cachexia. J Cachexia Sarcopenia Muscle (2011) 2:191-200.

[52] Coats AJS, Surendran J, Vangipuram SRKG, Jain M, Shah S, Irhfan ABH, Fuang HG, Hassan MZM, Beadle J, Tilson J, Kirwan AB, Anker SD. The ACT-ONE trial, a multicentre, randomized, double blind, placebo-controlled, dose-finding study of the anabolic/catabolic transforming agent, MT-102 in subjects with cachexia related to stage III and IV non-small cell lung cancer and colorectal cancer: study design. J Cachexia Sarcopenia Muscle (2011) 2:201-207.

Permissions

The contributors of this book come from diverse backgrounds, making this book a truly international effort. This book will bring forth new frontiers with its revolutionizing research information and detailed analysis of the nascent developments around the world.

We would like to thank Dr Rajunor Ettarh, for lending his expertise to make the book truly unique. He has played a crucial role in the development of this book. Without his invaluable contribution this book wouldn't have been possible. He has made vital efforts to compile up to date information on the varied aspects of this subject to make this book a valuable addition to the collection of many professionals and students.

This book was conceptualized with the vision of imparting up-to-date information and advanced data in this field. To ensure the same, a matchless editorial board was set up. Every individual on the board went through rigorous rounds of assessment to prove their worth. After which they invested a large part of their time researching and compiling the most relevant data for our readers. Conferences and sessions were held from time to time between the editorial board and the contributing authors to present the data in the most comprehensible form. The editorial team has worked tirelessly to provide valuable and valid information to help people across the globe.

Every chapter published in this book has been scrutinized by our experts. Their significance has been extensively debated. The topics covered herein carry significant findings which will fuel the growth of the discipline. They may even be implemented as practical applications or may be referred to as a beginning point for another development. Chapters in this book were first published by InTech; hereby published with permission under the Creative Commons Attribution License or equivalent.

The editorial board has been involved in producing this book since its inception. They have spent rigorous hours researching and exploring the diverse topics which have resulted in the successful publishing of this book. They have passed on their knowledge of decades through this book. To expedite this challenging task, the publisher supported the team at every step. A small team of assistant editors was also appointed to further simplify the editing procedure and attain best results for the readers.

Our editorial team has been hand-picked from every corner of the world. Their multi-ethnicity adds dynamic inputs to the discussions which result in innovative outcomes. These outcomes are then further discussed with the researchers and contributors who give their valuable feedback and opinion regarding the same. The feedback is then collaborated with the researches and they are edited in a comprehensive manner to aid the understanding of the subject.

Apart from the editorial board, the designing team has also invested a significant amount of their time in understanding the subject and creating the most relevant covers. They scrutinized every image to scout for the most suitable representation of the subject and create an appropriate cover for the book.

The publishing team has been involved in this book since its early stages. They were actively engaged in every process, be it collecting the data, connecting with the contributors or procuring relevant information. The team has been an ardent support to the editorial, designing and production team. Their endless efforts to recruit the best for this project, has resulted in the accomplishment of this book. They are a veteran in the field of academics and their pool of knowledge is as vast as their experience in printing. Their expertise and guidance has proved useful at every step. Their uncompromising quality standards have made this book an exceptional effort. Their encouragement from time to time has been an inspiration for everyone.

The publisher and the editorial board hope that this book will prove to be a valuable piece of knowledge for researchers, students, practitioners and scholars across the globe.

List of Contributors

Rajunor Ettarh
Department of Structural and Cellular Biology, Tulane University School of Medicine, New Orleans, USA

Christos Lionis and Elena Petelos
Clinic of Social and Family Medicine, Faculty of Medicine, University of Crete, Greece

Shahana Gupta
Department of Surgery, Medical College & Hospitals Kolkata, India

Anadi Nath Acharya
Department of Surgery, Institute of Post Graduate Medical Education and Research, Kolkata, India

Ingrid Flight
CSIRO Preventative Health Flagship, Australia

Carlene Wilson
Cancer Council South Australia and Flinders University, Flinders Centre for Innovation in Cancer, Australia

Jane McGillivray
School of Psychology, Deakin University, Australia

Hitoshi Okamura
Hiroshima University, Japan

Martina Perše
University of Ljubljana, Faculty of Medicine, Institute of Pathology, MEC, Slovenia

Karina Vieira de Barros, Ana Paula Cassulino and Vera Lucia Flor Silveira
Department of Physiology, Federal University of São Paulo, São Paulo, SP, Brazil

Vera Lucia Flor Silveira
Department of Biological Sciences, Federal University of São Paulo, Diadema, SP, Brazil

Federica Tramer and Sabina Passamonti
University of Trieste, Italy

Spela Moze
University of Ljubljana, Slovenia

Ayokunle O. Ademosun
Federal University of Technology, Ondo State, Nigeria

Jovana Cvorovic
University of Trieste, Italy

Seitz K. Helmut and Nils Homann
Department of Medicine (Gastroenterology & Hepatology), Salem Medical Centre, Centre of Alcohol Research, University of Heidelberg, Department of Gastroenterology, City Hospital Wolfsburg, Wolfsburg, Germany

Adam Naguib
Cold Spring Harbor Laboratory, USA

Laura J Gay
Queen Mary, University of London, UK

Panagiota N Mitrou
Medical Research Council Centre for Nutritional Epidemiology in Cancer Prevention and Survival, UK

Mark J Arends
Department of Pathology, Addenbrooke's Hospital, University of Cambridge, UK

Renata Dobrila-Dintinjana
Department of Radiation Oncology, Clinical Hospital Center Rijeka, University of Rijeka, School of Medicine, Croatia

Dragan Trivanović
General Hospital Pula, Department of Internal Medicine, Croatia

Marijan Dintinjana
Clinic of General Medicine Dr Dintinjana, Croatia

Jelena Vukelic
Department of Speech and Hearing Disorders Diagnostics and Rehabilitation, Clinical Hospital Center Rijeka, Croatia

Nenad Vanis
Division for Gastroenterology and Hepatology, Clinical Center University of Sarajevo, Faculty of Medicine, University of Sarajevo, Bosnia and Herzegovina

Printed in the USA
CPSIA information can be obtained
at www.ICGtesting.com
JSHW011423221024
72173JS00004B/646

9 781632 411365